PROMOTING HEALTH: KNOWLEDGE AND PRACTICE

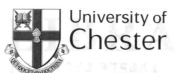

University of Chester

This book is to be returned on or before the last date stamped below. Overdue charges will be incurred by the late return of books.

This book forms part of the core text for the Open University course *Promoting Health: Skills, Perspectives and Practice* (K301) and a new qualification, The Certificate in Health Promotion. It has been produced with support from the Health Education Authority and Health Promotion Wales, although the content of the book is the sole responsibility of The Open University.

If you are interested in studying the course and gaining the new Certificate please write to the Information Officer, School of Health and Social Welfare, Walton Hall, Milton Keynes MK7 6AA, UK.

Other texts required for the course and also published by Palgrave Macmillan in association with The Open University are:

- the second core text, *The Challenge of Promoting Health: Exploration and Action,* edited by Linda Jones and Moyra Sidell
- the course reader, *Debates and Dilemmas in Promoting Health,* edited by Moyra Sidell, Linda Jones, Jeanne Katz and Alyson Peberdy
- the set book, *Health Promotion: Professional Perspectives,* edited by Angela Scriven and Judy Orme.

Promoting Health
Knowledge and Practice

Edited by

Jeanne Katz, Alyson Peberdy and Jenny Douglas
The Open University

The Open University

in association with

palgrave

First published 1997 by
MACMILLAN PRESS LTD
Houndmills, Basingstoke, Hampshire RG21 6XS and London
Companies and representatives throughout the world

Second edition 2000

ISBN 0–333–94930–7 paperback

A catalogue record for the book is available from the British Library.

This book is printed on paper suitable for recycling and made from fully managed and sustained forest sources.

10   9   8   7   6   5   4   3   2   1
06   05   04   03   02   01   00   99   98   97

Printed in the United Kingdom by The Alden Group, Oxford

13096B/k301b1p1i2.1

Contents

Preface

The Open University Team have perceived precisely one of the major challenges facing health care today. Through this book, they have approached the challenge with insight and inspiration. The increasing importance of health promotion means that promoting health has become the business of all those engaged in health and social care. This book will be invaluable for a wide range of practitioners, policy makers, academics and other lay and professional people interested in enhancing the nation's health. The text will prove to be particularly timely for large numbers of nurses in roles which actively embrace preventive care and the promotion of health.

This practice-led book illuminates the complexity of health promotion as a concept and focuses appropriately on key approaches to working in this area. Issues associated with ways of working and building collaborative relationships are carefully addressed. Readers are eased into examining the paradox between empowerment and the traditional medical model and lifestyle approach.

The principles of analysis and critique pervade the text and encourage innovation and progressive practice. Some deeply held assumptions about the definitions of ownership and control in health are challenged.

Emancipation and partnership are presented as key determinants of effectiveness and the need to evaluate rigorously health promotion activity is emphasised.

This book is itself a testimony to the value of collaboration and open-mindedness. Its content has been debated and vetted by a range of individuals and organisations. The Open University course, Promoting Health: Skills, Perspectives and Practice, of which this book and its sister publication *The Challenge of Promoting Health: Exploration and Action* form core texts, has evolved in partnership with potential consumers, the Health Education Authority and Health Promotion Wales.

Promoting Health: Knowledge and Practice truly breaks new ground. It provides the building blocks for progressive health promotion through skilfully helping readers to apply theory to practice. It offers exactly what is needed by all those charged with a responsibility to enhance health. It stimulates provocation and challenge to turn thinking into action.

Professor Jill Macleod Clark
The Nightingale Institute
King's College London

Acknowledgements

Grateful acknowledgement is made to the following sources for permission to reproduce material in this book:

Text

Boxes 1.2, 12.1[adapted from]: © Health Education Authority, 1995; Cooper, D. (1994) *Alcohol Home Detoxification and Assessment*, Radcliffe Medical Press, Oxford; 'To beef or not to beef...' *The Independent*, 6th December 1995; Boseley, S. (1995) 'Nutrition specialist warns against "BSE beef products"', *The Guardian*, 6th December 1995; Blakemore, C. (1995) 'Why we should all give up beef', *The Independent*, 7th December 1995; Extract from *Which*, May 1996; Box 17.4: Nutbeam, D. and Harris, E. (1995) *Health Promotion International*, 10, (1), Oxford University Press, reprinted by permission of Oxford University Press.

Figures

Figure 1.1: Naidoo, J. and Wills, J. (2000) *Health Promotion: Foundations for Practice*, 2nd edn, Baillière Tindall; *Figure 2.1: The Health of the Nation: A Strategy for Health in England* (1993) © Crown Copyright. Reproduced with the permission of the Controller of Her Majesty's Stationery Office; *Figure 3.2:* DHSS (1980) *The Black Report on Inequalities in Health*, © Crown Copyright. Reproduced with the permission of the Controller of Her Majesty's Stationery Office; *Figure 3.3:* Dahlgren, G. and Whitehead, M. (1991) *Policies and Strategies to Promote Social Equity in Health*, Institute for Futures Studies, Stockholm; *Figure 5.1:* Tones, B.K. (1996) 'The anatomy and ideology of health promotion: empowerment in context', in Scriven, A. and Orme, J. (eds) *Health Promotion: Professional Perspectives*, Macmillan Press Ltd; *Figure 5.2:* Downie, R.S., Fyfe, C. and Tannahill, A. (1993) *Health Promotion: Models and Values*, by permission of Oxford University Press; *Figure 5.3:* adapted from Beattie, A. (1991) 'A test case for social policy and social theory', in Gabe, J., Calnan, M. and Bury, M. (eds) *The Sociology of the Health Service*, Routledge; *Figure 5.4:* Caplan, R. (1993) 'The importance of social theory for health promotion: from description to reflexivity', *Health Promotion International*, 8, 2: pp.147–57, Oxford University Press; *Figure 6.1:* adapted from Seedhouse, D. (1988) *Ethics: The Heart of Health Care*, © 1988 by John Wiley and Sons Ltd. Reprinted by permission of John Wiley and Sons Ltd; *Figure 9.1:* Davidson, R. (1992) 'Facilitating change in problem drinkers', in Davidson, R. *et al.* (eds) *Counselling Problem Drinkers*, Routledge; *Figure 9.2:* Tones, K. (1995) 'Making a change for the better', *Healthlines*, **27**, November 1995, Health Education Authority; *Figure 10.1:* Tones, B.K. and Tilford, S. (1994) *Health Education: Effectiveness, Efficiency and Equity*, 2nd edn, Chapman and Hall; *Figures 13.1, 13.2, 13.3, 13.4, 14.2, 14.3, 14.4, 14.7:* Copyright © Health Education Authority; *Figure 14.1:* The design of the medical certificate of cause of death is © Crown Copyright and is reproduced with the permission of the Controller of HMSO and of the Office for National Statistics; *Figure 14.8:* Liverpool

Healthy City 2000 *Draft Liverpool City Health Plan: Summary Guide*, Liverpool City Council; *Figure 15.1:* McCarthy, M. (1982) *Epidemiology and Policies for Health Planning*, King Edwards Hospital Fund for London; *Figure 15.2:* Ewles, L. and Simnett, I. (1995) *Promoting Health: A Practical Guide*, 3rd edn, p.96, Scutari Press, by permission of the publisher W. B. Saunders Company Limited, London; *Figure 15.3:* Ong, B.N. and Humhris, G. (1994) 'Prioritising needs with communities: Rapid appraisal methodologies in health', in Popay, J. and Williams, G. (eds) *Researching the People's Health*, Routledge; Figure 16.1: adapted from Edwards, J. (1991) *Evaluation in Adult and Further Education: A Practical Handbook for Teachers and Organisers,* The Workers' Educational Association, © Judith Edwards, 1991; Figure 16.2: adapted from Feuerstein, M.T. (1986) *Partners in Evaluation: Evaluating development and community programmes with participants*, Macmillan Press Ltd.

Tables

Table 2.1: Blaxter, M. (1987) in Cox, B.D. *et al.* (eds) *The Health and Lifestyle Survey: Preliminary Report*, The Health Promotion Research Trust, © Mildred Blaxter; *Table 2.2:* Stainton Rogers, W. (1991) *Explaining Health and Illness: An Exploration of Diversity*, Harvester-Wheatsheaf; *Table 3.1:* Jones, L.J. (1994) *The Social Context of Health and Health Work*, Macmillan Press Ltd, © Linda J. Jones, 1994; *Table 3.2:* Jarman, B. (1983) 'Inequalities in health', *British Medical Journal*, **286**, pp. 1705–9, BMJ Publishing Group. Townsend, P. *et al.* (1985) 'Inequalities in health in the city of Bristol: a preliminary review of statistical evidence', *International Journal of Health Services*, **15**, (4) Baywood Publishing Company, Inc.; *Table 3.3:* adapted from *OPCS Decennial Supplements on Occupational Mortality 1971, 1978, 1986. OPCS Longitudinal Study* © Crown Copyright. Reproduced with the permission of the Office for National Statistics; *Table 4.2:* WHO (1977) *Health for All by the Year 2000*, World Health Organisation; *Table 4.3: The Health of the Nation: A Strategy for Health in England* (1993) © Crown Copyright. Reproduced with the permission of the Controller of Her Majesty's Stationery Office; *Table 5.1:* Ewles, L. and Simnett, I. (1995) *Promoting Health: A Practical Guide*, 3rd edn, p. 39, Scutari Press, by permission of the publisher W. B. Saunders Company Limited, London; *Table 10.1:* Tones, B.K. and Tilford, S. (1994) *Health Education: Effectiveness, Efficiency and Equity*, 2nd edn, Chapman and Hall; *Table 11.1:* Hubley, J. (1993) *Communicating Health: An action guide to health education and health promotion*, Macmillan Press Ltd; *Tables 12.1, 12.2:* OHE (1994) *OHE Briefing Health Information and the Consumer*, **30**, May 1994, Office of Health Economics; *Table 13.1:* © Health Education Authority; *Table 14.1:* OPCS (1992) *General Household Survey 1992* (1994), © Crown Copyright 1994. Reproduced by permission of the Controller of HMSO and the Office for National Statistics; Table 17.2: adapted from Aggleton, P., Moody, D. and Young, A. (1992) *Evaluating HIV/AIDS Health Promotion*, Health Education Authority.

The authors wish to acknowledge the K511 course team, whose work they have drawn on in Chapter 8.

General Introduction

This book is a response to the growing interest in health and health promotion issues over the last decade. Health has now become a major area of concern in professional circles and in self-help groups, in the media and among individual citizens. The 1985 World Health Organisation targets for 'Health For All' in Europe, which focused on both disease reduction and health promotion, have now to varying degrees been incorporated into health and local authority planning. National strategies for health in the UK now include specific illness reduction targets, health education goals and support for broader strategic approaches such as building 'healthy alliances' and working for 'health gain'. In several areas of health work, health promotion has become a higher priority. In nursing, for example, health promotion is a 'key characteristic' in the Higher Award and it features more significantly in the Project 2000 common foundation programme.

As a blend of critical review, evaluation of good practice and encouragement to innovate, this book will extend the debate about promoting health. Health and welfare professionals and all others involved in the wide-ranging activity of searching out and responding to health needs will find the book supports and informs their work. It will be particularly appropriate for health professionals completing under-graduate degrees but it should also attract other lay and professional groups involved in social service provision, education, environmental work, policy-making and planning. Its focus is not only on health sector policy and practice but on the wider range of agencies and activities that can influence health.

The search for health is not confined to the medical sphere and the promotion of health is not an activity exclusive to professional, specialist health promoters. Since health can be the business of anyone who cares to make it so, it seems increasingly important that it should not be left in the hands of any one group, profession or set of commercial interests. So this book is written for everyone who wishes to reflect upon and develop the health promoting potential of their own work and activities both professional and lay.

When we use the term 'professional' in this book it is in a generic sense which includes, for example, teachers, social workers, town planners and office managers, as well as those working within the health sector. In all of these spheres health promotion involves exploring new ways of carrying out existing roles by, for instance, creating partnerships between agencies and professional groups or providing the kind of information and supportive relationships that open up new possibilities for individuals. Teasing out what this process involves and what knowledge and skills it requires form a major concern of the authors of this book.

This is a challenging book which raises questions about some deeply embedded assumptions. The notion that promoting health is an activity extending well beyond the sphere of medical or health services implies a certain redistribution of power and control. This view of health promotion implies a willingness to take seriously a plurality of values and to entertain the possibility of a more open-ended and less predictable future. Yet it has also been argued that the more emancipatory aspects of health promotion can be seen as evidence of increasing surveillance, as a policing of everyday lifestyle in the name of health. So we suggest that health promotion is not one single project but has several competing strands which may be interpreted in very different ways.

The opening chapters of Part 1 focus on the meanings and values attached to health and health promotion. They explore how medical and lay accounts of health differ and how different 'models' of health give rise to conflicting priorities for practice. Investigation of the factors influencing health status highlights the connections as well as the tensions between a lifestyle and an environmental analysis. Discussion of the relationship between social, cultural and economic influences on health leads into a discussion of the emergence and character of health promotion and the shifting balance between prevention, health education and public policy.

Part 1 also introduces readers to debates about the health promotion movement. Recent history has seen a series of international and national conferences and charters presenting health promotion as a movement for social and political change. From this perspective health promotion is linked into a broader environmental movement which claims to prioritise sustainablility above economic growth and social justice above wealth creation. The role of health education within this movement is to raise people's consciousness and to empower them to work together to create healthier environments and press for healthy public policy. We ask how far this vision can be reconciled with a narrower lifestyles approach and a continued preoccupation with medical treatment. Drawing closer to home, the vision embodied in the Ottawa Charter provides a context for discussion and critical assessment of the more medically focused aspects of some of the UK health promotion strategies.

The second part of this book focuses on some of the debates relating to communication and education about health. The centrality of effective communication is undisputed in the world of health promotion, but the methods used arouse considerable debate and discussion. To ensure that there is a real rather than putative partnership between health professionals and their clients, communication needs to be facilitating and effective rather than a one-way process.

Counselling can be seen as one form of communication – the skills identified in the book highlight the conflicts inherent in this endeavour and suggest a number of ways to move forward some of these debates. The book firmly cites counselling as a central focus of contemporary health education. In Chapter 9 the history of health education is explored using

Tones' views that health education has two particular functions: influencing healthy choices, as well as seeking to empower the client as well as the professional. The different strands of health education are examined looking, for example, at the development of peer education and environment within which this has developed.

As has been particularly evident in the health scares of the mid-1990s in the UK, the role of the media in educating for health is crucial in terms of some of the strategies employed. This is clearly in contrast with the forms of health education discussed earlier as the immediate impact is more difficult to ascertain and it lacks potential feedback of interpersonal interaction. The different strands of mass media employ a variety of methods and these are examined in the light of the general purposes and strategies of health education raised earlier in the book.

Part 3 explores the variety of ways in which information about health is accessed and looks in depth at what counts as trustworthy evidence. The nature of health information is clearly complex and issues such as what constitutes evidence are addressed. Health scares about food provide good examples of the dilemmas professionals and lay people alike face in making health choices. The ground between professional and lay perspectives is shifting – health professionals' advice has much less impact than that of the mass media, and this in itself creates and fosters uncertainty regarding health choices. What information can be trusted, and which sources produce reliable data? This part continues to speculate about the impact of new technologies on access to health information; how can health promoters assist clients to make health choices when they are in competition with the plethora of contradictory information churned out on the world wide web?

Health information is created by a number of disciplines and readers will explore the development of demography and epidemiology, examining some of the methods used in these disciplines and teasing out the relevance for health promotion. The usefulness and hence the potential abuse of statistics in misleading the public about research data findings is explored. This information, and in particular the range of methods of ascertaining pertinent data, is developed in Chapter 15, which seeks to identify the kinds of information required in order to plan, implement and evaluate interventions.

Just as there are a variety of perspectives on health and promoting health so too there are debates about how best to evaluate health promotion. These are addressed in Part 4. Running through these debates are three connected issues. The first is the question of which values and standards are to be used as the basis for evaluation and who should decide. Often evaluation is presented as a value-free rational technical exercise, but this is simply to choose one set of values without even entering into the debate. The second is whether the kind of experimental design used in drug trials is appropriate to the evaluation of health promoting activities given their complex and open-ended nature. If it is not, then why and how is evaluation expected to provide evidence of effectiveness and/or cost-effectiveness? Finally, there is the question of how health promoting values such as partnership and critical awareness can be built into the process of evaluation It is argued that top-down pressure for monitoring and evaluation represents managerial interests in a way that may stifle creativity and divert attention away from the kind of evaluative questioning most likely to contribute to improved ways of working for health. Thus questions of how best to go about evaluation are closely linked with the differing perspectives on health and health promotion identified in the opening chapters of this book.

We want to emphasise that the future of health promotion lies very much in the hands of all who are engaged in promoting health and not simply with managers, health promotion specialists or 'expert' evaluators. We hope this book will help readers relate knowledge and practice in ways that will prove exciting and rewarding for all concerned.

Jeanne Katz and Alyson Peberdy
1st July 1996

Introduction to the 2nd edition

This second edition has been revised and updated to reflect recent changes in health promotion practice, policy and research, including the changes in UK government policy since 1997 and the European Health for All policy (Health 21). Central to these developments is the renewed emphasis on addressing inequalities in health, which has important implications for those involved in promoting health. This edition highlights the further developments that have taken place in the scope and application of health promotion, new debates and dilemmas that are emerging from current government policies, and the debates which continue to engage all those involved in promoting health.

Jenny Douglas
September 2000

PROMOTING HEALTH: KNOWLEDGE AND PRACTICE

Part 1
Exploring health promotion

Introduction

Health promotion starts from the premise that improving people's health is a worthwhile and important activity and one which should aim to enhance participation and equity and avoid being judgemental or victim-blaming. But this assumption inevitably prompts questions about health promotion work. How are health promotion interventions to be justified? Whose values should count? Is there one appropriate health promotion model to use? How are participation and equity to be ensured?

Part 1 responds to such questions by developing a critical awareness of concepts, models and values in health promotion. At the same time, it begins to build a systematic knowledge base and to address key heath promotion skills. Chapter 1 introduces health promotion as a diverse and contested field of action which involves lay people as well as professionals. Chapter 2 explores concepts of health and Chapter 3 discusses the social, economic and cultural factors influencing health status and health behaviour. Chapter 4 considers the frameworks influencing contemporary health promotion. Chapters 5 and 6 focus on central debates in health promotion about values and the relative merits of different health promotion models. In Chapter 7 readers are invited to review their own experience and draw out from earlier chapters the main components of the health promotion role. The exploration of key skills, knowledge and understanding needed for effective health promotion will then be developed in the rest of the book.

Chapter 1
Promoting health: everybody's business?

1.1 What is health promotion?

Health is a major focus of interest and concern in contemporary society. National surveys in the UK and in many other European countries have demonstrated that people are willing to spend more money on health services and that they rate good health as of central importance in living a full and satisfying life. This has been highlighted in the notion of health as 'the foundation for achievement' (Seedhouse, 1986). Attempts to develop a theory of human needs which can establish a set of rights, responsibilities and goals within contemporary UK welfare society have highlighted our basic need for and entitlement to health (Doyal and Gough, 1991).

Concern for health has most often prompted demands for more medical services to treat ill health. Indeed, the dominant definition of health in the western world has been 'absence of disease' or 'not ill' (Blaxter, 1990). Critics have labelled this the medical definition of health because it focuses not on health as a positive state but health as an absence of the manifestation of disease. In this view, health is when you are not classified as sick or in need of medical intervention.

But there has also been a significant investment in many countries in creating infrastructures and services to protect health and to prevent ill health. In most industrialising countries over the last 150 years public health regulations and health and safety legislation have been enacted to provide safeguards for the industrial workforce, to control pollution levels in rivers, to enforce proper sewage and drainage and so on, even if they have not always been enforced. In nineteenth century England sanitary reformers and radical politicians argued, on economic grounds, for ill health prevention through public policy interventions. Joseph Chamberlain, mayor of Birmingham, pushed through an ambitious improvement programme in 1875 by claiming that 'we may hope to see disease and crime removed' and that 'the cost of the goal, the hospital and the workhouse is infinitely greater than that of any sanitary improvement which the most extravagantly-minded man can devise' (Jones, 1995)

Slum clearance, the paving of city streets and other similar measures were seen as paying long term dividends in creating healthy and orderly communities run on hygienic principles (Jones, 1995). The argument that 'prevention was cheaper than cure' helped to persuade local authorities to extend health services beyond prevention of disease towards a notion of improving health through health education. For example, schoolchildren were taught hygienic principles and parents (in particular mothers) were instructed in hygiene, nutrition and childcare through home visiting (Lewis, 1980).

These various overlapping approaches – the doctrine of prevention, the public health movement, protective legislation and health education – are today most accurately characterised as elements of 'health promotion'. Their common concern is to improve health (as opposed to a focus on treating disease) and this is driven by an assumption that people's health is influenced not just by, or even principally by, the availability of medical treatment but by a range of measures in and outside the health sector (Lalonde, 1974). This suggests an initial definition of health promotion as actions and interventions to support and enhance people's health.

1.2 Changing priorities in health promotion

The origins of formal health promotion as a modern movement lie in the World Health Organisation declaration of 1946 that 'health is not merely the absence of disease, but a state of complete physical, mental and social well-being'.

Compare this statement with the notion of health as the 'absence of disease'. What are the advantages and drawbacks of adopting the WHO definition?

This idealistic statement conceptualises health as a positive state rather than a state of 'not being sick'. People are viewed not only in physical but in psychological and social terms and all-round health is seen as including well-being. Such a definition is a useful starting point for thinking about the components and parameters of health promotion. In focusing not just on absence of disease but on the attainment of a more positive and holistic state it presents a challenge to think more seriously about 'what makes for good health'. But moving the boundaries in this way raises difficult questions about what being healthy really involves. Can anyone hope to attain a state of complete health, judged in World Health Organisation terms?

Health education or health promotion?

The initial focus in the UK and the Republic of Ireland health services was on health education and for many health professionals providing information, advice, personal skills and support remains a key concern. In the UK a Central Council for Health Education was first established in 1927, financed by local authority public health departments. Its main tasks were to provide information which would persuade the public to change to healthier habits, in particular to safer sexual practices. The Health Education Council was created in 1968 in England as a non-governmental organisation with an objective to create 'a climate of opinion generally favourable to health education, develop blanket programmes of education and (target) selected priority subjects' (HEC, 1968). In addition to mass publicity campaigns the Council launched national programmes such as 'Look After Yourself' (LAY) which emphasised the links between personal behavioural changes and better health. Similiar health education agencies were set up in the other three countries of the UK, and in 1975 the Health Education Bureau was established in the Republic of Ireland (Hensey, 1998).

Fierce lobbying and political manoeuvring characterised the Health Education Council's history (Sutherland, 1987; Pattison and Player, 1991). Above all, the links between smoking and lung cancer and between poor diet and ill health, which had been well researched and were increasingly hard to ignore, pointed to the need to confront tobacco companies and even to try and influence food producers through the Department of Agriculture, Fisheries and Food. Yet pressure was exerted to ensure that the health messages targeted individual behaviour. *Prevention and Health: Everybody's Business* (DHSS, 1976), commenting on smoking-related diseases, alcohol misuse and other drug dependencies, obesity and its consequences, and the sexually transmitted diseases, saw all these as 'preventable problems' about which 'the individual must decide for himself'. The huge expenditure on advertising and marketing of health damaging products was at this stage not seen as a central health issue.

During the 1980s a flurry of reports indicated the need to take broader action on health. The Health Education Council and the Scottish Health Education Group increasingly tangled with government departments over the extent to which they should attempt to influence and change public policy. The National Advisory Council on Nutritional Education (NACNE, 1983) reported that the British diet was too high in saturated fats, sugar and salt and too low in fibre, and that this was adding to the burden of cardio-vascular and digestive tract diseases. The British Medical Association strongly backed a campaign against smoking (Action on Smoking and Health) which called for a ban on tobacco advertising and stricter regulation of sales.

The links between poverty, unemployment and poor health, which had been highlighted in many parts of Europe at the end of the nineteenth century, began to be 'rediscovered'. In the UK, for example, a major study of poverty (Townsend, 1979) and a government-sponsored report on health (*The Black Report on Inequalities in Health*, DHSS, 1980) both pointed to the close relationship between health and poverty. Social class gradients in health were identified: in other words, semi- and unskilled groups had much lower life expectancy and experienced more ill health than those in the non-manual and professional groups. A follow-up report sponsored by the Health Education Council indicated that in some areas the health gap had widened (Whitehead, 1987). This fuelled the call for a broader view of health and health services, which acknowledged how agencies outside the health sector might enhance or damage health, and a shift of resources towards prevention, health protective legislation and health promotion (Rodmell and Watt, 1986). We will focus on present government policy in Chapter 4.

Health For All by the Year 2000 (WHO, 1977, 1985), while endorsing health education, proposed a wider agenda which involved socio-economic change. There were calls to change health sector priorities and invest in health promotion and prevention rather than clinical and curative services. Health promotion embraced the community development approach which involved supporting local residents in actions to improve their health. By the mid-1980s it became more widely acknowledged that effective health education involved 'making healthier choices easier choices' by modifying the circumstances, environment and policy frameworks within which people lead their lives so that they have more opportunities to chose a healthier 'lifestyle' (WHO, 1986). This required health to be prioritised on the public policy agenda so that policy making in every sector became 'health promoting'.

In the Republic of Ireland the Department of Health produced a consultative statement entitled *Health – the Wider Dimension* (Department of Health, 1986). This document stated that 'the focus of health policy needs to be widened to take into account the many factors apart from health service which impact on health'. It also stated that emphasis should be placed on health promotion.

Creating environments that enable people to live healthier lives has now become a central concern of health promotion. Successive World Health Organisation conferences in the late 1980s and 1990s have emphasised 'healthy public policy' as a central part of promoting health. The contemporary public health movement – the *'new* public health' as it has been called – puts great emphasis on improving health through changing people's environments and living conditions (Ashton and Seymour, 1988). Its focus is largely on public policy change rather than individual behaviour. There has been a call to build on older public health traditions which improved people's health by tackling housing, sanitary and environmental causes of ill health (Draper *et al.*, 1991).

The Ottawa Charter for health promotion

The health promotion movement, through the *Ottawa Charter* (WHO, 1986), the Adelaide Conference (WHO, 1988), the 1991 Sundsvall Conference (WHO, 1991), and the Jakarta Declaration (WHO, 1997) has extended the discussion about environmental influences on health to encompass many of the ideas of the 'green' movement. This environmental approach to health promotion is expressed in the *Ottawa Charter for Health Promotion* (1986) as 'building healthy public policy' and in broader ecological terms as 'creating supportive environments' which will ensure global health (see Box 1.1).

Assess what definition of health lies behind the Ottawa Charter extract in Box 1.1. On what grounds can the Ottawa Charter approach to health promotion be criticised?

Box 1.1: Extracts from the *Ottawa Charter for Health Promotion* **(1986)**

Health promotion action means:

Build healthy public policy – putting health on the agenda of policy makers in all sectors and at all levels, directing them to be aware of the health consequences of their decisions and to accept their responsibilities for health.

Create supportive environments – systematic assessment of the health impact of a rapidly changing environment ... is essential. The protection of the natural and built environment and the conservation of natural resources must be addressed in any health promotion strategy.

Strengthen community action – health promotion works through concrete and effective community action in setting priorities, making decisions, planning strategies and implementing them to achieve better health. At the heart of this process is the empowerment of communities.

Develop personal skills – health promotion supports personal and social development through providing information, education for health and enhancing life skills.

Reorient health services – the role of the health sector must move increasingly in a health promotion direction, beyond its responsibility for providing clinical and curative services.

The definition of health promotion indicated in the Ottawa Charter is extremely broad, encompassing health education, public policy change, environmentalism and community action. This reflects the World Health Organisation pronouncement that health is about 'a state of complete physical, mental and social well-being' but goes beyond it in indicating how this state of health will be attained. There is a clear intention to link achievement of health with political, social and economic change. Behind this stands a definition of health which is the polar opposite of 'absence of disease'.

Promoting health is viewed not just as the business of professional health promoters within the National Health Service, nor even of health professionals in general. It is to some extent 'everybody's business', at a personal, community, societal and global level. Some of the most important measures to protect and promote health are to be taken outside the health sector by those with responsibility for economic and social policy, such as politicians, industrialists, retailers, educators, planners and economists. In addition, individuals – in their private and public capacity – can play a part in protecting their own and others health and can work together with others at a local organizational and national level to change 'unhealthy' practices and policies. 'Healthy' people are to be empowered within their communities as individuals, as full contributors to and as participants in social life and decision making. All public policies need to become 'healthy' and, beyond this, health is linked to a 'healthy' planet, where sustainable development is achieved through environmental protection and conservation.

A critical comment ...

The Ottawa Charter can be criticised for creating a 'catch-all' framework for health promotion in which priorities are unclear. Empowering communities, for example, means attending to their agendas for change which may be in tension with demands to build healthy public policy and supportive environments. Developing personal skills implies that, once in place, people will opt for healthier lifestyles. Yet people are often sceptical about health information and offering them more may not alter this. Research into public perceptions regarding diet, cholesterol control and heart disease drew comments that:

I think your body's the best judge.

If everyone is telling you different things, you have got to assess them for yourself. And your body is sure going to tell you when something is going wrong.

It frustrates me because the pattern through my life is that [doctors] tell you it is good for you, then they tell you it is not. They tell you to do this, then they tell you not to. So you wonder who do you believe? And I guess basically you have to think, everything in moderation.

(Focus group members, in Lupton and Chapman, 1995: 488)

For some critics, health and ill health are determined by socio-economic and political structures and relationships so that attempts to change personal behaviour through empowerment are essentially misconceived (Tesh, 1988). For others the concern lies in the requirement that health should be prioritised by agencies, governments and individuals, who may have other valid priorities:

Lifestyle interventions and social engineering are disruptive to people's lives and raise the political question – do people want to be healthy? This is not a facetious question, as there is always a price to be paid for health. For some people health is not a top priority. Some actively seek high risk pastimes such as rock climbing, fast driving or excessive drinking. Alternatively, health may be accorded a relatively low priority by individuals suffering psychological difficulties or social deprivation. In such circumstances we must ask whether people have a right not to experience interference, and whether health promoters are in danger of becoming a 'safety police'.

(Kelly and Charlton, 1995: 223)

The broad, all-encompassing agenda in the Ottawa Charter extends health promotion into yet more parts of social life – global governance, communities, relationships, self-care – a trend that Armstrong (1993, 1995) has termed 'the rise of surveillance medicine'. Surveillance critics claim that health promotion acts as a form of social regulation by shaping people's thinking about their bodies, relationships and 'lifestyles' (Nettleton and Bunton, 1995). It builds on a longer-standing critique of the medicalisation of everyday life, which highlighted how doctors were regarded as authorities not just on medicine but on lifestyle and behaviours (Zola, 1972).

And a rejoinder ...

You may have voiced some of these views, and certainly health promotion is unlikely to escape criticism either from those who see it as part of the offending 'nanny state' of 'health police' undermining people's liberty (Anderson, 1986) or who argue that structural change rather than personal skills or community action is the only legitimate way to create health (Tesh, 1988). Health promotion specialists would respond to the latter criticism by arguing that 'health can't wait for the revolution'! In other words, action at a personal, local and organisational level, provided it is ethically sound and respects people's freedom of choice, is better than waiting for social and economic transformation to happen. Besides, there is no reason why campaigning for policy change should not also be a priority, as in the Ottawa Charter.

When accused of being 'health police', health promotion specialists respond in three ways: attack, rejection and an appeal to history. First, it is pointed out that those who sell ill-health do so without compunction, often through mass media persuasion as in tobacco advertising. To combat this, health promotion can legitimately use marketing techniques in the much more justifiable attempt to improve health.

> Look at the techniques that the tobacco industry have used to sell what is after all a mass produced known carcinogen. So I've got no problem with people adopting techniques used by the tobacco industry... because our primary objective is improving people's health and quality of life, whereas theirs is manifestly selling a product which kills people and their primary motive is profit.
>
> (Interview with Maurice Swanson, Director Of Health Promotion Services, Western Australia, on 15 December 1995)

Second, it is argued that since health promotion accepts personal autonomy within its framework of intervention, people's right to free choice can always be safeguarded. The earlier comment that 'if everyone is telling you different things, you have got to assess them for yourself' is not a residualised lay view but a central part of current health promotion orthodoxy. We'll explore this argument further in Chapter 6. The third response concerns a re-examination of the record of curative medicine and the shifting burden of disease, which is discussed in the next section.

1.3 Why promote health?

Human health may be improved by treating disease, by minimising or preventing the onset of sickness and enhancing the health of those who are already reasonably healthy: for example, older or disabled people (who have often been labelled as unhealthy). In addition, health maintenance for those who are sick – the concept of 'healthy ill people' – has become increasingly important (Milz, 1992). Contemporary health promotion would see itself as having a major part to play in all these areas.

A critique of medicine

For much of the twentieth century it seemed that medical advances would be sufficient to bring about health for all but there has also been acute questioning of the effectiveness and the costs of clinical medicine (Dubos, 1959; Cochrane, 1971; McKeown, 1976). In the UK the establishment of the welfare state in the 1940s, and in particular of a National Health Service, was seen as the beginning of the end of the waste of life and health in the population. Free treatment, though it might initially be expensive to the state, would be both curative and preventive. As people were able to get early treatment and could afford to visit the doctor when they first felt ill, disease would gradually be eradicated and demand for health care would plateau out. The virtual elimination of some of the worst killers of urban industrial populations – typhoid, diphtheria, measles, scarlet fever, tuberculosis – served to reinforce the role of medicine in creating a healthy population. As life expectancy evened out and people attained their natural life span, morbidity was becoming compressed into the last years of life, prompting the claim that the 'medical and social task of eliminating premature death is largely accomplished' (Fries, 1980).

But by the mid-1960s it had become clear in most of the western world that the costs of modern medicine would go on rising to cope with new technologies and therapies and with rising demand for health services. The burden of disease was shifting from acute towards more intractable and long-term degenerative illnesses such as cancers, mental disorders and strokes. These were expensive to treat and treatment made only a small difference compared with the more dramatic breakthroughs of the early part of the twentieth century. The role of medicine in reducing infectious diseases was questioned and nutrition, birth control and rising living standards were seen as crucial in explaining declining death rates (McKeown, 1976). The 'compression of morbidity' theory was challenged by evidence that there was no sign of age-specific decline in conditions such as hip fracture or cancers. In addition the evidence linking poverty with poor health in older people remained strong (Marmot and McDowall, 1986). In this situation prevention and health promotion appeared to offer a potentially cost-effective strategy for maintaining health and preventing disease.

Multicausality and lifestyle

Another factor in the shift towards health promotion was the acknowledgement of the multifactoral origins of disease, in particular chronic diseases. Multicausal theories highlighted the potential for a range of social-psychological as well as physical factors to influence the production of disease. The person's own health status or mental state played an important part in the episode; host, co-factors and invading organism became seen as part of a dynamic interaction (Dubos, 1959; Engel, 1977). This directed attention to lifestyle and environmental influences on health although it did not offer much assistance in determining precise responsibility for disease. 'The equal weighting of causes ... means that those who have something to lose from prevention programmes can insist that the factor for which they have no responsibility is the real cause' (Tesh, 1988).

The first outcome of multicausal theorising in health policy terms was a focus on 'lifestyles'. In the UK this meant official acceptance of evidence that chronic diseases such as cardiovascular disease and cancers could be prevented through appropriate behavioural changes (DHSS, 1976). If health educators transformed the lifestyle of the population – diet, physical activity levels, use of alcohol and tobacco – it seemed possible to effect a dramatic improvement in health status.

Such claims about the 'simple steps' needed to change behaviour were criticised from the start, not least as potentially victim-blaming (Crawford, 1977; Rodmell and Watt, 1986). The Ottawa Charter itself emphasised the social and environmental influences on human health by insisting that building healthy public policy and supportive environments should be central features. Health promotion endorsed multifactoral theories and accepted that personal health choices were influenced by wider socio-economic and structural factors. Nonetheless, it remains difficult to focus on both lifestyle and environment at the same time; strategies which focus on reducing risk and targeting behavioural change tend to understate the environmental causes of disease (Davison *et al.*, 1992).

1.4　Who promotes health?

Specialist services

In the UK, co-ordination of health promotion is a specialist activity within most health services. There are four national agencies in the UK: the Health Development Agency (successor to the Health Education Council and Health Education Authority) for England, National Assembly for Wales: Health Promotion Division (successor to Health Promotion Wales), the Health Education Board for Scotland and the Health Promotion Agency for Northern Ireland. The Health Development Agency was established in April 2000 and Health Promotion England was also created in April 2000 with responsibility for mass media campaigns. At a national level these specialist agencies advise government departments, run a wide range of national- and community-based health initiatives involving public, voluntary and private sectors, undertake research and development work, and training and professional development. They publish regular surveys of health-related attitudes and behaviour (see Box 1.2) and of epidemiology (the incidence and prevalence of disease in populations).

In the Republic of Ireland the national agency is the health promotion unit, which took over from the Health Education Bureau in 1988 and is part of the Department of Health. The HPU continued the work of the HEB in terms of education and information disseminations and also acting as an executive as well as a policy-making unit with close links to the health boards. The HPU commissions research such as the National Health and Lifestyle Survey (Centre for Health Promotion Studies, 1999) and develops some national programmes. All eight health boards have some kind of explicit health promotion policy overseen by a health promotion officer who holds a senior management position within the board.

Box 1.2: A health and lifestyles study

In 1995 the Health Education Authority for England published a report on the health and lifestyles of just over 5,000 people aged 16–74 in the UK. This aims to provide comprehensive baseline data of habits and attitudes towards issues that are central to the Health of the Nation initiative. For example, people are asked about their perception of their general health and mental health status, their health behaviours (such as physical activity levels, sexual behaviour and diet), their smoking behaviour and attitudes to smoking, and their awareness and feelings about cancer.

The findings indicated that people were less fearful about cancer than in the past and that 90 per cent thought early detection gave a good chance of recovery. Significant class gradients were discovered, for example in uptake of services such as screening and in smoking. Emerging and worrying trends, such as the increase in young women smokers, were confirmed as were encouraging signs, such as the very high levels of

---

support for a total ban on smoking in most public places (but not workplaces, restaurants and pubs). The important role of the family doctor in giving advice that was listened to and often acted upon became clear, as did the current fairly restricted use of practice nurses in health promotion work. The report is part of an ongoing survey of health which will be repeated over the years to provide a comprehensive data set for each of the areas within the Health of the Nation.

(HEA, 1995)

Within the National Health Service some health promotion specialists in public health departments advise health authorities on the health needs of local populations. Health promotion units may be based in NHS hospital and community trusts, health authorities in England or health boards in Scotland. Health promotion services might include counselling and advisory work, support for groups with special needs, work with community health projects and indirect health promotion through campaigning and linking with other agencies and sectors. Health promotion specialists may use all kinds of interventions to reach ordinary people and encourage them to think about their health in a more positive way. In 1988 West Birmingham Health Authority, for example, opened a 'health shop' in a local high street where passers-by could drop in without an appointment for a range of services, such as a blood pressure reading, eye testing, a cholesterol test, and for free health information and advice.

The setting of health targets has been the basis for local health initiatives and has provided a clear focus for the work of health professionals. For example, the main Health of the Nation targets for England were for the reduction of coronary heart disease and stroke, cancers, mental illness, HIV/AIDS and sexual health and accidents (DoH, 1992). These influenced the work of nurses, midwives and health visitors (see Box 1.3), the professions allied to medicine and, through changes in contract, general practitioners. In the Republic of Ireland, health promotion targets were identified in the report 'Shaping a Healthier Future' in the broader context of health and social gain.

Box 1.3: A smokers' advisory service in Southampton

A smokers' advisory service was piloted by two health visitors who had been involved for some time in a range of smoking cessation activities. They decided that better continuity between hospital and community and better use of scarce skills in the promotion of stop-smoking policies was required. The initiative relates to lung cancer reduction and is being evaluated. The pilot service provides:

- an advice and drop-in centre in an outlying hospital (now only 8.30am–5.00pm but under review)
- one-to-one counselling on an appointment basis

- assistance for introduction of no-smoking policies

- referrals of in-patients who have been advised to stop before admission

- referrals from antenatal clinics

- regular visits to schools

- *ad hoc* talks to groups such as women's groups

- providing information related to stopping smoking.

(DoH, 1993b: 46–7)

The new strategy for health in England, *Saving Lives: Our Healthier Nation* (DoH, 1999) has set targets for the reduction of coronary hearts disease and stroke, cancers, mental illness and accidents. The main aims of Saving Lives will be discussed in Chapter 4.

Healthy alliances

The UK health strategies of the early 1990s also called for the creation of 'healthy alliances' to create 'health gain' reaching outside the formal health sector into the wider public, voluntary and private sectors (DoH, 1992; 1993a). At a national level this has been carried forward by the creation of government-level task forces and working groups on specific aspects of health, such as physical activity and workplace health.

Alliances between health sector and other professionals, such as teachers, urban planners, leisure services workers, youth leaders and so on, are growing in importance (Scriven and Orme, 1996). The settings approach highlights the ways in which work with health promotion programmes for particular population groups can be organised. In the course of their work teachers in schools may give their pupils information about diet and exercise, youth leaders may offer information on smoking and other drugs, leisure service workers may promote sport and physical fitness and planners may create local environments which encourage walking and cycling and improve people's quality of life.

The Wellness Forum, launched in 1992, is an instructive example of a healthy alliance. It brings together large employers and health organisations with an interest in providing health promotion services for their employees, and is represented on the Department of Health workplace task force. The aim of the Wellness Forum (1995) reflects its main concern with improving efficiency and productivity and provides an interesting parallel with arguments from some nineteenth century employers that business efficiency and the welfare of the employees reinforced each other (Jones, 1995).

[Members have] the common interest of developing the health of employees through prevention measures to better morale, reduce absenteeism and improve performance

(Wellness Forum briefing paper, 23 August 1995).

Box 1.4: A workplace health initiative

Workers at a metal processing factory in the West Midlands found noise levels on the factory floor a major problem. Some of the longer serving employees felt that the decibel level was above the prescribed level and that their hearing had been affected. After discussing this with their union, support was gained from the Birmingham-based Health and Safety Advice Centre to train a union representative to carry out hearing tests which could provide solid evidence of the extent and degree of hearing loss and support claims for compensation. One consequence of this was that negotiations began with the employer to develop a noise reduction strategy.

(interview with Tommy Harte, Health and Safety Advice Centre, reported in The Open University, 1992: Workbook 2: 98)

The UK health strategies in the late 1990s have built upon this approach and further developed it in terms of 'partnerships'.

Assess the differences between the health promotion initiatives outlined in Boxes 1.2, 1.3 and 1.4. Draw out and discuss what this reveals about the focus of health promotion work in the UK.

These initiatives are concerned with different aspects of health promotion and represent very different approaches. The Health and Lifestyles survey (HEA, 1995) provides data to underpin work with clients and guide national campaigns, whereas the health visitors' smoking advisory service is a direct service. Both, however, were initiated by health 'experts' – the researchers and the health visitors – in contrast to the workplace health initiative which was started by the workers themselves. It is not clear whether there was a clearly expressed demand for a smoking advisory service. The goals were professionally focused: that is, 'better continuity' and 'better use of skilled resources'. The Health and Lifestyles survey was also a response to professional requirements, in this case a need to establish baseline data for Health of the Nation. The workplace initiative was lay-led, although to gather support it had to coincide with the agenda of the employer.

These brief reports give a flavour of the variety of contemporary health promotion. The emphasis on underpinning research is much stronger than it was in the early 1990s and reflects government requirements to show 'value for money' by enabling health promotion initiatives to be systematically evaluated and to be evidence-based. The focus on a national disease reduction target – lung cancer – is also typical of much health promotion work. By contrast, the workplace initiative demonstrates current interest in a settings approach to health promotion. This has been argued for on the grounds that using settings enables health promotion specialists to create an integrated health programme for a chosen group rather than focusing on disease targets in a fragmented way (Tannahill, 1994).

Characteristics of professional-led work

Much of the visible health promotion in the UK is expert-led and some of it has been criticised for giving too little attention to ordinary people's concerns and priorities. One issue that often arises is the availability of the service. The health visitors seem to have recognised this by reviewing their drop-in centre opening hours. Another is the poor targeting of health promotion messages which research such as the Health and Lifestyles survey is designed to help overcome. Research into health education messages in South Wales, for example, suggested that they were less effective because they were 'quite seriously out of step with popular culture in those areas' (Davison *et al.*, 1992). The researchers recommended that the content of the messages needed reworking so that they emphasised 'probability rather than certainty' about lifestyle and disease links and acknowledged the limits to lifestyle explanations: 'some fat smokers really do live till advanced old age and some svelte joggers really do fall down dead'.

Three case studies cannot reproduce the variety of contemporary health promotion and tend to overemphasise new initiatives, so it is important to remember that routine work can be health promoting. Indeed it is one of the central arguments of this book that promoting health is about seizing existing opportunities and transforming existing practices. An occupational therapist might make an assessment of a client with multiple sclerosis which results in the provision of a downstairs toilet or taps and switches for kitchen appliances which make them easier to use and help prevent accidents. These adaptations to the home can transform people's ability to manage their own lives and remain independent. This in turn can free up time for leisure activities and have an important influence on their physical and mental health, and perhaps that of their family or other carers.

Lay-led health promotion

While health education by health professionals has an important contribution to make to promoting people's health, other formal and informal sources, such as parents, friends and teachers, may also be a

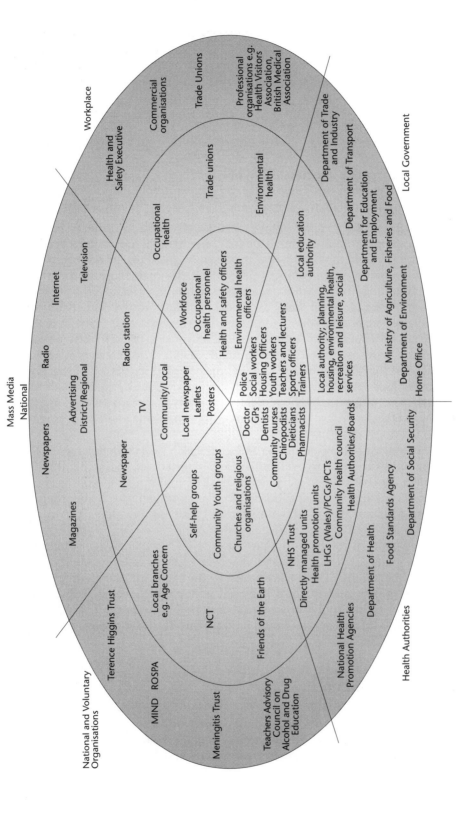

Figure 1.1 UK agencies involved in promoting health (adapted from Naidoo and Wills, 2000). LHG = local health group; PCG = primary care group; PCT = primary care trust.

valued source of health advice and support. One of the most significant movements of the 1980s in the UK was the rise of the community health movement, with its focus on local collective action for health by lay people (Watt and Rodmell, 1993; Beattie, 1990a; Smithies and Webster 1998).

Promoting health is an activity in which ordinary people are often involved, as parents, informal carers, and as individuals protecting and promoting their own health. Most parents, for example, think it important to teach their children about how to protect their health. This might range from teaching about brushing teeth, eating a balanced diet and getting plenty of sleep to training children in the safe use of their local area, why not to talk to strangers and how to act in dangerous situations. As individuals most of us spend a considerable time cleansing, grooming, exercising, feeding and resting our bodies. Not all of this by any means is directed towards promoting its health, but some of it is and this amount is probably increasing. *The Health and Lifestyle Survey: Seven Years On* (Cox *et al.*, 1993), which updated a major survey of health and lifestyles undertaken in 1985, indicated that young manual workers in particular thought their diet had improved over the last seven years and evidence from their records of food intake suggested that they were probably right. Using the government guidelines on healthy nutrition the respondents were eating less fat and sugar than at the time of the first survey.

1.5 Conclusion

By now it should be clear that health promotion is a complex and controversial activity. From relatively narrow origins in health education and a primary focus on changing people's health behaviour it has become a broader, some would say all-encompassing, movement which aims to work at the level of individuals, communities, organisations, governments and through international agencies (see Figure 1.1). In the chapters that follow you will be exploring the scope and significance of actions to promote health and the skills that are needed.

This chapter has covered a good deal of ground. It has introduced you to some key elements of health promotion – prevention, health education, public health, healthy public policy, community action, and creating supportive environments. It has briefly explored some different ways of thinking about health and the implications of these for health services, noting why modern medicine has been increasingly supplemented by health promotion work. Some of the key skills needed to promote health, such as an understanding of advice work, community level action, epidemiology and evaluation, have been introduced. One or two of the fundamental dilemmas in promoting health have been noted. In doing so, it has suggested why health might indeed be seen as 'everybody's business'.

Chapter 2
What is health?

2.1 Introduction

Health promotion is unlikely to improve health and to bring about change unless health promoters have developed an understanding of why and how people's ideas about health differ and can adjust health priorities and actions to meet the expressed needs of different social groups. Those who would promote health may themselves have strong views about health and may implicitly or explicitly seek to impose their views on the groups with whom they work. So there is also a need for self-awareness about health concepts. Health educators have sometimes worked within a narrow view of health, emphasising the need for 'patient compliance' in changing behaviours. In this approach 'good health' is equated with the avoidance of health damaging behaviours (Calnan, 1984). Individuals receiving the health advice are assumed to be 'empty vessels' waiting to be filled. If people do not co-operate they might then be blamed, with little consideration given to their own views of health or their ability to modify their lifestyles (Naidoo, 1986; Davison *et al.*, 1992).

This chapter starts from the premise that an understanding of health concepts is central to health promotion. It explores definitions of health, disease, illness and sickness and highlights the diversity of contemporary views about health. It suggests why there are differences in the way individuals and social groups define health and how these arise from everyday experiences and life events. It assesses alternative ways of accounting for health and their implications for health promotion practice.

2.2 Defining and measuring health

Definitions of health contain within them complex ideas about what it is to be healthy, whose responsibility it is to maintain health and how illness and disease should be interpreted. They may project officially sanctioned ways of viewing health which have passed into public circulation and become part of popular thinking. The 'absence of disease' view noted in Chapter 1 sends powerful signals that health is not about feeling well, at ease, energetic, or even necessarily about not feeling ill; it is about not having a disease. It derives from a medical concept of disease as a pathological state which can be diagnosed and categorised, or as deviation from measurable biological variables which represent 'normal' parameters in the 'healthy' body. Some evidence of the extent to which health is viewed as 'an absence of disease' is provided by *The Health and Lifestyle*

Survey (Cox *et al.*, 1987). In this survey of 9,000 adults in England, Scotland and Wales, 30 per cent of respondents offered a definition of health as 'not ill' or 'no disease'.

By contrast, defining health as 'a state of complete physical, mental and social well-being' (WHO, 1948) projects the view that freedom from disease is not health; real health is viewed as the transformation of no disease-type health into all-round well-being. Health becomes a personal struggle and a goal to be worked towards on a community, national and global level. The WHO Working Group Report on health promotion defined health rather more cautiously as:

> ... the extent to which an individual or group is able, on the one hand, to realize aspirations and satisfy needs and on the other hand, to change or cope with the environment. Health is therefore seen as a resource for everyday life, not the objective of living: it is a positive concept emphasizing social and personal resources as well as physical capabilities.
>
> (WHO, 1984: 23)

Evaluate this definition of health (WHO, 1984). What advantages and drawbacks does it have compared with the 'well-being' and 'absence of disease' accounts?

This definition emphasises that health is embedded in the processes and actions of people's everyday lives. It relates health to ability to cope and adapt within a particular environment. Unlike the earlier WHO definition it deliberately avoids viewing health as an object, seeing it instead as 'a resource for living'. It signals that health might be understood in different ways by different individuals and groups, and emphasises the dynamic interaction between individuals and their environment. This has considerable advantages because it directs attention to the 'embedded' nature of health and to the potential contribution to health not just of individual biology and medical services, but of conditions in the wider natural, social, economic and political environment.

On the other hand there are also advantages in seeing health as absence of disease. It has enabled us to take minor complaints in our stride; we can have aching feet, period pains, a bad cold, back ache, and still see ourselves as healthy. But the medical focus on disease conditions has resulted in the labelling of people with disabilities and chronic conditions as inevitably 'sick' or 'diseased' when they are otherwise healthy. This kind of thinking, together with the measurement of health in terms of avoided or delayed death, has left lay people and professional health workers alike with a rather negative view of health.

Disease, illness and sickness

The terms disease, illness and sickness are frequently used interchange-ably, although they describe several different states. Illness is the subjective state of feeling ill or unwell. This draws attention to the fact that illness is mediated through the individual: in other words, illness is about how people feel. A doctor may break the news to one patient that she has a high blood pressure score or reassure another that he doesn't have bronchitis. The doctor's words may not change how either feels. The first patient may feel just as well after her blood pressure test as she did before and, in spite of the assurance that he doesn't have bronchitis, the other patient may feel just as ill.

Sickness is reported illness, and is about going to the health centre for treatment of some kind and becoming a medical statistic. Hannay (1971) identified what he termed an 'illness iceberg', in that only a proportion of illness ever gets reported and officially recorded. People treat themselves, ask advice from friends, or just put up with feeling ill. Sickness rates are calculated from the use of health services and absence from work records. Neither are very reliable measures of the extent of disease because both are influenced by individual circumstances and different methods of record-ing and reporting sickness across the country (Whitehead, 1987).

The essential point about disease is that it refers to a specific condition of ill-health or pathological state in a patient. From a viewpoint of modern scientific medicine this can usually be identified as an actual change (lesion or abnormality) on the surface of, or inside, some part of the body. Diseases are created as a medical reality by being entered in the International Classification of Diseases (ICD) index. In theory a specific disease condition should characterise every episode of reported sickness. In practice, health workers treat patients and sign them off work in some cases where no disease can be identified; some disease categories, such as repetitive strain injury or post-viral fatigue syndrome (ME), are still hotly contested.

Apply these definitions to ill-health episodes that you have experienced recently. What criteria did you use to define yourself as sick, ill or as having a specific disease?

Among the criteria you may have selected some were probably intrinsic, such as the nature and severity of the symptoms and how long they had persisted, and others situational, such as whether others were also suffering, what deadlines you had and whether you had experienced similar symptoms in the past. Such factors are likely to determine whether you reported sick and how you presented your state of health to others. 'Flu', for example, is a familiar, widely experienced and vague condition which isn't generally seen as a disease. People may classify themselves as ill – feeling awful but keeping going – but if symptoms persist (or if they can take time off work or family responsibilities) they may self-report or register as sick. This may in turn give them 'permission' to be ill. There is often a complex pathway from illness to sickness, mediated by people's state of knowledge, mental attitude, personal relationships and by social factors (Calnan, 1987).

Measuring health through mortality and morbidity

In the West health has been defined and measured most often in terms of disease and death. Differences in health between various groups in society are calculated by means of the standardised mortality ratio (SMR), which measures the relative chances of death at a stated age. Mortality (death) statistics began to be collected and published by the British government in the 1840s, although official estimates of death rates go back long before this. All deaths (and births and marriages) had to be notified to the local registry office, so that the Registrar General's office in London was able to build up detailed information on death rates and causes of death. This work is still carried on by the Office for National Statistics in the UK (formerly known as the Office of Population Censuses and Surveys) and by the Central Statistics Office in the Republic of Ireland (see Figure 2.1).

By the 1890s Medical Officers of Health (MOH) in towns all over the country were producing quite sophisticated analyses of mortality by cause and of the pattern of morbidity (sickness) in their populations. For example, the Medical Officer of Health for Birmingham, Alfred Hill, reported in 1896 on child mortality in different wards of the city. He demonstrated that the death rate in the 'unhealthy', inner area wards was nearly twice that of the 'healthy' wards and argued that diseases such as whooping cough and measles, though not in themselves killers, became so through neglect:

> due to ... uncleanness and bad feeding, lack of clothing, lack of fresh air [and] poverty ... With poverty as such the Sanitary Authority is, of course, not officially concerned [but] with the provision of fresh air and removal of filthy conditions it is directly concerned.
>
> (MoH Annual Report, 1896: 9)

There are obvious advantages in measuring health in terms of mortality and morbidity, because it is generally relatively easy to record reported sickness and actual death. Moreover, reducing the burden of ill health consequently increases the level of health in a population. The national health strategies for the UK in the 1990s were framed in terms of 'reducing' and 'preventing' disease and sickness, partly because it is still much more feasible to set targets for reduction of ill health and death than to set targets for improving health. For example, coronary heart disease and stroke was justified as a key area 'because of the scope for preventing illness and death from these conditions, and because reductions in risk factors ... would also help to prevent many other diseases'. Cancers were selected 'because of the toll that cancers take in ill-health and death'

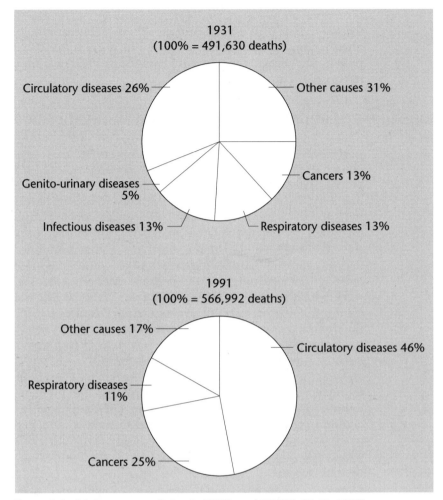

Figure 2.1 **Major causes of death (1931 and 1991*)** (DoH, 1992)

* Data for 1991 exclude deaths of those aged under 28 days
Percentages do not add up to 100 due to rounding

(DoH, 1992). In contrast, recording 'health', as you may have begun to realise, is rather problematic.

Positive measures of health

Mortality and morbidity are still widely used today as proxies for health, and lowering morbidity is equated with improving the nation's health. Mortality statistics have been used to measure health standards in terms of potential years of life lost (PYLL). Improved health is still frequently measured in terms of life expectancy but other approaches have been developed which attempt to measure aspects of health and quality of life rather than just quantity. Measures of health status such as the Nottingham Health Profile (Hunt *et al.*, 1986) allow respondents some scope to make subjective assessments of their health by recording scores in a range of categories selected by the researchers, including physical mobility and emotional reactions.

Health promotion has focused on the objective of adding 'life to years' as well as 'years to life' to signal the priority it accords to quality of life. A whole range of different scales and questionnaires have been developed to measure quality of life (Bowling, 1991), the most contentious being the QALY – quality adjusted life year (Gudex, 1986). This research tool, refined by health economists at York University, measures people's quality of life in terms of their relative freedom from disability and distress as well as the years of life added. In doing so it makes judgements, based on a range of professional and lay (non-expert) views, about the relative importance of types of disability and distress.

2.3 Exploring concepts of health

Health is subject to wide individual, social and cultural interpretation. We experience health and illness as individuals yet it is through influences such as culture, class and gender that these are shaped. Images of health are built on media messages and prevalent ideas about health rights, levels of service, access, awareness and so on. These include social expectations about what it means to be healthy in a particular society and historical time. For example, studies have suggested that older people are more likely to view health in terms of resilience and coping than fitness (Williams, 1983; Blaxter, 1990). Young people frequently define it in terms of fitness, energy, vitality and strength, emphasising positive attainment and a healthy lifestyle. The notion that health is about physical fitness and being in peak condition often reflects a broader view that responsibility for health lies with the individual.

People's views about health and illness, both the public, officially sanctioned ideas and more hidden personal beliefs, are diverse and complex. Popular 'folk' beliefs about the causes of health and illness have always existed, reflecting a range of social and cultural experiences. Research into lay beliefs about colds and fevers in an English suburb in the 1970s resulted in a series of explanations of these illnesses in terms of the natural world. This demonstrated how the popular phrase 'feed a cold, starve a fever' is underpinned by a more elaborate classification of colds and fevers in terms of 'hot' and 'cold', 'wet' and 'dry' symptoms (Helman, 1986).

These ideas link to much older beliefs about health and the body, in particular to ideas of correspondence between the individual human being and the universe. This supposes that the features of the natural world are reflected in human physical and mental characteristics. To varying degrees

Chinese medicine, Indian Ayurvedic beliefs, and Humoral medicine all emphasise how nature – the cycle of life and death, seasonal change, and so on – influences human health. Properties and characteristics of nature, such as wind, water and heat, are viewed as properties of human bodies which need to be kept in balance if health is to be maintained (Open University, 1992). Alternative accounts of health, such as homeopathy, also emphasise the importance of balance and wholeness. They focus on the whole person as an essential partner both in diagnosis and in restoring health (Aakster, 1993).

Beliefs about health and illness

The uncovering of contemporary beliefs about health and illness has focused on classifying people's accounts, pointing to their diversity and to the conflicts between them. It is not just that different groups of people make different responses – for example, working-class and middle-class, men and women, black and white people, young and older people. It is also that the same person may use several distinctive explanations or stories to make up a complete account. In a classic study Herzlich (1973) investigated the beliefs of mainly middle-class people in Paris and Normandy, and identified three different conceptions of health:

1 'Health in a vacuum'– the lack or absence of illness.
2 'Reserve of health' – a quality someone has, making them able to resist illness.
3 'Equilibrium' – which she calls 'real' health, in which someone is active and aware of their body.

These findings have been echoed to varying degrees by other researchers. In particular, the notions of health as a reserve of strength (the result of a good constitution or inner strength or fitness), as the capacity to function fully, and as absence of disease have been identified (Williams, 1983; Blaxter and Pattison, 1982; Blaxter, 1990, McClusky, 1989). The Health and Lifestyles Survey (Cox *et al.*, 1987) asked a representative sample of 9,000 adults about their health beliefs and attitudes. Among the questions asked were ones about describing 'someone you know who is healthy' and 'what it is to be healthy yourself' (see Table 2.1).

> **Study Table 2.1 which identifies concepts used to describe what health is. What patterns can you identify in these responses?**

People in this survey offered a range of definitions of health which are differentiated in Table 2.1 by age, gender and whether they are describing themselves or someone else. In describing someone else most chose either 'never ill, no disease' or 'fit, strong, physically active' but in describing

Table 2.1   **Concepts used in the attempt to describe what 'health' is**

Concept of health used for describing someone else	Males Age 18–39	40–59	60+	Females 18–39	40–59	60+
			Percentage			
Never ill, no disease, never see a doctor	26	39	37	45	51	37
Fit, strong, energetic, physically active	46	28	13	30	21	11
Able to do a lot, work, socially active	13	16	22	14	18	20
Has healthy habits (eg not smoking, taking exercise, taking care of health)	24	18	14	27	17	14
Psychologically fit (e.g. relaxed, dynamic, contented, able to cope)	9	9	6	11	8	5
In good health for their age (applied to an older person)	2	8	15	3	8	17
Mean no. of concepts used	1.2	1.2	1.1	1.3	1.3	1.1
Concept of health used for describing what it is to be healthy oneself						
Never ill, no disease, never see a doctor	15	17	16	12	10	11
Fit, strong, energetic, physically active	25	18	12	36	28	14
Able to do a lot, work, get out and about	18	18	27	18	25	31
Feel psychologically fit (e.g. good, happy, able to cope)	55	60	54	58	62	54
Can't explain, or don't know what it is to be healthy	8	7	8	6	6	10
Mean no. of concepts used by those offering any	1.3	1.3	1.2	1.4	1.4	1.3
Base = 100%	*1668*	*1240*	*997*	*2150*	*1596*	*1352*

Multiple answers possible

(Cox *et al.*, 1987)

themselves people overwhelmingly emphasised 'psychological fitness'. This may be because it is easier to judge physical fitness than psychological fitness in other people. However, when age and gender are taken into account the pattern is more complex. Younger men and women emphasised physical fitness more, but women applied this more to themselves whereas men used it in describing someone else. For women at all ages the category 'never ill' was most in evidence when describing someone else. Reviewing the findings, Blaxter (1990) has commented that 'it is the individual's own perceived health status which appears to determine the way in which health is defined'.

There are other factors likely to influence definitions of health, one of which is cultural identity. A secondary analysis of the health and lifestyles data identified that people of African-Caribbean background were more likely than matched white respondents to see health in terms of physical fitness and energy (Howlett *et al.*, 1991: Ahmad, 1993). By contrast, respondents of Asian background frequently offered a functional definition of health: that is, as the ability to do things.

Mounting evidence of the complexity of lay explanations of health and illness has led to the claim that people are weavers of stories making 'artful use of language to make sense of the world' and drawing on rich and varied experiences and insights (Stainton Rogers, 1991). Her research identified eight such accounts which differed considerably from each other in their approach, priorities and types of explanations (see Table 2.2). Respondents did not necessarily frame their explanations in terms of one account but selected from 'one text and then another, gradually weaving a narrative that makes sense'. People's accounts are both general and particular, making ideological statements which define their 'social fitness' and statements about personal dilemmas 'which exemplify their claims to being ill or healthy' (Radley and Billing, 1996).

Compare Stainton Rogers' categories with the findings of Herzlich and the Health and Lifestyles Survey and consider which of these categories of explanation you would endorse.

All three researchers found more conventional medical-influenced views of health and illness: the 'body as machine', 'health in a vacuum', and 'health as never ill, no disease'. They also unearthed more positive concepts. These may be about deep personal feeling, as in 'equilibrium', 'psycho-social well-being', and 'will-power', for example. Or they may be more concerned with various types of external influences, such as 'the modern way of life', 'external environment' or 'body under siege'. There are links between Herzlich's category of 'reserve of strength', Stainton Rogers' 'robust individualism' and the 'functional' approach cited in the Health and Lifestyles Survey (Cox *et al.*, 1987). In addition, all three have emphasised the multiple dimensions and shifting combinations of lay

Table 2.2 **Lay accounts of health**

1 The 'body as machine' account, in which illness is accepted as a matter of biological fact and modern biomedicine is seen as the only valid type of treatment.	2 The 'body under siege' account, which sees the individual as under constant threat from germs, diseases, stresses and conflicts of modern life.
3 The 'inequality of access' account, which accepts modern biomedicine but is concerned about unequal access and treatment.	4 The 'cultural critique' of medicine account, which highlights how western biomedicine has oppressed women, minority groups and colonial peoples and which emphasises its 'social construction'.
5 The 'health promotion' account, which emphasises the importance of a healthy lifestyle and personal responsibility although it also sees health as a collective responsibility.	6 The 'robust individualism' account, which emphasises the individual's right to live a satisfying life and their freedom of choice.
7 The 'God's power' account, which views health as righteous living and spiritual wholeness.	8 The 'will-power' account, which emphasises the moral responsibility of individuals to use their will to maintain good health.

(Stainton Rogers, 1991)

ideas, which might have been endorsed in your review of your own view of health.

Explaining health and illness

Popular health beliefs are not unitary, one-dimensional or simplistic. This has important implications for those engaged in promoting health, where directive lifestyle messages remain prominent. Many respondents do emphasise personal behaviour as a major cause of disease, citing smoking and drinking as significant factors in lung cancer, heart attacks, chronic bronchitis and other conditions. But they also explain ill health partly in terms of 'the unhealthiness of modern living' (Herzlich, 1973; Blaxter, 1990). They refer to factors beyond their control, such as heredity, the external environment, and to psycho-social influences, especially 'stress'. There is both widespread awareness of the contribution of personal behaviour and some scepticism about whether doing the 'correct' healthy things will make much difference.

It doesn't matter what you do, you could go out and jog every day and have a heart attack for no reason. You know? I mean, you've got to live life the way you want to and the way you feel you can push yourself.

The way I look at it, if you're going to die of cancer or anything else, you're still going to die of something. You can't be a health fanatic all you life, can you?

I smoked more when I was carrying Sally, and yet she was the biggest of the four ... I was doing about sixty a day ... [The girls] said, 'The way you're smoking, Mother, you'll have a yellow baby'. You know? Because I was, literally, one after the other. And yet she turned out the biggest of the lot and nothing wrong with her.

(Cornwell, 1984: 165-7)

These comments, recorded in the 1980s, are very similar to those from respondents in the early 1990s who were asked about causes of coronary heart disease (Davison *et al.*, 1992). They stressed heredity, environment, luck, fate, randomness and chaos as well as personal behaviour in the distribution of disease, reflecting the complex, multifactoral theories of disease causation that currently exist. This prompted the conclusion that 'popular belief and knowledge concerning the relationship of health to heredity, social conditions and the environment may be more in step within scientific epidemiology than the lifestyle-centred orientation of the health promotion world' (Davison *et al.*, 1992). If official models of health explanation are over-simple they not only mislead but risk being ignored – and not only by lay people. One of the health service commentators on the Open University course *Health and Wellbeing* acknowledged:

In my professional life I know the facts about health-damaging behaviour. But in my everyday life I think – I'm young. I don't need to worry about it. At this stage in my life, money is all important, and it dominates other factors.

(Open University, 1992: Workbook 1: 34)

Explanations of health and illness are embedded in people's life experiences and influence their attitudes and actions. They are also intricately bound up with values. It cannot be assumed that everyone will be able to or wish to value their health highly, simply because health promoters do. For both these reasons health promoters need to uncover and understand the health beliefs of those groups with whom they are working. In relation to this it may be difficult to uncover the complex private beliefs that people have about their health (Cornwell, 1984; Radley and Billing, 1996). People may be giving researchers the answers they think they want to hear rather than revealing their private thoughts about health and illness. For example, working class respondents are more likely to give simpler, unidimensional responses to questions about health. This is particularly likely when using survey techniques (Cornwell, 1984). But given more time and space to respond, the respondents become more descriptive and expansive in their accounts (Calnan, 1987).

2.4 Accounting for health

Accounts of health not only 'weave stories' about beliefs but also about practices. In the eighteenth and nineteenth centuries, as scientific medical knowledge developed and challenged older ways of thinking about health, medical power also grew (Foucault, 1973). Doctors exerted increasing control over the human body, creating a whole regulatory framework of observation, diagnosis, categorisation, treatment and segregation. Healthy people became those with 'normal' functioning (as measured within a defined range) and with no evident pathology. By the early twentieth century medicine had consolidated its power base within the health field and was able to influence the training of other health professionals, so that medical concepts and practices became generalised and normalised. Foucault termed this a 'discourse'; that is, a comprehensive framework of conceptualising (seeing) and practising (doing) health work.

The medical model of health

This 'medical model' of health is the most powerful and influential discourse about health and, as we have seen, one which defines health quite narrowly. Treating disease in individuals is the central activity, underpinned by an explanation of the causes of ill health which privileges physical features (see Table 2.3). This view of disease has come to dominate western thinking about health during the past two centuries. It is linked to the rise of clinical pathology and the scientific investigation of disease by a growing body of specialist doctors and researchers, and to the emergence of health work as a formal, professionalised area of expertise (Friedson, 1970). This is underpinned by a set of power relations between patients and doctors in which patients are conceptualised as largely inactive recipients of expert knowledge and intervention.

> Assess the medical model in Table 2.3 in relation to health promotion, suggesting which aspects of this approach are of value and which create difficulties.

If health promotion views health in a positive way as a 'resource for living' it sees people as being in dynamic interaction with their social, economic and physical environments. It focuses on whole populations or groups and seeks to enhance health by preventing disease before it strikes or in its early stages. This is difficult to reconcile with a medical view concerned with physical health and normality, which focuses mainly on individual patients, treatment and cure of disease. The medical model, therefore, seems less relevant for health promotion.

Table 2.3 **The medical model**

- Health is predominantly viewed as the 'absence of disease' and as 'functional fitness'.
- Health services are geared mainly towards treating sick and disabled people.
- A high value is put on the provision of specialist medical services, in mainly institutional settings.
- Doctors and other qualified experts diagnose illness and disease and sanction and supervise the withdrawal of patients from productive labour.
- The main function of health services is remedial or curative – to get people back to productive labour.
- Disease and sickness are explained within a biological framework that emphasises the physical nature of disease: that is, it is biologically reductionist.
- It works with a pathogenic (origins of disease) focus, emphasising risk factors and establishing abnormality (and normality)
- A high value is put on using scientific methods of research (hypotheco-deductive method) and on scientific knowledge.
- Qualitative evidence (given by lay people or produced through academic research) generally has a lower status as knowledge than quantitative evidence.

(adapted from Jones, 1994)

There are, however, three important ways in which health promotion has identified with the medical model:

- health promotion also puts a high value on using scientific methods of research and scientific knowledge, and has tended to give a lower status to qualitative evidence. Many epidemiological studies and baseline studies of health status and behaviour have been produced over the years, whereas most qualitative research has been produced outside the field by social scientists (eg. Cornwell, 1984; Sidell, 1995)
- health promotion has focused on medical risk factors as a basis for developing campaigns and projects aimed at specific 'at risk' groups in the population. A significant part of health promotion deals with prevention and risk reduction strategies and the contribution these can make towards the improvement of health. The publication of the UK health strategies and the focus on health targets make such an approach more justifiable, even though health promotion specialists are attempting to broaden this by developing a programmes and settings approach (Tannahill, 1994)
- it is only since the 1980s that health promotion experts at an international level have systematically developed strategies to share power with lay people through community action, healthy cities projects and health alliances. Such initiatives are underway but it will

remain difficult to ensure that lay people's voices and their expressed needs are heard (Smithies and Adams, 1990; Kelly and Charlton, 1995).

As health promotion becomes a broader activity undertaken by professionals and lay people in and outside the health sector the shortcomings of the medical model are more generally perceived. Social work has found it difficult to work within a disease and abnormality framework. Other professional groups in the health field have also been critical; occupational therapists, for example, work with a more positive model of occupational performance. Doctors, particularly public health physicians and some general practitioners, have called for a reorientation of health services and a redistribution of resources towards public and primary health and there is, of course, a strong tradition within medicine that is concerned with public health improvement and prevention of disease. Nursing education now explores the health–illness continuum and the potential for health despite disease.

A 'salutogenic' approach

The medical model is pathogenic, focusing on why people fall sick and on treatment (Dubos, 1959). It labels risk, stressors and disruption as invariably 'bad'. Antonovsky's research (1993; 1987) had the opposite focus: on what keeps people healthy. He argued that working within this 'salutogenic' (health producing) framework focused attention for almost the first time on why some people remained healthy and emphasised that stressors and disruption were unavoidable aspects of life rather than the demons they are portrayed to be in the pathogenic account. The salutogenic paradigm suggests that the normal state of affairs is one of entropy, of disorder, and of disruption of homeostasis so that most people are neither diseased nor healthy but somewhere along a 'health-ease disease' continuum.

The central focus is on 'behavioural immunology': that is, successful coping with adverse conditions in life. Among other groups studied by Antonovsky were concentration camp survivors from the Second World War. These studies of survivors suggested that people were enabled to cope by having developed by early adulthood a feeling of confidence that the world had meaning and was predictable, that they had the resources to cope with the challenges they faced and that these challenges were worth responding to. He suggested that these three components – comprehensibility, manageability and meaningfulness – together created 'a sense of coherence' which he defined as:

... a global orientation that expresses the extent to which one has a pervasive, enduring though dynamic feeling of confidence that:

(1) the stimuli deriving from one's internal and external environments in the course of living are structured, predictable and explicable;

(2) the resources are available to one to meet the demands passed by these stimuli; and

(3) these demands are challenges worthy of investment and engagement.

(Antonovsky, 1987: 19)

Salutogenic research explores, in any given setting, how changes can be made so that the sense of coherence is strengthened, rather than blaming the victims who fall sick. In the workplace, for example, people's sense of coherence will be enhanced if they have work that is meaningful, not over-stressful, and if a sense of autonomy and participation is fostered (Antonovsky, 1984; Cooper and Payne, 1988). The investigation of why people cope and remain healthy emphasises the dynamic relationship between people and their environment. Managing depends not just on personal resources but on relationships, social support and supportive environments.

A social model of health

The concept of salutogenesis is a useful bridge from the medical approach to health to what has been termed the 'social model', an approach that adopts the logic of multicausal theories of health and sees health as influenced by political, economic, social, psychological, cultural and environmental as well as biological factors. That is not to say that the social model of health dispenses with modern medicine; far from it. But there is a fundamental assumption that a medical model is only part of the answer. Modern medicine is mainly concerned with alleviating suffering – pulling people out of the river downstream (Zola in McKinlay, 1979). It is so preoccupied, in fact, that there is no time to move upstream and see why they keep falling into the river! A social model of health proposes that to improve health requires a refocus upstream on the origins of ill health in individuals and groups – the socio-economic pressures that are pushing them into the river of ill health in the first place. Built into the social model, therefore, are assumptions about the importance of reducing inequalities in health and creating equity.

Another central concern is to 'start where people are at' – to understand and value the views of lay people and to recognise that their ideas and concerns about health and illness may not necessarily coincide with professional views and priorities. A good example of this relates to housing. In strictly 'scientific' terms it has taken years to prove the adverse impact of damp housing because of the intervening variables which make precise measurement very difficult. But ordinary people living in poor housing had a very clear and detailed understanding of the impact of housing on their families' health, for example on childhood asthma (Hunt et al., 1986). For them better housing was a central priority, whereas smoking was of marginal importance (except perhaps as a way of coping with poor housing conditions). Intervention based on a social model would respond to people's expressed priorities rather than professional-led priorities for change, and would recognise how people's behaviour is shaped by structural factors.

It might also embrace examples of practical interventions outside the formal health sector. By the late-1980s the National Council for Voluntary Organisations had recorded information about more than 10,000 local health projects. The Health Education Authority local projects database had also recorded thousands of local initiatives. Many projects, such as the Pilton Community Health Project in Edinburgh, use a self-help approach which is conceptualised in terms of a social model.

> We are working with a social rather than a medical model of health. So we believe that health is as much affected by damp housing as diet or exercise. This means, for example, that although we would agree that diet affects a person's health, we would also think that proximity to good shops, cost, advertising and government subsidies were also important. We might also want to explore people's feelings about food and what it represents to them.
>
> (Open University, 1992, Workbook 1: 30)

On the run-down Pilton estate local residents acted together on projects which would improve their health. A high level of participation was achieved and residents operated a fruit and vegetable co-operative, a stress centre and a 'big woman' club on the estate.

At first glance, the social model seems to provide a much more accommodating framework for health promotion. Its underlying philosophy is that the health of individuals and social groups is the result of complex and interacting material-structural and behavioural-cultural factors. This fits in well with the multicausal theory of health which, as we noted in Chapter 1, underlies contemporary health promotion.

The most frequently stated guiding principles of the social model are a commitment to empowerment, to local participation, to equity in health, to accountability, and to co-operation and partnership with other agencies and sectors (Open University, 1992). This in turn creates distinctive objectives: to work to improve adverse features of the environment, such as pollution, bad housing or poor working conditions; to reduce health inequalities; to work with groups such as older people and women, whose health needs may be overlooked. Priorities vary but most programmes which claim to project a social model of health will use World Health Organisation targets and UK targets for disease reduction. In other words the social model does not abandon a medical model but adds to it a greater concern for identifying and ameliorating the social and environmental framework within which health and ill health arise.

A dissenting view

People involved in promoting health, however, have found some difficulty in pinning down what types of actions and interventions would be indicated by working with a social model of health. It is a broad 'umbrella' concept underneath which several different sets of priorities have sheltered, variously emphasising large-scale statutory intervention, small-scale self-help, lay power and shared lay and professional leadership. Health promotion projects, public health programmes, local health projects and campaigning groups have all used its rhetoric (Open University, 1992). The phrase has been used to describe:

- a set of underlying values – a philosophical approach to health
- a set of guiding principles to orientate health work in a specific way
- a set of practice objectives.

As the philosophy is turned into principles and then action it has become characterised differently by groups with different priorities and interests. One assumption has been that the social model is focused on local 'communities' even though community is an ill-defined concept which projects a vision of social solidarity and mutual interest which rarely exists in the late twentieth century. Large-scale health projects, such as those aimed at influencing change within a whole region or city, have also embraced the social model but the types of changes they have planned are ambitious and structural, making it difficult to respond to lay views and needs.

Beyond (and to some extent within) the health promotion field there have been criticisms of the social model, particularly by sociologists. One criticism has focused on the perceived failure of this new approach to replace the epistemology (way of knowing about knowledge) of the medical model (Kelly and Charlton, 1995). At the heart of the social model, it is argued, is an expert discourse about social causes of disease and social system breakdown that is analogous to the medical model's focus on biological cause and malfunction. Health promotion specialists are also accused of committing the 'ecological fallacy'. This means that they blame social structures for causing disease (in the same way as doctors blame germs) although what epidemiological evidence is actually demonstrating is that there is a correlation between, say, low social class and high rates of disease.

> In the medical model the pathogens are microbes, viruses or mal-functioning cellular reproduction. In the social model they are poor housing, poverty, unemployment and powerlessness. The discourse may be different but the epistemology is the same. The social model is not, in our view, an alternative to the discredited medical model. It is a partner in crime...
>
> (Kelly and Charlton, 1995: 82)

Another criticism of the social model as a new model of health concerns its imperialism, its success in taking over the whole of life. The social model is particularly culpable, because its approach is so much broader than that of the medical model. In this view health now encompasses all contexts, structures and cultural styles. It has now been 'dispersed into non-medical surveillance and maintenance systems that target behaviours and beliefs, norms and mores and blur the boundaries between public and private, individual and social life in the name of "wellness"'. (O'Brien, 1995: 204).

Evaluate the potential of the social model of health as an approach to health promotion in the light of this explanation and criticism.

The social model of health is one among several philosophical approaches to health. Like others, it sets down principles and priorities for action. There is a danger that such a broad-brush approach will deliver an equally vague set of outcomes. Linking everything to health could simply mean that health loses its meaning and the messages of health promotion are discarded.

But the dangers of a narrow approach to health promotion are surely greater? The dominance of the medical model of health, unchallenged, will perpetuate risk factors, narrowly defined 'high risk' groups, notions of normality and the marginalising of broader socio-economic influences on health and disease. It is possible to focus on social and economic influences on ill-health without claiming a cause-and-effect relationship where there is none. Health promotion specialists are well aware that not everyone who gets a virus will therefore become sick, even if they do live in inadequate housing or have poor working conditions. But if health promoters are really going to listen to lay people's views about the causes of poor health then they will have to find a way to reconcile expert discourse about correlations and coefficients with – for example – lay beliefs that bad housing makes you sick (Martin *et al.*, 1987).

2.5 Conclusion

We have only given you a flavour of these debates and we'll return to them later. The values of a social model of health underpin World Health Organisation approaches to promoting health. It carries within it a clear commitment to social and political change, focusing attention on socio-economic factors influencing health. It sits uncomfortably in some ways with a medical model which concentrates on treating presented sickness. But there is also considerable overlap between the two views of health and they have a shared interest in prevention, risk and health targets.

The social model places a greater emphasis on positive health and on broader structural and strategic interventions to improve people's health. It emphasises the need for health authorities, government agencies, voluntary and commercial organisations to work together to improve health. But to some extent – and critics would say to a great degree – analyses of the factors influencing ill health, and assessment of the action required to reduce ill health and promote good health, are not always reflected in interventions or evaluation processes. Failure may be attributed to individual incompetence or backsliding rather than to unchanged features of the environment.

If the causes of ill health lie partly outside individual control any intervention would need to respond at several levels: by treating the resultant ill health, by giving advice and support to individuals and households, and by taking wider action such as alerting the primary health care team, networking with other community workers, tackling housing departments, organising a residents' campaign, helping to start a self-help group and so on. Behind this lie some of the central messages of *Health For All by the Year 2000* (WHO, 1977) and the Ottawa Charter (WHO, 1986) about building healthy public policy at all levels and working to create supportive environments.

Chapter 3
Behavioural and environmental influences on health

3.1 Introduction

Chapter 2 suggested that a wide range of meanings is attached to health and that a 'social model' may offer a useful framework of understanding to use in health promotion practice. By exploring socio-economic, environmental and cultural influences on health, health promoters can view health in a more holistic way. But how far is health status to be explained by reference to these wider influences? What, for example, is the contribution of an individual's behaviour in the health/disease balance scales?

This chapter examines some major influences on mortality and morbidity, drawing on research into patterns of health and health behaviour. It indicates that explanations which target people's behaviour and those which emphasise social and environmental explanations are not discrete but are in various ways interlinked. It suggests that a failure to understand and act on this will limit success in health promotion.

3.2 Influences on health and disease

Multicausal explanations highlight the complex ways in which disease is produced and this is acknowledged in the 'social model' of health, as we noted in Chapter 2. The social model directs attention to the interaction between people and their total environment – biological, psychological, social, political, economic, cultural, environmental – putting a particular emphasis on structural and material influences on health. In this way it builds on the influential Lalonde Report, produced in 1974 by the Canadian government, which argued that

> the health care system ... is only one of the ways of maintaining and improving health (and) for the environmental and behavioural threats to health, the organised care system can do little more than serve as a catchment net for the victims.
>
> (Lalonde, 1974: 5)

This report identified four 'fields' within which health could be promoted which it termed: environment, biology, health services and lifestyle. It suggested that most attention had so far been paid to health care and medical interventions, but that it was within the environment and lifestyle fields that there were most opportunities for promoting health in the future (Figure 3.1).

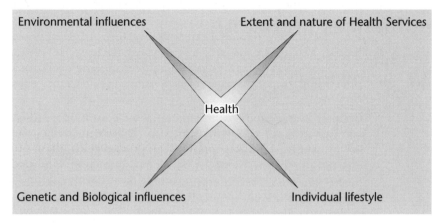

Figure 3.1   **The health field concept**   (Lalonde, 1974)

The 'health field' concept was influenced and endorsed by multicausal theories which emphasised the multifactoral nature of disease. 'States of health or disease are the expression of the success or failure experienced by the organism in its efforts to respond adaptively to environmental challenges' (Dubos, 1959). If people's dynamic interaction with their total environment was the focus, it followed that only a multi-field prevention and health promotion strategy could respond effectively (Lalonde, 1974).

Such thinking has influenced our current understanding of contemporary disease causation and of appropriate responses. It has underpinned the health promotion enterprise (Parish, 1995). In coronary heart disease, for example, a wide range of risk factors has been identified. These include not only physiological indicators such as raised blood pressure and high levels of blood cholesterol, but also related 'lifestyle' features such as smoking and obesity which are linked to these physiological indicators. Beyond this there are psycho-social and environmental factors such as stress, housing tenure, regional location and social class (Rose and Marmot, 1981; Shaper *et al.*, 1985). Applying a health field analysis involves shifting from a treatment focus to a focus on these lifestyle issues and on contributory environmental factors; in other words, addressing the underlying behaviours and contexts that influence heart disease.

Lifestyle or environment?

The health field approach is not without its critics but the report set the terms on which more recent debates about health promotion have developed (Parish, 1995). Within health promotion in the UK, for example, a main focus for debate has been the relative contribution of 'lifestyle' and the 'environment': that is, between individual and social responsibility for ill health. It is argued on the one hand that 'having a healthy diet', 'taking enough exercise' or 'not smoking' are individual lifestyle choices. They are about the exercise of personal decision-making power, which everybody can and should undertake. Successive government reports have emphasised that targeting people's personal behaviour is a key goal for health promotion policy (DoH, 1976, 1987, 1992, 1999).

On the other hand it is pointed out that some decisions – about food pricing, marketing, transport provision and access, pedestrian safety, provision of open spaces, and so on – are made at a wider social level, largely beyond the control of individuals, although acting with others they may be able to influence this decision-making. Some groups in society tend to have consistently poorer health than others, even if differences in lifestyles are taken into account (Townsend *et al.*, 1988). It is also suggested that some social groups may find it easier to accept health messages than others because they have greater autonomy, job security, higher levels of educational attainment and so on (Blaxter, 1990). The next two sections look in turn at the evidence about lifestyles and environment.

3.3 The rise of 'lifestyles' accounts

Lifestyle is a central focus for health education and health promotion. One prominent justification has been that although in the nineteenth century people died of diseases of poverty, in the twentieth century they have died mainly of diseases of affluence – coronary heart disease, lung cancer and strokes – which are largely caused by an unhealthy lifestyle (DHSS, 1976, 1987). By the 1970s smoking behaviour, eating habits and levels of physical activity, which were hitherto thought of as largely private concerns, became public issues and the focus for professional health action. They joined other aspects of people's lifestyle, such as their sexual habits and alcohol consumption, which had already been subject to scrutiny or official regulation.

The Lalonde Report (1974) endorsed significant interventions in the environment, for example legislative change to enforce the wearing of seat belts. But subsequent attention focused on lifestyle as the area in which intervention by health promoters seemed most possible. In the UK lifestyle aspects have received most attention from governments in recent decades. In the 1970s a government document, *Prevention and Health: Everybody's Business*, commented that 'to a large extent though, it is clear that the weight of responsibility for his own health lies on the shoulders of the individual himself' (DHSS, 1976). In 1987 the British government published *Promoting Better Health* in which behavioural change was highlighted:

> Much distress and suffering could be avoided if more members of the public took greater responsibility for looking after their own health ...

family doctors and primary health care teams should increase their contribution to the promotion of good health ... [they] are very well placed to persuade individuals of the importance of protecting their health; of the simple steps needed to do so; and of accepting that prevention is better than cure...

(DHSS, 1987: 3)

Such conclusions were based on evidence indicating that semi-skilled and unskilled workers had higher rates of smoking than those in skilled non-manual and professional occupations and that evidence of a 'healthy diet', as measured in terms of, for example, eating wholemeal bread, was more widespread in higher occupational groups (Black Report, 1980). Studies in the 1990s in the UK and Republic of Ireland have reported similar differences in behaviour. *Variations in Health*, a report commissioned by the Chief Medical Officer's Health of the Nation Working Group, noted that cigarette smoking was still more widespread among semi-skilled and unskilled groups in the UK population. It also reported that the incidence of lung cancer was much higher among these groups, as were mortality rates (DoH, 1995). Expenditure on tobacco by the poorest 25 per cent of families was nearly three times as great as that of the wealthiest quartile (Benzeval *et al.*, 1995). While expenditure by the latter group had fallen by two-thirds between 1980 and 1992, the poorest households were still spending in real terms as much in 1992 as in 1980.

From a narrow lifestyles perspective it can be argued that such evidence demonstrates both the unhealthy choices being made by semi-skilled and unskilled groups and their responsibility to change their behaviour so that their health improves (Anderson, 1986). Indeed, the claim that people have the choice about whether to pursue an unhealthy lifestyle or not is reflected in public opinion. Pill and Stott (1982) reported that women blamed themselves for their inability to eat a more 'healthy' diet even though their failure was seen by the researchers as largely the result of material factors such as lack of money, time pressures and so on. In spite of considerable research which has highlighted the relationship between poverty and ill health (Townsend *et al.*, 1988; Blackburn, 1994), there is widespread support from surveys for the view that personal lifestyle is the main influence upon health. Or rather, respondents expressed their thoughts about health and the way to achieve better health in personal rather than environmental terms. Cornwell (1984) noted that although illness tended to be seen by people in East London as a separate entity which 'happened' to them and for which they were not responsible, they believed that health (as an ability to function) was maintained by having 'the right attitude'. 'The moral prescription for a healthy life is in fact a kind of cheerful stoicism, evident in the refusal to worry, or to complain, or to be morbid'.

On the other hand, it is difficult to tell how far people's responses to researchers represent what they feel they ought to accept or what they *really believe*. Smaller-scale, more intensive contextual studies have provided stronger evidence of people's belief that environmental factors, styles of living and social relationships influence their health (Calnan, 1987). How far are people offering a public, officially sanctioned view of health and keeping their private opinions to themselves? Blaxter has commented:

> There is a high level of agreement within the population that health is, to a considerable extent, dependent on behaviour and in one's own hands... at least it is recognised that these are the 'correct' and 'expected' answers to give.
>
> (Blaxter, 1990: 162)

Respondents in *The Health and Lifestyle Survey* (Cox *et al.*, 1987) echoed this view, although there was also some support for the view that housing and poverty influenced health as well. The Health Education Authority-sponsored health and lifestyles survey (1995c) found that lifestyle factors were the single most important group of factors which respondents saw as influencing their health, although, as in the 1987 survey, other factors were mentioned. Black and minority ethnic respondents reported stress at home, unemployment and crime as having a bad effect on health. But 61 per cent of respondents in the main survey reported 'that they currently did something to improve their health', mainly some type of physical activity or dietary change.

Lifestyle approaches have received support as one element in the 1984 WHO Health For All targets for Europe and have also been endorsed by UK government reports (DoH, 1992; Scottish Office, 1993, 1999; Welsh Office, 1990; DoH Ireland, 1993). Many health professionals have also welcomed the idea of a strategic framework and the setting of health targets. All the UK health strategies identified several aspects of individual behaviour as risk factors, including smoking, diet, alcohol consumption and drug use. They set 'risk factor targets' for the reduction of unwanted types of behaviour and consumption. This is not the only concern of the reports and they do not view lifestyle change as a purely personal matter but as providing targets which a range of agencies will support. Another element in the UK strategies is for central and local government, individuals, statutory and voluntary agencies, and health professionals to work together to meet these targets.

Individual behaviour plays some part in many diseases. The connection between lung cancer and smoking is well established, for example (Doll and Peto, 1981), and dietary factors are thought to be significant in relation to circulatory disease and in some cancers (COMA Report, 1984). So working to persuade people to change risky aspects of their lifestyle seems appropriate. Indeed, developing such preventive strategies at national, organisational and local level is currently a major part of the work of health promotion specialists. If clear targets and priorities are set, progress can be closely monitored and strategies adjusted if the hoped-for changes fail to materialise.

Limits to lifestyle approaches

There are practical and ethical doubts about an approach which mainly targets individual lifestyles (Breslow, 1994). There is still debate about how far health can be improved through targeting personal behaviour. In some instances such campaigns can be effective. A national campaign to prevent cot deaths, for example, which did concentrate on persuading people to change what might be quite well established habits, was highly successful (HEA, 1994). In other contexts, such as those in which lifestyle choices are bound up with a valued cultural identity, change may be much more difficult to achieve. This has long been claimed as the case in relation to some forms of drug-taking, where people learn to enjoy the drug as part of their initiation into a particular sub-culture (Becker, 1971). A study of young people's behaviour also indicated that 'there seemed to be certain lifestyle factors that underpinned risk-taking behaviours' and identified smokers and drinkers as those who 'tended to go out to discos, parties and pubs, and to have a boy/girlfriend' (HEA, 1992).

> **What do you see as possible problems or pitfalls in an approach which focuses mainly on individual behaviour?**

Making changes in many types of personal behaviour can be very difficult. The five-year study of working-class mothers in South Wales indicated that although half of the women had made a change in their behaviour at some point in the study, most fairly quickly relapsed (Pill and Stott, 1982, 1985, 1986). Although the women tended to blame themselves for their relapses, many of the explanations for failure were to do with pressure from domestic or work circumstances and from partners and children. Attempts by women to change themselves and their families to a more healthy type of diet were often resisted by male partners (Pill and Parry, 1989).

This raises a second point, about the ethical basis of a lifestyles approach. If many of the impediments to change are related to social circumstances, to the constraints imposed by income, housing, childcare demands or social pressure from partners or peer group, how justifiable is it to target personal behaviour? Targeting individual lifestyle can come close to 'blaming the victims' if people are in a position where change is very difficult or even impossible, and yet are made to feel guilty for not making a change. Pill (1990) commented that 'some were only too ready to blame themselves' and their 'lack of willpower' and for a few 'this led to loss of self-esteem and strong guilt feelings'. This may not be the intention of the intervention but it is a risk, especially in working with individuals and groups who have very few options for change. It is one reason why the health promotion movement acknowledges the importance of creating environments and policies which support people in making healthier choices (WHO, 1988; WHO, 1992).

The targeting of behaviour is bound up with a wider discussion about the relative merits of types of preventive strategies: 'high risk' and 'whole population' (Jacobson *et al.*, 1991). A 'high risk' approach involves identifying only sections of the population which are at risk of disease or ill health and offering treatment or programmes aimed at changing their behaviour. In one sense this can been seen as victim blaming, but it has also been defended on the grounds that it offers people the freedom to refuse. It could also be more beneficial for the individuals identified than a population strategy which targets everyone and will not necessarily offer much help to at-risk individuals (Rose, 1981). The 'whole population' strategy has also been seen as authoritarian since people are unable to avoid it (Jacobson *et al.*, 1991). Fluoridization of tap water is one example of a whole population strategy, although in the UK its implementation has been left to the discretion of local authorities. This leads into a discussion about the contribution of environmental influences to human health and how far health promoters should focus on whole-population interventions.

3.4 Environmental influences on health

The other main way of explaining patterns of ill health is by examining environmental influences. The major factors which have been explored are social class, poverty, gender, 'race', housing, employment, place of residence and access to health services, and this section will highlight some of their interconnections. With the coming of the Welfare State in Britain in the 1940s, and the right to free, needs-based medical treatment in the new National Health Service, it was thought that health status would gradually be equalised. But the Black Report (DHSS, 1980) indicated that, although health was improving for the population as a whole, health inequalities were still widespread.

Health and social class

The Black Report arose within the wider framework of concern for welfare needs. In 1978 David Ennals, the Secretary of State for Social Services, echoed the concern of many health professionals by drawing attention to differences in life expectancy between high paid professionals and low paid unskilled workers:

> ... the crude differences in mortality rates between the various social classes are worrying. To take the extreme example, in 1971 the death rate for adult men in social class V (unskilled workers) was nearly twice that

of adult men in social class I (professional workers) ... When you look at death rates for specific diseases the gap is even wider.

(David Ennals, reported in Townsend *et al.*,1987: 1)

A working group was set up to examine the issue under the leadership of Sir Douglas Black, president of the Royal College of Physicians. In particular it reported that between the 1950s and the 1970s the mortality rates for both men and women aged 35 and over in occupational classes I and II (professional and non-manual groups) had steadily declined, whereas those in classes IV and V(semi-skilled and unskilled manual) were the same or marginally worse (Figure 3.2).

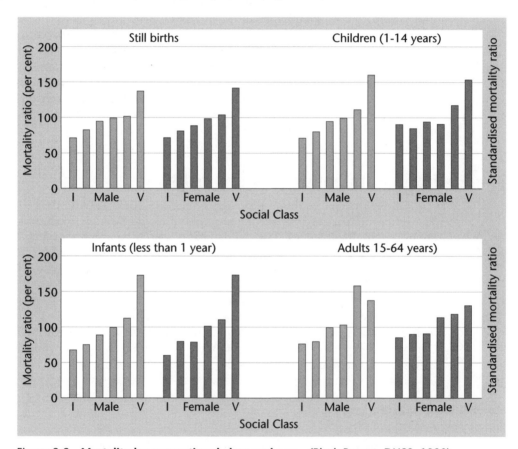

Figure 3.2 **Mortality by occupational class and age** (Black Report, DHSS, 1980)

Occupational class represented the major, though not the only, means by which health inequalities were measured in the Black Report. Although the use of occupational class tends to marginalise women's work, it is a widely used and relatively reliable long-term indicator not only of differences in income, occupational status and living standards but also of relative levels of deprivation. As the report commented, 'undoubtedly the clearest and most unequivocal – if only because there is more evidence to go on – is the relationship between occupational class and mortality' (Townsend *et al.*, 1988). In addition, there was other evidence indicating, for example, that black and minority ethnic groups suffered differentially high rates of heart disease, that regional variations and sex differences were widespread, and that disease risks linked to household type, with owner occupiers having the lowest risk of premature death.

Study Table 3.1 which is a summary of the main recommendations of the Black Report (DHSS, 1980). What are seen as the major priorities? In your view, are these still relevant priorities now?

The main feature of its recommendations was a series of measures to end child poverty and 'give children a better start in life' by halting the 'inadequately treated bouts of childhood illness' that 'cast long shadows forward' (Townsend *et al.*, 1987). The report came down firmly on the side of universalist benefits such as Child Benefit as the most effective means of fighting health inequalities. It called for the increase of Child Benefit, the introduction of child benefits for older children, an increase in the maternity grant and the gradual introduction of an infant care allowance.

Table 3.1   **The Black Report: summary of recommendations**

1   The abolition of child poverty should be adopted as a national goal for the 1980s, by:
   •   Increasing the maternity grant and child benefit
   •   Introducing an infant care allowance for under fives
   •   Ensuring adequate local authority day care for under fives
   •   Providing nutritionally adequate school meals for all
   •   Mounting a child accident prevention programme.

2   The introduction of a comprehensive disability allowance for people of all ages.

3   Draw up minimally acceptable and desirable standards of work, security, conditions and amenities, pay and welfare or fringe benefits.

4   Shift resources more quickly towards community care and primary health care, to improve child health services, expand home help and nursing services for disabled people and extend joint care funding and programmes.

5   Set national health goals after consultation and debate.

6   A substantial increase in local authority spending and responsibilities under the 1974 Housing Act.

7   Establish a Health Development Council.

8   Improve research and statistical data relating to health, such as statistics on child health, income and health inequalities.

(Jones, 1994)

It made increased spending outside the health service a priority, recognising that social and economic factors like income levels, work, environment, housing, transport, education and 'lifestyle' choices influenced health. Other recommendations included the development of comprehensive disability allowances and more state spending on council housing. It argued that an inter-sectoral approach, and a greater concentration upon vital areas such as child health services were needed. But its findings, and the call for extra spending, were rejected in favour of a focus on individual 'lifestyle' change as the route to better health (Townsend *et al.*, 1988).

Poverty, deprivation and health

In spite of the failure to get its most costly recommendations implemented, the Black Report had a significant if gradual effect on the health work field. A study of 'health inequalities' became incorporated into nurse education courses and other health work training programmes. Throughout the 1980s the lines of research highlighted in the report were developed, with many local studies of health and poverty being undertaken in which the impact of poverty on health was revealed. *The Nation's Health*, an authoritative survey of the state of UK health first published in 1988, and a strategic policy document for health in the 1990s, commented that:

> While we may still lack knowledge of the exact mechanisms through which [risk] factors operate, this does not put their contributory role in doubt... Income is clearly associated with health. The evidence is clear that the death rates of old people are affected by changes in the real value of state pensions, and also that as occupations move up or down the occupational earnings rankings they show a corresponding and opposite movement in the occupational mortality rate. The implication is that income – perhaps the major determinant of standard of living and of life-style – has a direct effect on health. It is also clear that health is more sensitive to small changes in income at lower than at higher levels.
>
> (Jacobson *et al.*, 1988: 116)

The report documented research highlighting the links between unemployment and health, pointing out that mental ill health was linked to the 'material disadvantages' which unemployment creates. It also pulled together the research into diet, commenting that consumption patterns 'almost certainly reflect income and cost considerations as well as differences in culture or education' (Jacobson *et al.*, 1988). In this, it reflects one main consequence of a decade or more of research into 'class and health': a more open acknowledgement of the complex interconnections between 'lifestyles' and structural, 'environmental' factors. The report comes down heavily in favour of a broadly based approach to tackling poverty, pointing out that risk factor reduction may accentuate deprivation unless it takes place within a much wider framework of economic action to increase wealth and redistribute resources, community development to promote autonomy and self-esteem, and education of the community.

The Nation's Health, while it emphasised the importance of reducing 'socio-economic disadvantage' as a prelude to tackling specific risk factors and promoting community action, stopped short of including the kinds of welfare targets in its recommendations which ensured that the Black Report was sidelined. Not only was there little commitment by government to pursue the kind of broad assault on poverty sought by Black; a survey by Castle and Jacobson (1988) which analysed the strategies and policies of regional health authorities for promoting health and preventing disease concluded that a commitment to the reduction of inequalities in health 'was not prominent'. A survey in 1990 indicated that Health For All targets, prominent among them targets to reduce inequalities in health, were being only slowly addressed at district health authority level (Beattie, 1990b).

The Health Divide (Whitehead, 1987), a follow-up survey of research into health inequalities, confirmed the Black Report's findings about 'class gradients' in health as well as documenting other differences in health chances and in access. Having reviewed the findings made by researchers in the 1980s, it commented:

> The results of these studies, taken together, give convincing evidence of a widening of health inequalities between social groups in recent decades, especially in adults. In general, death rates in adults of working ages have declined more rapidly in the higher than in the lower occupational classes, contributing to the widening gap. Indeed in some respects the health of the lower occupational groups has actually deteriorated against the whole background of a general improvement in the population as a whole. While death rates have been declining, rates of chronic illness seem to have been increasing, and the gap in the illness rates between manual and non-manual groups has been widening too, particularly in the over-65 age group.
>
> (Whitehead, 1987: 266)

'Race' and health

Black and minority ethnic groups have higher risks of mortality from a range of diseases, such as diabetes, liver cancer, tuberculosis, stroke and heart disease (Whitehead, 1987). Infant mortality, in particular perinatal death, has been highlighted as a problem, as have the higher rates of mental illness (especially diagnosis of schizophrenia) among African-Caribbean men. It is, however, difficult to assess the causes of these variations. Medical intervention has tended to focus on aspects most amenable to behavioural change, such as cultural practices. But there is acknowledgement also of the part played by poverty and unemployment.

The Coronary Prevention Group (1986) highlighted poor working conditions, unemployment and stress as major influences in coronary heart disease.

Experience of racism can also affect health (Ahmad, 1993). First, epidemiological studies and psychological experiments have demonstrated that the 'experience of discriminatory treatment occasioned by racism can have a direct and negative impact on health' (Smaje, 1995). In the following example from maternity care the patient feels blamed for non-attendance at the ante-natal classes by midwives who took no account of cultural barriers to take up of health services or of the possible impact of their judgements.

> At that moment, I was mad... the pain was unbearable... they were shouting ... why you never took the ante-natal classes ... you should have, then there wouldn't be that much problem for you and for us.
> (Pakistani woman in Glasgow, reported in Bowes and Meehan Danokas, 1996: 45)

In a more indirect way, racism influences the socio-economic position of minority ethnic groups. Past discriminatory treatment influenced the ability of ethnic minority groups to get decent housing and satisfactory (or any) employment and these groups still experience discrimination today. This has created particular spatial and socio-economic divisions which will have an impact on successive generations (Smaje, 1996). In this way social class, poverty, place of residence and access may interact with 'race' to influence health status. This has been explored in a study which attempts to examine the effects of 'race', class, poverty and gender, and to establish new approaches to this field of research (Nazroo, 1997).

Developing social indicators

During the 1980s and early 1990s there was a considerable amount of new research which focused on health status and inequalities at a local and regional level, and which demonstrated that there were often wide variations within quite small areas. Researchers began to develop social indicators which could be used to assess health by measuring levels and risks of deprivation (see Table 3.2).

Study Table 3.2. Do you think that all the indicators listed here are likely to be equally reliable and valid as measures of deprivation?

The Jarman index, developed for general practitioners, combines direct measures of deprivation – overcrowding, poor housing, unemployment – with indirect measures of numbers of people 'at risk' of deprivation – ethnic minorities, children under five, single-parent households, elderly living alone, and so on. The indirect measures have been criticised on the grounds that not all people in such 'at risk' groups are deprived, so that too great a reliance on indirect measures can produce a distorted outcome

Table 3.2 **Social indicators used to assess health in other area-based studies**

Jarman Index (1983, 1984) Underprivileged Area Score

Children aged under 5

Ethnic minorities

Single-parent households

Elderly living alone

Lower social classes

Highly mobile people

Non-married-couple families (indicating less stable family groups)

Overcrowding factor

Poor housing factor

Unemployment

Townsend *et al.* (1986) Bristol study

Households with fewer rooms than persons

Households lacking a car

Economically active persons seeking work (or temporarily sick)

Children aged 5–15 who receive school meals free

Households experiencing disconnection of electricity

(Whitehead, 1987)

(Thunhurst, 1985). For example, the Jarman index indicates that seven out of ten of the most deprived local authority areas are in London. But it has been argued that this arises largely because of the disproportionately high numbers of one-parent families and ethnic minority households in London, which skew the figures (Thunhurst, 1985). The greatest concentration of material deprivation can be found in the North of England and Scotland (Whitehead, 1987). Another index of deprivation, developed by Townsend and other researchers (1986) tried to avoid this criticism of indirect indicators by using direct measures. It calculated deprivation in terms of levels of unemployment, overcrowding and ownership of key household goods. The research team argued strongly that 'it is we believe mistaken to treat being black, or old and alone, or single parenthood as part of the definition of deprivation... the point is to find out how many are deprived rather than operate as if all were in that condition' (Townsend *et al.*, 1987).

A strategic response to inequalities?

To critics it seemed as if evidence presented on health inequalities in the UK was consistently being marginalised (Public Health Alliance, 1992). The development of national health promotion strategies, however, gave some recognition to inequalities or what became known in the Health of the Nation (1992) strategy as 'variations' in health. The health promotion strategy for Wales called for 'affirmative action... to enable the disadvantaged to reach their full health potential' (HPW, 1990) and the Northern Ireland strategy noted the 'clear evidence of inequalities in health status' and the need for 'an equitable response to need' through which such inequalities would be identified and addressed (HPANI, 1992). The then Scottish strategy gave similar recognition to the evidence of variations in health (HEBS, 1992). In the Republic of Ireland 'the achievement of equitable health services' was identified as a key principle underpinning the health strategy. Shaping a Healthier Future (1994) and the links between lower socio-economic status and the association with higher rates of mortality, morbidity and psychological stress was explicitly stated in the *Health Promotion Strategy* (DoH, Republic of Ireland, 1995).

Table 3.3 **Mortality of men aged 15–64 at death by social class (based on occupation): standardised mortality ratios for England and Wales**

Social class (based on occupation	1959–63	1970–72	1979–83*	1976–81	1982–85	1986–89
I Professional	76	77	66	69	61	67
II Managerial	81	81	74	69	78	80
IIIN Skilled, non-manual	100	104	93	103	98	85
IIIM Skilled, manual	100	104	103	95	101	102
IV Partly skilled	103	114	114	109	113	112
V Unskilled	143	137	159	124	136	153

Columns 1–3 from Decennial Supplements; columns 4–6 from OPCS Longitudinal Study (of a 1 per cent sample followed prospectively from 1971.)

* Men aged 20–64, 1979–80 and 1982–83

1 A standardised mortality ratio is used to compare the mortality of a particular sub-group of the population *relative* to a standard, adjusting for differences in population age structures. *Where different standards are used for different periods (as in the above table) it is only possible to show changes in relative differences over time, not changes in absolute differences or absolute values.*

2 The Decennial Supplement for 1979–83 records a very high SMR for social class V. The social class V figure may be artificially raised as a result of reclassification of occupation and numerator-denominator biases.

The Chief Medical's Officer Working Group on the Health of the Nation
Sub group on Variations in Health (DoH, 1995)

There was a further review of inequalities in health and the impact of environmental factors, supported by Sir Donald Acheson (former Chief Medical Officer of Health), who concluded: 'although in general the nation's health had continued to improve, inequalities between the social groups had persisted as a serious and almost certainly increasing problem.' (Acheson, in Benzeval *et al.*, 1995). The review gathered together evidence from the UK and across Europe of wide inequalities in health related to unemployment, poor housing, poverty and manual, unskilled work. It noted that these inequalities had widened in the 1980s and reviewed the explanations offered by the Black Report of 1980. Table 3.3 demonstrates the social class gradients in mortality in the mid-1980s among children and adult men and women.

In 1994 a sub-group of the Chief Medical Officer of Health's Health of the Nation Working Group was established to examine variations in health. Its 1995 report emphasised the need to address the 'marked differences by occupational class, sex, region and ethnicity, in life expectancy, healthy life expectancy, and incidence of and survival from a range of diseases' (DoH, 1995). It commented on the marginalisation of work to combat health variations in health authorities and called for more systematic measures and evaluation of those measures, not as special projects but as part of 'mainstream work'. Each health authority and GP purchaser should develop a plan, working in alliance with other bodies, for identifying and tackling variations and monitoring its progress.

Following the election of a new Labour Government in July 1997, the Secretary of State for Health appointed Sir Donald Acheson to lead an independent inquiry into inequalities in health. The aim of this inquiry was to review and summarise inequalities in health in England and to identify priority areas for the development of policies to reduce them. In November 1998 the report was published. It made 39 recommendations underpinned by a broad analysis of the social, economic and environmental determinants of health inequalities in the areas of:

- poverty, income, tax and benefits
- education
- employment
- housing and environment
- mobility, transport and pollution
- mothers, children and families
- young people and adults of working age
- older people
- ethnicity
- gender
- the National Health Service.

The report identified three areas as crucial:

1　all policies likely to have an impact on health should be evaluated in terms of their impact on health inequalities
2　a high priority should be given to the health of families with children
3　further steps should be taken to reduce income inequalities and improve the living standards of poor households.

These areas formed the basis of the first three recommendations.

The Acheson Report was influential in Scotland too, where it helped to inform the White Paper 'Towards a Healthier Scotland' (Scottish Office, 1999). Speaking of 'a sustained attack on inequality, social exclusion and poverty', the White Paper identified 'life circumstances' at one of three action levels for better health (along with 'lifestyles' and 'health topics') and stressed that 'the government agree that tackling inequalities has such importance that it should be regarded as an overarching aim'.

3.5　Interconnections between lifestyles and environment

Explaining health inequalities

Four possible explanations for inequalities in health have been discussed: artefact, social selection, behavioural, and material and social circumstances (see Box 3.1). It concluded in the Black Report (1980) that material and social circumstances were probably most heavily implicated because people's behaviour largely arose from the circumstances and environments in which they had to live. It saw the most productive way forward as large-scale legislative action and intervention.

Black and later investigators (Whitehead, 1987; Benzeval, 1995) dismissed the artefact explanation on the grounds that, while there is some evidence that social classes IV and V have shrunk over the last 30 years, there is no hard data suggesting that this can explain more than a small percentage of the measurable health differences between the lowest and highest classes. Increasingly, epidemiologists group social classes IV and V together and compare them with classes I and II, thus minimising any distortion.

Social selection, while not dismissed out of hand, is not seen to account for more than a small proportion of health differences. There is evidence of upward as well as downward mobility, although the latter is more common, but there are no data suggesting routine and systematic downward social mobility in the post war UK (Whitehead, 1987). The two explanations that have been favoured by most recent investigators

---

Box 3.1: Possible explanation for inequalities in health

Artefact:

This proposes that the inequalities are an artefact of the way the statistics are produced, and that biases and changes in the composition of different social classes over time have made the evidence unreliable.

Social selection:

This proposes that inequalities are a result of social mobility. Those in good health move up the social scale whereas those in poor health slip down.

Behaviour:

Health inequalities are the result of people engaging in health-damaging behaviour and those in the lower social classes are more likely to exhibit such behaviours.

Material and social circumstances:

Poverty, poor living, pollution and poor environment, weak social networks and many other material and social factors influence health and largely create health inequalities.

---

have been behaviour and material and social circumstances. But as we have seen, the interrelationships between these factors are now recognised more fully, as is the possible contribution of other factors. The *Variations in Health* report (DoH, 1995), for example, noted the complex interrelation-ships between environments, behaviour, genetic endowment and health services – the four fields originally identified by Lalonde.

> While socio-economic, gender, regional and ethnic differences are widespread, and are observable in all countries, the magnitude of these differences is not fixed; differences are recorded within and between countries and over different time periods. It is likely that cumulative exposure to health damaging or health promoting physical and social environments is the main explanation for observed variations in health and life expectancy, with health related social mobility, health damaging or health promoting behaviours, use of health services, and genetic or biological factors also contributing.
>
> (DoH, 1995: 1)

This suggests that, although environmental determinants are of central importance, behaviour, social selection, service usage and genetic inheritance also play some part.

Environmental influences on lifestyles

The two major lines of research inquiry into the formation of health chances – one focusing on structural health inequalities, and the other on health behaviour – have developed alongside each other in recent years.

There have been considerable tensions between them, but there is an increasing recognition that they are not mutually exclusive but interdependent (Whitehead, 1987).

Health research increasingly suggests that behavioural and cultural factors on the one hand and material, environmental, and structural factors on the other are interrelated and interdependent. If behaviour cannot easily be separated from its social context then an attack targeted at how people behave, unless it also addresses the social, material and cultural environment in which that behaviour takes place, will have little chance of success. Work on young working class women with children under five who are regular smokers indicates that their smoking behaviour arises largely from their social circumstances (Graham, 1988; Graham and Blackburn, 1993). Smoking became the one activity that the women could choose to do 'for themselves'; it gave them a little time and personal space during a day filled with housework and responding to children's demands. This suggests that wider material and structural changes – perhaps in child care provision, the availability of part-time work, educational provision – might be as useful, or more useful, in improving health as targeting individual behaviour. On the other hand, supporting behaviour change can be effective, as we noted in Section 3.3. Where adequate support, individual commitment and reliable information are available, as in the case of gay sexual behaviour changes in response to HIV/AIDS, then change can be highly significant in health terms (see Part 2 on health education).

Child accidents provide another example (Whitehead, 1987). The higher incidence of childhood accidents in lower social groups could be explained, she suggests, in terms of personal risk-taking and parental neglect, but it could equally well be seen as the result of unsafe local environments which create supervision problems for parents. 'In the latter view, the environment is dictating the behaviour of both mother and child'. This latter interpretation implies the need for a shift of emphasis in practice from seeing parents and children as solely responsible to seeking ways to make the physical environment safer for children. Research into child accidents on the Corkerhill estate in Glasgow identified significant differences between professionals' and parents' allocation of blame for accidents and suggestions for change. Planners, health visitors and accident prevention officers emphasised 'educating the parents, obviously, with a lot of reinforcement' and 'a scheme of paid instructors for training child pedestrian skills'. Parents, while they accepted some responsibility, also emphasised environmental change:

> I'd start with a play area, and a one way street ...

> ... And sleeping policemen on the street.
>
> (respondents in Roberts *et al.*, 1993: 458-9)

Researchers have also highlighted the interconnections of lifestyle and environmental factors, suggesting that action was required to combat inequalities at various levels: strengthening individuals, strengthening communities, improving access to essential facilities and services and encouraging macroeconomic and cultural change (Benzeval *et al.*, 1995). The analysis of health inequalities in the Black Report was revisited and, as with Black, the artefact explanation was rejected: 'the size and consistency of evidence suggest that the artefact explanation can be largely discounted.' Similarly social selection was 'only likely to account for a small proportion of the mortality differences between social groups.' The interaction between behaviour and material and social circumstances was noted as of central importance and the distinction between them as needing care. Blaxter's view (1983), that 'there is no doubt that behaviour is implicated, but it is behaviour which is inevitable in certain circumstances,' expresses the dilemma and the connections very well. Figure 3.3 highlights the range but also differentiates between factors determining people's health.

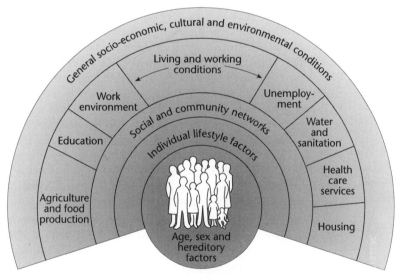

Figure 3.3   **The main determinants of health**

(Dahlgren and Whitehead, 1991)

Look at Figure 3.3 which shows the main determinants of health. What ideas about the causes of ill health are indicated here?

Figure 3.3 offers a multifactoral analysis of the determinants of ill health. It differentiates between individual and social factors, offering an onion-like diagram which we can peel away. The core consists of inherited attributes which are largely fixed, although medical science can ameliorate some debilitating genetic conditions, such as sickle-cell disease which affects the children of one in ten of the African-Caribbean community

(Anionwu, 1993). Medicine can also treat or prevent bacterial and viral diseases and individuals can take action to influence their weight, cardiac function and so on.

The inner layer suggests that health is partly determined by individual lifestyle factors, such as patterns of smoking, physical activity and diet. Moving outwards, the diagram draws attention to relationships with family, friends and significant others within their local community. The next layer focuses on working and living conditions – income levels, housing, employment, access to services and so on. The outer layer highlights broader socio-economic forces such as economic development, shifts in welfare systems, political change, social forces and structures. Although it is not really shown in the diagram, there is the potential for influences from layer to layer. Social support networks, for example, are important in maintaining people's health and well-being (Berkman and Syme, 1979) and may help to offset the adverse effects of unemployment on health. Conversely, cutbacks in welfare might adversely affect people's access to adequate housing and thus influence their health.

It remains difficult to disentangle the relative importance of behaviour and environment in creating health chances. For example, there is evidence that middle-class households consume more of what are considered to be healthier foods than do working-class households (Townsend et al., 1988). It may be argued that this is due to their greater willingness to modify their behaviour, to 'act responsibly' and rationally, and to think more seriously about their health. In this view, it is the attitudes and behaviour of working-class people which need to be modified so that they too 'act responsibly'. On the other hand, it is clear that in some respects middle-class people, with higher living standards and greater material security, are able to make 'healthy choices' more easily than people from poor working-class backgrounds. A diet that meets national nutritional guidelines (NACNE, 1983) by including brown bread, lots of fresh vegetables and fruit, low fat spreads and lean meat is more expensive to maintain than a nutritionally unsatisfactory diet of white bread and sugary or salty foods (Graham, 1986). It may be that working class people are acting responsibly and rationally – by buying the cheapest, most filling foods available to feed their families.

Claims about what is rational behaviour also seem to be class biased: it is the lower social classes who are seen as the problem. But it is likely that middle-class people are just as liable to be influenced by 'peer group pressure' as others; witness the spectacular spread of jogging, aerobics, health clubs and fitness training with the attendant mass middle-class consumption of appropriate clothing and footwear. This may be a result of individuals making 'healthy choices'. Alternatively it may be the consequence of multi-million pound advertising campaigns and promotions which create fashions and persuade people that they must jog and work-out to keep up with their peers (Jones, 1994).

3.6 Conclusion

During the 1970s and 1980s the focus on lifestyles sometimes threatened to marginalise environmental issues completely. It seemed as if health education had only to persuade people to modify their behaviour and their health status would be transformed. The growing awareness of the interconnections between lifestyles and environment which health researchers have documented, and the now explicit commitment to tackling health variations, have brought this approach into question.

There is now more understanding of the significance of health beliefs held by different cultural and social groups, how they are embedded in values and ways of life and how likely it is that they will prove resistant to change. Health promoters, at least in rhetorical terms, acknowledge the need to challenge and change structures and policies for health, so that 'healthy choices' are made easier and people are supported and enabled to make informed choices in health matters. Nonetheless, a lifestyle focus is still a significant feature of health promotion policy.

Chapter 4
The rise of health promotion

4.1 Introduction

This chapter explores the development of health promotion and discusses its main components: prevention, health education and healthy public policy. In doing so it builds on previous chapters which have begun to tease out the ideas and assumptions that underlie terms such as health, health behaviour, 'models' of health and, of course, health promotion itself.

Chapter 1 opened the discussion about why promoting health had become a more prominent feature of contemporary social life, highlighting how both priorities and participation had shifted over time. One marked feature has been the concern to extend health promotion beyond the health sector to embrace community action and healthy alliances between lay people, professionals, employers and the voluntary sector. A related development has been increasing public interest in health matters. Chapters 2 and 3 indicated both that health has a wide variety of meanings which reflect people's fundamental beliefs and values, and that there are conflicting explanations of health variations and of how good health can best be achieved.

This chapter suggests that there is no single account of 'what health promotion is' and what its processes and outcomes should be. It argues that much of health promotion will be about working in new ways but in traditional roles. It introduces health promotion as a contested area in which medical, social and political approaches jostle for position. This argument is then developed through the analysis of health promotion models that follows in Chapter 5.

4.2 The origins of health promotion

In 1977 *Health For All by the Year 2000* was launched at the 30th World Health Assembly. This policy initiative formulated a range of performance indicators by which progress towards better health might be judged, such as reductions in rates of disease, increased levels of nutrition and improved primary health care. As we have noted, it built on earlier work, in particular the Lalonde Report (1974), which had emphasised that changes in lifestyle and the wider environment would be needed to improve people's health.

This was reinforced and extended by the Alma Ata Declaration (1978) which highlighted the contribution that agriculture, education, housing, industry and other sectors of the economy might make to improving health. In Alma Ata, where the focus was primarily on the developing world, there was a strong emphasis on the role of health education and the importance of primary health care. It called for 'education concerning prevailing health problems and the methods of preventing and controlling them' to enable people to change their behaviour and for education to enable people to participate in decision-making about primary care services. Within this approach, it emphasised basic health and medical services, including preventive and sanitary services, provided by primary health workers rather than highly qualified doctors. Alma Ata also introduced the concept of equity and health and commented on the need to reduce gross inequalities between rich and poor peoples and countries.

Table 4.1 **Health promotion: a brief UK and international chronology**

1974 Lalonde Report, *A New Perspective on the Health of Canadians*

1976 *Prevention and Health: Everybody's Business* (DHSS)

1977 *Health For All by the Year 2000*, launched at 30th World Health Assembly

1978 Declaration of Alma Ata

1980 *The Black Report on Inequalities in Health* (DHSS)

1984 Healthy Toronto 2000, launched in Canada

1985 World Health Organisation: 38 Targets for Health in the European region

1986 *Ottawa Charter for Health Promotion* (WHO)

1987 Healthy Cities project launched

1987 *Promoting Better Health*: The Government's Programme for Improving Primary Care (DHSS)

1988 Adelaide Conference on Healthy Public Policy

1991 Sundsvall Conference on Supportive Environments

1990–3 Publication of: *Health For All in Wales, Health of the Nation* (England), *Scotland's Health: A Challenge to Us All, A Health Promotion Strategy for Northern Ireland*

1990 *NHS and Community Care Act*

1991 WHO Revised *Health For All* targets

1992 Rio Earth Summit: Agenda 21

1997 Jakarta Declaration on Health Promotion into the 21st Century

1997–9 UK Government's White Paper *Saving Lives: Our Healthier Nation, Towards a Healthier Scotland, Better Health Better Wales, Well into 2000 (Northern Ireland)*

1998 Health 21 – the Health for All policy for the WHO European Region: 21 targets for the 21st century.

2000 Fifth Global Conference on Health Promotion (Mexico) *Health Promotion: Bridging the Equity Gap*

From the mid-1980s, the role of health promotion as a movement for social and political change was elaborated in a series of health promotion conferences and charters (Table 4.1). Greater emphasis was placed upon building healthy public policy and developing intersectoral collaboration so that all agencies were working together with health as their priority. In 1985 The World Health Organisation produced 38 targets for achieving Health For All in Europe which included the call that by the year 2000:

> the actual differences in health status between countries and between groups should be reduced by at least 25%, by improving the health of disadvantaged nations and groups.
>
> (Target 1, WHO, 1985)

The reduction of inequalities in health was the first target and under-pinned all the following targets. This explicit, though less well known, philosophy, linked the improvement of health inextricably with political and social change (Table 4.2). It was not expected that the health sector working alone could hope to establish these prerequisites and perhaps for this reason the WHO targets have been given greater prominence. But the philosophical commitment of Health For All to peace, equity and equalising opportunities is undoubted. The Healthy Cities initiative of the mid-1980s represented a modest attempt to put these principles into action through demonstration projects in European cities.

Table 4.2   **World Health Organisation: Health For All prerequisites**

- Freedom from the fear of war
- Equal opportunity for all
- Satisfaction of basic needs:
  - adequate food and income
  - basic education
  - safe water and sanitation
  - decent housing
  - secure work
  - a satisfying role in society
- Political will and public support

(WHO, 1977)

What do you see as the implications of accepting the Health For All prerequisites listed in Table 4.2? To which account of health discussed in Section 2.4 do they most closely relate?

To accept these prerequisites is to link health promotion with politics and with political systems which allow peaceful participation, foster equality of opportunity and meet the basic needs of their citizens. This effectively broadens its scope and positions it as a potential force for social change to create healthier public policies. In one sense the Health For All prerequisites demonstrate the effective limits of health promotion. It cannot compensate for political instability, social inequality, war and poverty. But some of the targets in *Health For All* (WHO, 1985) do assume that health promotion has an important role to play in creating equal opportunity and meeting basic needs. The prerequisites may have reminded you of the 'social model' of health discussed earlier which emphasised lay participation and the importance of environmental interventions to improve health. In the 'salutogenic' approach to health a satisfying role in society and at work were seen as protective of health (Antonovsky, 1987).

4.3 The response of the health sector

The countries in Europe who were signatories to the Charter, including the UK, responded to Health For All targets to varying degrees. By 1990 nearly thirteen of the 33 European member states had produced a national strategy for health. Lack of commitment, conflicting priorities, structural complexity and intellectual confusion have been held responsible for the slow move from 'rhetoric' to 'reality' (Parish, 1995).

The UK was among those whose response was slow, perhaps because Health For All was treated as an international issue and fell within the International Division of the Department of Health (Scott-Samuel, 1992).

Elsewhere, countries such as Germany, Sweden and Denmark established national targets for health in the late 1980s and regional and local authorities adapted these targets to local health needs. Inspired by the launch of Healthy Toronto 2000 in Canada, WHO initiated a Healthy Cities project which by 1989 included 30 cities around the world. Copenhagen entered the project in 1988 and its plans reflected the Health For All vision of and national targets for action, while giving priority to local problems (Copenhagen Plan, 1994/97). Commenting that the health profiles showed 'Copenhagen citizens engage in substance abuse to a larger extent than is seen in the rest of the country' the action plan had a particular focus on building supportive networks and offering counselling and information services to enable people to cut down their drinking and smoking.

The UK response

In the UK several cities joined a Health For All network and began to adapt Health For All targets to local needs. Liverpool, one of the fifteen cities in the official WHO Healthy Cities project (1987), launched an ambitious intersectoral action programme supported by the City Council which stated:

Most of the major influences on health lie beyond the scope of health services. Despite this fact, there has been little real shared development between agencies at central or local levels of plans and strategies for promoting public health. We acknowledge the need for genuine joint planning for health for all; this must start from a consideration of the health needs of the people and 'work backwards' to the institutional means of meeting them. Such a joint approach to public health is required both between government departments and between local agencies and groups.

(City of Liverpool, 1988: 1)

Liverpool's notion of joint working was ambitious and initial attempts to develop structures and alliances were not initially very successful (Green, 1992) although the 1994–97 City Plan became more focused and realistic in its approach to joint working. In a more general sense, such an unambiguous declaration of government responsibility for creating healthy public policy, which was endorsed by other healthy city projects, sat uneasily with free market and New Right political philosophies which emphasised 'consumer sovereignty' and the need to retreat from the 'nanny state' (Open University, 1992). It was, in part, the political implications of health promotion that hindered its development. UK Government reports to WHO argued that Health For All was primarily a concern for regional and local health authorities (Parish, 1995).

In the early 1990s the four countries of the UK each produced a national health plan. 'Health For All in Wales' was published in 1990 and the 'Health of the Nation' strategy consultation document for England followed, with publication in 1992. 'Scotland's Health: A Challenge to Us All' and 'A Health Strategy for Northern Ireland' appeared in 1993. All the national strategies endorsed the target-setting approach, focusing on major target areas such as coronary heart disease, cancers, mental illness, HIV/AIDS and sexual health, suicide and accidents. But the commitment to Health For All philosophy was more evident in some plans than others. In 'Health of the Nation', for example, the philosophy was discussed in an appendix, but the main concern of the report lay elsewhere (DoH, 1992).

'Health of the Nation'

The health strategy for England aimed to ensure that 'action is taken, whether through the NHS or otherwise, to improve and protect health' (DoH, 1992) and recognised that this required action at various levels. First, the Department of Health was given a lead role in implementing the health strategy through inter-departmental committees within central government, through inter-sectoral collaboration and through healthy alliances with non-governmental agencies at all levels. It was an important step in strategic thinking about health because it recognised the extent to which improvements in health depended on change outside the health sector. It also represented an acknowledgement by central government of its strategic responsibilities for health promotion at a time when it was creating an 'internal market system' in health care.

Second, it commented on the relative contribution of the state and the individual in health matters. There was an acknowledgement that government should 'eliminate and minimise threats to the individual' but this was tempered by the comment that 'people cannot be forced to behave sensibly' and a concern that people should have the 'freedom to exercise choice'. It noted that variations in health existed but, commenting that 'these are by no means fully understood', it focused more specifically on individual risk behaviours. In this sense the report projected a fairly circumscribed model of health promotion which did not envisage major public policy changes to promote health. This was interesting in view of the fact that some policy measures – for example seat belt wearing and breathalising of car drivers – had been very successful.

Third, it set out national targets for improving health on which the whole health sector could focus.

While 'Health of the Nation' had a clear focus on specific, measurable targets it was difficult to see how the broader WHO targets were to be achieved. For example, while most health promoters would endorse the claim that 'people should have the basic opportunity to develop and use their health potential to live socially and economically fulfilling lives', it is difficult to translate this into action. In a similar way to the Ottawa Charter (Box 1.1) and the Health for All prerequisites (Table 4.2) the WHO targets represented very ambitious, radical political philosophies. The Health of the Nation document, by contrast, was geared towards specific goals where measurement was possible. Its supporters claimed that in setting realisable targets it was practical and politically astute, and was an evolving policy framework within which health promotion could be developed.

It is difficult, however, not to agree with critics who have characterised this strategy as indicating a view of health that is very much in line with health as 'absence of disease': that is, a preventive medical approach. It proposes risk modification strategies that could result in blaming those who are unable, for whatever reason, to change their lifestyles. It says relatively little about socio-economic influences on health, and 'health inequalities' are not acknowledged.

Critics of the Health of the Nation strategy have commented on the over-emphasis on individual lifestyles, the predominance of medical and disease reduction targets and the marginalising of discussion about socio-economic, environmental and political influences on health (PHA, 1992; Nettleton and Bunton, 1995). The report was in some ways a disappointment to specialist health promoters, who saw it as a missed opportunity to embrace the WHO approach (Adams, 1994). Although socio-economic variations in health were mentioned, far more attention was paid to individual risk behaviours such as smoking, heavy drinking and poor diet. Target setting was made the central approach in the strategy rather than taking its place alongside environmental interventions and policy change.

Opportunities to create supportive environments for health, for example through a ban on tobacco advertising, were largely ignored (Williams *et al.*, 1993). Also excluded were less specific targets, such as improving 'opportunities for people with disabilities' and developing 'health potential'. 'The main philosophical and practical thrust of Health of the Nation was much more consistent with a traditional model of preventive health education than with the more radical ideology of the World Health Organisation and *'Health For All by the Year 2000'* (Tones and Tilford, 1994).

On the other hand, there are difficulties in getting to grips with the more general targets and abstract approach of Health For All. The Healthy Sheffield project, for example, began by working within this strategy but 'in trying to relate these to Sheffield they found it difficult to progress beyond generalities'. They devised appropriate local targets which concentrated on meeting the health needs of the main groups of people in the city and this formed the basis for health promotion planning (Office for Public Management, 1992).

There is also sound evidence, such as that from the North Karelia smoking cessation project in Finland, that target setting accompanied by well targeted health education can work (Puska *et al.*, 1989). The number of male smokers in North Karelia declined from 44 per cent to 31 per cent compared with a 4 per cent reduction across the rest of Finland.

4.4 Health promotion and radical change

In the 1990s, health promotion consolidated and extended itself as a movement concerned not just with outcomes but with the process by which these outcomes should be achieved. New issues were added to the health promotion agenda. In the early part of the decade health promotion incorporated ideas from the environmental movement, in particular the notion of 'sustainability': the careful use and replacement of natural resources so that the life of future generations was not compromised (WHO, 1991). By mid-decade there was a stronger emphasis on how economic development could enhance health. The Jakarta Declaration (WHO, 1997a) identified a revised list of prerequisites for good health: 'peace, shelter, education, social security, social relations, food, income, empowerment of women, a stable eco-system, sustainable resource use, social justice, respect for human rights and equity'.

Compare the Jakarta Declaration list with the pre-requisites set out in Table 4.2 above. What do you see as the key differences?

There are some quite significant differences. As we noted above, sustainability is a new entrant (stable eco-system and sustainable resource use) but so are 'respect for human rights', 'social justice' and the 'empowerment of women', although the 1977 language of 'equal opportunity' might embrace these ambitions. The other new entrant is 'social relations', which highlights the concern of health promotion with process as well as outcome.

Process had already figured strongly in health promotion, for example in ideas about inter-sectoral working, partnership and community action. Jakarta marked the commitment of the health promotion movement to the building of 'social capital': the creation in localities of 'norms, networks and trust' (Putnam, 1995) that bound the inhabitants together and sustained meaningful social relationships. This building of social capital, through strengthening social networks, civic involvement and social support, has been seen as the means by which health status can be enhanced (Hawe and Shiell, 2000). It might also play a part in combating health inequalities. The Jakarta Declaration, having commented that, 'above all, poverty is the greatest threat to health', stated:

> Health promotion, through investment and action, has a marked impact on the determinants of health so as to create the greatest health gain for people, to contribute significantly to the reduction of inequities in health, to further human rights and to *build social capital*.
>
> (WHO, 1997a, p. 1)

Health 21

In 1998 the Health 21 strategy replaced the 38 regional targets of the HFA (Europe) strategy with 21 targets for the European region. It had two main aims:

- to promote and protect people's health throughout their lives
- to reduce the incidence of the main diseases and injuries, and alleviate the suffering they cause.

The strategy reaffirmed the principles of Alma Ata that health was a fundamental human right. It emphasised equity, solidarity within and between countries, and the need for participation and accountability at all levels for continued health development.

Table 4.3   **Health 21 Targets (Source: WHO, 1998)**

Adopted by the WHO Regional Committee for Europe at its forty-eighth session, Copenhagen, September 1998

TARGET 1 – Solidarity for Health in the European Region By the year 2020, the present gap in health status between Member States of the European Region should be reduced by at least one third.

TARGET 2 – Equity in Health By the year 2020, the health gap between socioeconomic groups within countries should be reduced by at least one fourth in all Member States, by substantially improving the level of health of disadvantaged groups.

TARGET 3 – Healthy Start in Life By the year 2020, all newborn babies, infants and pre-school children in the Region should have better health, ensuring a healthy start in life.

TARGET 4 – Health of Young People By the year 2020, young people in the Region should be healthier and better able to fulfil their roles in society.

TARGET 5 – Healthy Aging By the year 2020, people over 65 years should have the opportunity of enjoying their full health potential and playing an active social role.

TARGET 6 – Improving Mental Health By the year 2020, people's psychosocial wellbeing should be improved and better comprehensive services should be available to and accessible by people with mental health problems.

TARGET 7 – Reducing Communicable Diseases By the year 2020, the adverse health effects of communicable diseases should be substantially diminished through systematically applied programmes to eradicate, eliminate or control infectious diseases of public health importance.

TARGET 8 – Reducing Noncommunicable Diseases By the year 2020, morbidity, disability and premature mortality due to major chronic diseases should be reduced to the lowest feasible levels throughout the Region.

TARGET 9 – Reducing Injury from Violence and Accidents By the year 2020, there should be a significant and sustainable decrease in injuries, disability and death arising from accidents and violence in the Region.

TARGET 10 – A Healthy and Safe Physical Environment By the year 2015, people in the Region should live in a safer physical environment, with exposure to contaminants hazardous to health at levels not exceeding internationally agreed standards.

TARGET 11 – Healthier Living By the year 2015, people across society should have adopted healthier patterns of living.

TARGET 12 – Reducing Harm from Alcohol, Drugs and Tobacco By the year 2015, the adverse health effects from the consumption of addictive substances such as tobacco, alcohol and psychoactive drugs should have been significantly reduced in all Member States.

TARGET 13 – Settings for Health By the year 2015, people in the Region should have greater opportunities to live in healthy physical and social environments at home, at school, at the workplace and in the local community.

TARGET 14 – Multisectoral Responsibility for Health By the year 2020, all sectors should have recognized and accepted their responsibility for health.

TARGET 15 – An Integrated Health Sector By the year 2010, people in the Region should have much better access to family- and community-oriented primary health care, supported by a flexible and responsive hospital system.

TARGET 16 – Managing for Quality of Care By the year 2010, Member States should ensure that the management of the health sector, from population-based health programmes to individual patient care at the clinical level, is oriented towards health outcomes.

TARGET 17 – Funding Health Services and Allocating Resources By the year 2010, Member States should have sustainable financing and resource allocation mechanisms for health care systems based on the principles of equal access, cost-effectiveness, solidarity, and optimum quality.

TARGET 18 – Developing Human Resources for Health By the year 2010, all Member States should have ensured that health professionals and professionals in other sectors have acquired appropriate knowledge, attitudes and skills to protect and promote health.

TARGET 19 – Research and Knowledge for Health By the year 2005, all Member States should have health research, information and communication systems that better support the acquisition, effective utilization, and dissemination of knowledge to support health for all.

TARGET 20 – Mobilizing Partners for Health By the year 2005, implementation of policies for health for all should engage individuals, groups and organizations throughout the public and private sectors, and civil society, in alliances and partnerships for health.

TARGET 21 – Policies and Strategies for Health for All By the year 2010, all Member States should have and be implementing policies for health for all at country, regional and local levels, supported by appropriate institutional infrastructures, managerial processes and innovative leadership.

Comment on the balance in these targets between the more traditional 'disease reduction' targets associated with medicine and broader targets related to a 'social model' of health.

Health 21 demonstrates just how far the health promotion movement in Europe had moved towards a radical 'social model' agenda for health action. While there is still considerable concern with disease and illness reduction (Targets 6–10, 12), the emphasis on promoting health and enhancing health potential – and therefore on policy change – is striking. Some of the means to achieve this – equity, environmental safety, partnerships, solidarity across the European region, health promoting policy, research – highlight the wide-ranging ambitions and radicalism of the movement. A major challenge remained, of course, the translation of these ambitious targets into action at international, national, regional and local level.

The breadth of the movement's ambition was also reflected in the 1999 international health promotion conference, *Health Promotion: Bridging the Equity Gap*. This focused on the key themes such as promoting social responsibility for health, increasing investments for health development, increasing community capacity and re-orienting health systems and services. It demonstrated the growing concern of health promotion to link health development with economic growth and development, a philosophy which underpins many present day national health promotion strategies.

4.5 The agenda for change in the UK

By the late 1990s, the public health agenda across the UK was dominant (see Table 4.4). New Labour, coming to power in May 1997, saw community development and participation, tackling social exclusion, and fostering partnership and integration as integral to policy development. In using the term 'social exclusion', the government acknowledged social divisions (such as class, race, gender and disability) which resulted in people's unequal experience of, and access to, welfare provision and which reinforced social inequalities in health. Strategic developments in England, Wales, Scotland and Northern Ireland were focused on policies to assess and reduce inequalities in health. At the same time, developments in the NHS heralded a move away from the internal market and the purchaser–provider split towards structures which promote co-operation, quality and performance, with an emphasis on a primary care led NHS. Government reforms in local authority functions emphasised greater integration of health and social services. In an attempt to demonstrate a commitment to public health, the new government appointed a minister for Public Health in England and produced a range of health-related strategies.

Table 4.4 **Health strategies 1997–2000**

1998 Independent Inquiry on Inequalities in Health (Acheson)

1998 Smoking Kills: A White Paper on Tobacco

1999 Social Exclusion Unit Report on Teenage Pregnancy

1999 Reducing Health Inequalities: An Action Report

1999 Food Standards Agency Bill

1999 Health Act

2000 The National Plan for the new NHS

These White Papers reflected both the government's adoption of a multi-agency approach to health and the link between social exclusion and health. In England, a social exclusion unit tackled sensitive issues such as reducing teenage pregnancy. The emphasis was on 'a wide range of linked programmes including measures on welfare-to-work, crime, housing and education as well as health'.

Other white papers on the modernisation of health services in each country proposed the development of primary care groups, health action zones, and healthy living centres in England and local health groups in Wales.

In England, The White Paper *Saving Lives: Our Healthier Nation*, replaced the 27 targets of the Health of the Nation with four targets: to reduce heart disease and stroke, accidents, cancers and poor mental health (see Table 4.5). In Scotland, the White Paper *Towards a Healthier Scotland* was produced in February 1999. Wales produced *Better Health: Better Wales* (March 2000) and Northern Ireland published *Well into 2000*. Although each of the documents was quite different, the underlying philosophy of each health promotion strategy was to address social inequality and social exclusion. Each document outlined a number of organisational changes for health promotion structures in each country.

Table 4.5 *Saving Lives: Our Healthier Nation* targets (DoH, 1999)

By 2010:

- **Cancer**
  reduce the death rate from cancer in people under 75 by at least a fifth – saving 100,000 lives

- **Coronary heart disease and stroke**
  reduce the death rate from coronary heart disease and stroke and related diseases in people under 75 by at least two fifths – saving 200,000 lives

- **Accidents**
  reduce the death rate from accidents by at least a fifth and to reduce the rate of serious injury from accidents by at least a tenth – saving 12,000 lives

- **Mental health**
  reduce the death rate from suicide and undetermined injury by at least a fifth – saving 4,000 lives

The challenge of health inequalities

In *Saving Lives*, the Government proposed a 'contract for health' – a partnership between Government and other national agencies, local communities and individuals to improve health. The strategy professed to provide a 'third way' which moved beyond 'individual victim blaming' and 'nanny state social engineering' and attacked inequalities. However, it delegated responsibility for tackling inequalities in health to local initiatives such as developing health improvement programmes, piloting health action zones and creating a network of healthy living centres.

The strategy's two key aims were:

- To improve the health of the population as a whole by increasing the length of people's lives and the number of years people spend free from illness.

- To improve the health of the worst off in society and to narrow the health gap

(DoH, 1998: 5)

Compare the aims of *Saving Lives: Our Healthier Nation* with the Health 21 aims on pages 66–67. What main differences are there?

Whereas Health 21 aimed to protect health and reduce disease, *Saving Lives* added a commitment to 'narrow the health gap'. The government claimed this acknowledgement of the 'social, economic and environmental causes of ill health' (DoH, 1998: 57), with its recognition of the link between poverty and ill health, as a major advance from the *Health of the Nation*. However, critics have argued that the return to area-based initiatives such as health action zones cannot address underlying fundamental inequalities in health unless there are national strategies to address poverty in a meaningful way (Shaw *et al.*, 1999). *Saving Lives* does not make health inequalities a national priority. Health Action Zones and Healthy Living Centres are funded by short term monies that must be bid for competitively, and hence there is not widespread reallocation of resources to all areas that are economically deprived. Thus only a small percentage of the budgets of health and social services are allocated to these special projects, while there is no change to mainstream funding and mainstream provision. Nonetheless, the strategy has encouraged local action:

> It is important to acknowledge that tackling health exclusion in poverty requires a radical restructuring of social and economic policy to reduce income inequalities and unemployment, and to promote better access to housing, education and childcare. At the same time there is a need to maintain a sense of what front-line practitioners can do to reduce health exclusion in poverty. Community practitioners are uniquely placed to collect and disseminate information on poverty and health exclusion, and to use it to shape responses which help households to avoid and cope with the worst aspects of health exclusion and which challenge policies that promote and maintain health exclusion. Responding to poor health in poverty is the major challenge facing health professionals at the present time. There is growing evidence that some practitioners are building pro-active responses to tackle health exclusion in poverty. However, an overwhelming conclusion arising out of the literature on professional practice is that there is still a long way to go to refocus practice away from its overriding concern with individual behaviour towards responses that acknowledge the structural causes of health exclusion.

> (Blackburn, 1999)

4.6 'Mainstreaming' health promotion?

In the late 1980s quite large sums of money began to be directed into health promotion and education. National campaigns were extended, in particular those directed at changing attitudes towards HIV/AIDS and heart disease. *Promoting Better Health* (DHSS, 1987) encouraged the incorporation of health promotion into primary care. Health promotion checks, it stated, should be carried out by GPs and linked to targets and financial incentives. In spite of setbacks, the relatively stronger position of GPs in the health care market and the new GP contracts in the early 1990s resulted in a wider array of GP-based services and a specific remit for health promotion. A GP-led model of prevention and health promotion emerged, which emphasised risk factors, screening and lifestyle advice (Williams *et al.*, 1993). However, the 1997 NHS reforms and the move to a more primary care led NHS offered opportunities for a more holistic approach. In England, the development of primary care groups and potential primary care trusts provided an opportunity for health promotion activities to become much more integral to primary care.

What types of health promotion services are now offered by your own GP?

You may have mentioned blood pressure checks, cervical smear reminder letters, the extension of minor on-the-spot surgery, and other services. Older people are offered an annual health check. Most doctors now have practice nurses who may run stress clinics, anti-smoking and immunisation services and offer advice on exercise and diet. But in the future a much wider circle of practitioners might become involved, including social workers, health visitors (seen as 'public health nurses') and workers in voluntary agencies.

From specialists to generalists?

In some ways, then, health promotion has become more mainstream in the health service. Public health and health promotion specialists have always provided a range of epidemiological and public survey research data which feed into the needs assessment process and influence purchasing decisions. The NHS and Community Care Act in 1990, divided the NHS into purchaser and provider units. This affected specialist health promotion units – with some becoming part of purchasing authorities. Specialist health promotion units were also operating as part of acute hospitals or community health trusts (Dix, 1995), having a strategic role in setting targets for health gain and influencing contracts with providers, or a provider role in contracting for programmes of training, education and other services to communities, users and health and welfare professionals.

The fragmentation in specialist health promotion services following the purchaser–provider split brought new challenges. Contracts increasingly became 'specific, targeted and time-limited' (Dix, 1995). Health promotion specialists felt by the mid-1990s that the contract culture had significantly weakened their ability to develop the more radical Health For All oriented strategies (SHEPS, 1993a). With the change of emphasis in the Government's priorities since 1997, and the move away from the internal market, there has still been continuous re-organisation, change and uncertainty for health promotion services. In England, specialist health promotion services are positioned in health authorities, NHS acute and community trusts, and now increasingly services are being devolved to primary care groups. In Scotland and Wales the picture is different, with health promotion services being part of Health Boards in Scotland; and following the review of health promotion in Wales in 1999, all health promotion units were relocated to become part of Public Health Departments.

With the change of emphasis to health improvement and health development, many agencies are appointing health promotion practitioners with titles that range from health development officers, to health improvement officers to public health practitioners. This reflects the growing debate on the role of health promotion and public health specialists

In the 1990s national health promotion agencies were restructured as well. The Health Education Authority, for example, was in the position of bidding for contracts against other competitor agencies, before being changed to become the Health Development Agency in April 2000. With devolution, the Welsh Health Promotion Agency became the Health Promotion Division of the National Assembly for Wales. The role of the national agencies changed to become more strategic.

In addition to the work of the primary health care team and specialist services, however, there was the growing emphasis within the health promotion movement on 'enabling people to increase control over, and to improve, their health' (*Ottawa Charter*, WHO, 1986). This positioned health promotion not as a specific, discrete sphere of activity but as a *process* in which all those in and outside the health sector can (and should) take part. The implication was also that health promotion could take place with all groups of people in any state of health. Thus health promoters are people who work in new ways within their traditional roles, whether lay or professional. Such work could involve the identification of ways to support carers more effectively by tailoring services to their individual social and cultural circumstances, providing more practical help, respite care, information about services or someone to talk to. It might be by adding a new dimension to an existing service, for example providing more information and support for young people leaving care (Jones and Rose, 2001). This would involve responding to young people's concerns about health rather than giving standard information about health risks.

4.7 Components of health promotion

This section discusses the main components of health promotion: prevention, health education and healthy public policy. All of them have already been introduced in Section 4.2 and, while they overlap to some extent and have changed over time, they have recognisably different priorities.

Look back through Section 4.2 and gather evidence indicating what constitutes 'prevention', 'health education' and 'healthy public policy'.

Prevention is associated with public health measures, for example improved sanitation mentioned in Alma Ata (WHO, 1978), and also with preventive medical measures in general practice such as immunisation which have been emphasised in the 1993 GP contract. It could also include health protective legislation, for example on wearing seat belts, but this intervention generally takes place outside the health sector. The second, health education, was conceptualised in Alma Ata (and in North Karelia) as educating people to change their behaviour, and most of the UK health strategies also had a concern to modify personal lifestyles (Nettleton and Bunton, 1995). This version focused on professionals informing lay people, but the 'empowerment' view of health education (Tones and Tilford, 1994) is concerned with raising ordinary people's awareness, developing their potential and responding to their expressed health needs.

The third component, healthy public policy, is a feature of the Health For All targets and prerequisites, of the Ottawa Charter and of the Healthy Cities movement, but until recently has played a less significant part in the UK health strategies. It is about policy change to enhance health and prevent disease and may include health protection measures, alliances between different agencies to work for health, community action, government inter-departmental strategies and joint planning. The sections below look at each of the components in more detail.

Prevention

Prevention is generally understood to be action to stop ill health before it starts, but in fact the term is used more broadly than this. In the twentieth century preventive medicine has included policies for health protection aimed at whole populations as well as defined 'at risk' groups, for example vitamin fortification. Preventive medicine partially subsumed the earlier public health tradition of environmental protection through measures such as adequate sewage, drainage and a clean water supply. In doing so public health priorities became marginalised in favour of a medical model of prevention (Ashton and Seymour, 1988).

Three levels of prevention have been identified: primary, secondary and tertiary. Primary prevention can be seen as the attempt to eliminate the possibility of getting a disease and immunisation is an obvious example of this. Health education directed at healthy people, such as advice about hygiene or contraception, might also be seen as a type of primary prevention (Lambert and McPherson, 1993). By changing people's health behaviour, it is argued, their chances of contracting diseases are minimised. This has been a major justification for large-scale campaigns to persuade people to stop smoking, wear condoms or eat less fat.

Primary prevention has a clear health promoting role but 'secondary' and 'tertiary' prevention are more medically driven. In secondary prevention people are caught in the early stages of a disease through early detection so that symptoms can be alleviated and if possible eliminated. Alternatively a pre-symptomatic change may be detected, as in raised blood pressure. Tertiary prevention refers to the control and reduction, as far as possible, of an already established disease and is not clearly distinguishable from medical care. However, recent discussion of health promotion and chronic illness has highlighted the health promotion potential of tertiary prevention by suggesting that those experiencing arthritis or heart attacks can be enabled to take control over and improve their health (Kaplan, 1992).

> From whatever point one starts in life, whether as a healthy baby or as somebody who has already gone through many life crises and has become chronically ill, health and well-being can be enhanced and developed.
>
> (Kickbusch in Kaplan, 1992: 8)

Comment on examples of primary, secondary and tertiary prevention from your own experience.

You will probably have been immunised as a child and, if you travel by car, you will generally wear a seat belt. Both represent primary prevention. You might have been on the receiving end of screening for early signs of breast or cervical cancer and these would fall into the category of secondary prevention (see Table 4.6). A chiropodist might be involved in secondary prevention by treating an early-stage ingrowing toe nail – a painful condition which if allowed to develop can seriously impede someone's mobility. An occupational therapist or social worker making an assessment of a client might pick up signals about stress or fatigue which indicate an early-stage disease. In a primary care context, a practice nurse offering advice sessions on how to cope with raised blood pressure would be engaged in secondary prevention. By contrast, examples of tertiary prevention might include mastectomy, rehabilitative classes for people who have had a heart attack, or the provision of false teeth.

Table 4.6 **Primary, secondary and tertiary prevention**

Primary prevention	Secondary prevention	Tertiary prevention
Aims to prevent the onset of disease	Aims to detect and cure a disease at an early stage before it causes irreversible problems	Aims to minimise the effects or reduce the progression of an already established irreversible disease
Examples:	*Examples:*	*Examples:*
Immunisation	Cervical cancer screening	Hip replacement surgery
No-smoking areas	Stress management	False teeth

Prevention and health protection

Health legislation or voluntary codes of practice are designed to protect the public against such dangers as polluted water or contaminated food products, which in the nineteenth century were the concern of the medical officers of health. Responsibilities are currently divided between public health medicine, government agencies and local authority departments of environmental services, who monitor pollution levels, carry out inspections and ensure that legislation is enforced. For example, the enforcement of industrial safety standards is the concern of the Health and Safety Executive, and food industry regulation is the concern of the Ministry of Agriculture, Fisheries and Food. Bans on smoking in many public places have come about as a result of local authority moves or decisions of transport providers or retailers rather than government legislation. But in some other areas government departments have taken a stand: for example, the acceptance by the Department of Health of the need for needle exchange to slow down the spread of HIV/AIDS. Although its origins lie in public health medicine, protection is now most appropriately included as part of a healthy public policy approach.

Health education

Health education is frequently defined as the process of giving information and advice and of facilitating the development of knowledge and skills in order to change behaviour. Most health promoters will already have some type of formal or informal health education role, most probably offering advice or helping someone talk through a difficult issue. The reconceptualisation of health education in WHO philosophy, however, emphasises it as a two-way process of critical consciousness raising, clarifying values, exploring attitudes, educating policy makers and taking control over one's own health (WHO, 1986; Tones, 1996). This is a much more radical approach to health education and one response to those critics who have dismissed it as narrow and victim-blaming (Rodmell and Watt, 1986).

Contemporary exponents of health education emphasise its potential to empower clients while also drawing attention to evidence of its power to achieve change. Major changes in health-related behaviours, such as the decline of smoking and the slow-down in the rate of spread of AIDS, can only be fully explained, it has been argued, in terms of the positive impact of health education campaigns (Tones and Tilford, 1994). They also claim that carefully constructed, individual-focused support programmes can result in quite high rates of change (Rowe and Macleod Clark, 1993).

Healthy public policy

Healthy public policy, with its focus on structural change, was emphasised in the 1986 Ottawa Charter on Health Promotion and the Adelaide Charter (WHO,1988). The Charters set out an agenda for achieving Health For All by the Year 2000 and responded to world wide expectations for a new public health initiative.

Box 4.1: Understanding Healthy Public Policy: Statement on Healthy Public Policy in the Adelaide Charter (1988)

'Healthy public policy is characterised by an explicit concern for health and equity in all areas of policy and by an accountability for health impact. The main aim of Healthy Public Policy is to create a supportive environment to enable people to lead healthy lives. Such a policy makes healthy choices possible or easier for citizens. It makes social and physical environments health-enhancing. In the pursuit of Healthy Public Policy, government sectors need to take account of health as an essential factor when formulating policy. They should pay as much attention to health as to economic considerations.'

(WHO, 1988)

The Ottawa Charter and the Adelaide recommendations on healthy public policy spelled out its value base in a much more explicit way, specifying that legislation, fiscal measures, taxation and organisational change in different combinations would be needed (see Box 4.1). Ottawa made an explicit reference to developing health, income and social policies 'that foster greater equity' and concluded that 'the aim must be to make the healthier choice the easier choice for policy makers as well'. The Adelaide conference also emphasised health as a fundamental social goal which could not be achieved without public participation and co-operation between all sectors of society.

> **Compare this approach with the other aspects of health promotion that have been discussed. What overlaps are there?**

Healthy public policy includes a good measure of health protection and prevention and builds on public health traditions. The main distinction is the emphasis on getting the health sector to work with other sectors and agencies. Health protection measures have not generally been the result of co-ordinated action by different agencies but rather the work of particular government departments.

The language of healthy public policy

The development of national health strategies, WHO strategies and the new public health movement has created a bewildering new language which can be rather disempowering for those engaged in trying to promote health. These include 'health gain', 'healthy alliances', 'supportive environments' and 'intersectoral collaboration' for health (see Box 4.2). Most have less than precise meanings and there are overlaps: for example, intersectoral collaborations and healthy alliances are closely related.

Some terms, such as 'health gain', have both a particular and a more general meaning. Integral to the notion of health gain are the dual goals of 'adding years to life' and 'adding life to years'. In health promotion terms gain is about length of life as well as quality of life, but the main driver has been a narrower strategic aim of reducing potential years of life lost and increasing life expectancy. In some areas, for example road accidents, potential years of life lost are high because the highest rates of accidents are for young male car drivers in their twenties and thirties and young pedestrians, especially young children and teenagers. Thus cutting accidents would have large spin-offs in health gain.

As health commissioning authorities analyse and plan how to meet health needs in their local populations, however, health gain is beginning to be seen in much broader terms. One issue is about how targets for health gain in their populations can be built into contracts and frameworks, such as those negotiated between the authorities and the acute hospital trusts. Another, arising from the new consortia arrangements to oversee health work education, is about the need to train appropriate health workers. A key issue is about partnerships: how health authorities can work, with others, across the health and welfare sectors to respond to health-damaging environments and situations, such as poor housing and high unemployment levels.

Box 4.2: Healthy Public Policy: related terms and concepts

Health gain: any advantage to health that may be gained through rethinking health policies, reorienting and restructuring health services, working collaboratively with other sectors (e.g. social services) to improve mental health.

Creating supportive environments: working to transform physical, social, resource and political environments so that health can be more easily protected and improved; e.g. improving air quality (physical), combatting racism (social).

Mediating structures: intermediate structures (meso structures) between political-administrative systems (macros) and individual citizens (micro) which can mobilise for health action; e.g. trade unions, community health networks, pressure groups.

Intersectoral collaboration: alliances between organisations and agencies in different sectors to work for health; e.g. joint health and social services planning for community care; employer, union and health action to improve workforce health.

Partnership: refers to joint action between partners (national and local agencies and the public). It implies the equal sharing of power (Naidoo and Wills, 2000: 157)

Healthy cities: World Health Organisation project to develop new ways of promoting health in urban settings. Goals are to mobilise citizens, encourage community participation, intersectoral links and participative public policy making.

Settings: focus on locations where there is potential to improve health. The World Health Organisation has launched several projects of this kind; e.g. the European Network of Health Promoting Schools, the Health Promoting Hospital Network.

Intersectoral collaboration and healthy alliances are really interchangeable in that they both involve working across sectors to achieve improvements in health. For example, a strategy to improve mental health in an English city might ideally involve not just the health sector but social services, recreation, leisure and housing departments of local authorities, voluntary sector agencies, employers and pressure groups. In the Copenhagen Healthy City project intersectoral collaboration is a cornerstone of the approach and the sectors to be involved are listed as 'schools, the social sector and the health sector as well as urban and traffic planning, environment and housing' (Healthy City Plan, 1994). Partnerships are now central to the development of primary care groups, health action zones and healthy living centres.

4.8 Conclusion

This chapter has suggested that promoting health potentially involves a cluster of related activities, ranging from disease reduction to primary prevention and health enhancement. The methods that may be employed depend partly on health sector directives, such as those in the GP contract which expanded the primary health contribution to primary prevention, but also on the settings and levels through which health is promoted. Here, promoting health has deliberately been discussed as a broad-based multi-faceted activity but it could be questioned whether health promotion should include disease reduction and prevention at all.

These types of interventions have been included in the discussions above for two reasons. First, because the title of this book is 'promoting health' rather than 'health promotion' and the view taken here is that promoting health also involves the reduction of ill health, particularly inequalities in health. Second, if promoting health is to be undertaken by a wide range of people in and outside the health sector they need to connect to health promotion at some concrete and practical level. For many workers in or outside the health sector, undertaking health promotion as part of their regular counselling, advice, regulatory, caring, investigative or other normal work will be the most important contribution they make. It will involve doing their usual work but within a health promotion framework and in a more health-promoting way.

Chapter 5
Theories and models in health promotion

5.1 Introduction

Health promotion, it has been suggested, is a contested area. This is partly because it is a very broad field of action and its focus has changed over time. Some of the terms used, such as 'health education' and 'public health', have shifted their meaning. There is no easy consensus about the underpinning ideas which inform health promotion, in particular ideas about 'what health is' and what the principal health goals should be. Health promotion is not neutral and value free; its protagonists hold very different ideas about priorities and strategies which reflect their underlying values.

These differences can be seen as creative conflicts through which those who promote health can battle towards a clearer understanding of their work. They can also be seen as destructive, as essentially a distraction from the main business of pragmatically 'doing the work'. This chapter will take the former approach. It suggests that there can be constructive debate over differences without disempowering those who promote health. It also argues that unless those who work for health build an understanding of how health promotion connects to broader social, political and cultural values it will prove difficult to advance their practice.

It is true, however, that the attempt to conceptualise health promotion more abstractly by comparing different approaches raises the whole debate about 'models' and indeed about the status of health promotion as a field of study. Why are theories and models important in health promotion? Should health promoters assume that different approaches and models will always exist? In what ways do different models assert core values and principles of practice? How far is the use of certain approaches pragmatic, determined by work role or organisational objectives rather than ideology? Can different approaches to health promotion and health education be used alongside each other or are they mutually incompatible? These questions open up central and important debates in health promotion.

5.2 The growth of health promotion models

Health promotion, like health itself, has been defined in varied ways. The word 'promotion' is an ambiguous term and is used in relation both to raising someone's status (a promotion at work) and to advertising or other campaigns to sell something (Dines and Cribb, 1993). In the mid-1980s Tones characterised health promotion as 'any activity designed to foster health' (Tones, 1985) but more recently he has argued that 'health promotion = health education × healthy public policy' (Tones and Tilford, 1994). There is also continuing debate about whether health promotion should include disease reduction, prevention and health protection or whether it should be concerned solely with positive health. French (1990) has questioned why disease management should not be included, whereas Downie *et al.* (1990) specifically excluded curative and acute medical services. Such haggling over the territory, which we noted in Chapter 4, has been a feature of the history of health promotion.

Models have been numerous and popular in health education and health promotion perhaps because the terrain has been dauntingly large, imprecisely defined and constantly evolving. For example, the term 'health education' has shifted in meaning over time so that several distinct and even conflicting approaches are in use together. Health education started as an offshoot of the environmental work of Medical Officers of Health and focused on information-giving and home visiting to instil housekeeping and mothering skills. In the twentieth century new interpretations of the causes of ill health shifted the emphasis from environmental to inter-personal interventions. Health education advice warned of the dangers of social contact in relation to diseases such as tuberculosis, measles and (especially in wartime) venereal disease. 'Maintaining a clean mouth and clear breathing, and ... abstaining from spitting, sneezing, coughing and shouting at each other' were proposed by the Chief Medical Officer of Health in 1920 as ways of promoting personal health (quoted in Armstrong, 1993).

By the 1950s health education was associated with broad programmes of popular education and then with mass publicity campaigns and adult education classes designed to persuade people to change their behaviour, to 'look after themselves' and 'take greater responsibility for their own health' (HEC, 1978). But by the 1980s the rhetoric of 'making healthy choices easier choices' had drawn attention to environmental influences on lifestyle choices and laid down a challenge to earlier traditions. Health education designed to persuade individuals to change their personal behaviour, as we noted in Chapter 4, sits somewhat uneasily with health education aimed at empowering people to make autonomous decisions.

One response to this confusion was to identify and map discrete 'approaches' to practice. A model of practice offered a way of representing 'a more complex reality' (Seedhouse, 1997) so that practitioners could review, understand and take forward key issues. In the 1980s, as the complexity grew, Rawson and Grigg (1988) identified seventeen types of health education model in the UK, suggesting that there was no consensus on core activities. Perhaps this is because health promotion is 'a magpie profession'(Seedhouse, 1997), adopting techniques, models and theories from a variety of disciplines – medicine, education, sociology, psychology, politics, economics, epidemiology and statistics. As new interpretations of health education emerged they were added on to existing accounts. In some cases normative judgements were made about the 'right' way to undertake health education but in others the accounts were presented side by side in a seemingly neutral way, leaving the health promoter to make the choice.

Models: neutral or normative?

In this sub-section we examine some of the conceptual models of health promotion. An influential example of the mapping of health education practice was developed by Ewles and Simnett in 1985 and then further refined (1992, 1995 and 1999) to create five approaches to health promotion (Table 5.1). These ranged from 'medical' interventions to encourage patient compliance and persuade people to seek early treatment across to a 'societal change' approach which focused on action to 'change the physical/social environment'. In between lay three different types of health education activity: teaching attitude and behaviour change; informing and educating people about health issues; and empowering clients to set their own agendas in health. Different types of health promotion activity were seen as important in each approach. In the behavioural approach, for example, the focus of activity was 'attitude and behaviour change to encourage adoption of "healthier" lifestyle', whereas in the client-centred approach it was 'working with clients' identified health issues, choices and actions'. In developing this framework the authors commented:

> In our view, there is no 'right' aim for health promotion, and no one 'right' approach or set of activities. We need to work out for ourselves which aim and which activities we use, in accordance with our own professional code of conduct (if there is one), our own carefully considered values and our own assessment of our clients' needs.
>
> (Ewles and Simnett, 1999: 41)

Table 5.1 **Five approaches to health promotion**

	Aim	Health promotion activity	Important values	Example – smoking
Medical	Freedom from medically-defined disease and disability	Promotion of medical intervention to prevent or ameliorate ill-health	Patient compliance with preventive medical procedures	*Aim* – freedom from lung disease, heart disease and other smoking-related disorders *Activity* – encourage people to seek early detection and treatment of smoking-related disorders
Behaviour change	Individual behaviour conducive to freedom from disease	Attitude and behaviour change to encourage adoption of 'healthier' lifestyle	Healthy lifestyle as defined by health promoter	*Aim* – behaviour changes from smoking to not smoking *Activity* – persuasive education to prevent non-smokers from starting and persuade smokers to stop

| Educational | Individuals with knowledge and understanding enabling well-informed decisions to be made and acted upon | Information about cause and effects of health-demoting factors. Exploration of values and attitudes. Development of skills required for healthy living | Individual right of free choice. Health promoter's responsibility to identify educational content | *Aim* – clients will have understanding of the effects of smoking on health. They will make a decision whether or not to smoke and act on the decision

Activity – giving information to clients about the effects of smoking. Helping them to explore their own values and attitudes and come to a decision. Helping them to learn how to stop smoking if they want to |
| --- | --- | --- | --- | --- |
| Client-centred | Working with clients on the clients' own terms | Working with health issues, choices and actions with which clients identify. Empowering the client | Clients as equals. Clients' right to set agenda. Self-empowerment of client | Anti-smoking issues are only considered if clients identify them as a concern. Clients identify what, if anything, they want to know and do about it |
| Societal change | Physical and social environment which enables choice of healthier lifestyle | Political/social action to change physical/social environment | Right and need to make environment health-enhancing | *Aim* – make smoking socially unacceptable, so it is easier not to smoke

Activity – no-smoking policy in all public places. Cigarette sales less accessible, especially to children, promotion of non-smoking as social norm. Limiting and challenging tobacco advertising and sports sponsorship. |

(Ewles and Simnett, 1999: 43)

Although the different approaches are seen as having distinctive priorities and objectives, and as reflecting very different views of patients/clients, there is an underlying assumption that if health promoters are acting in good faith any of these approaches is valid.

Test out the strengths and weaknesses of this framework with examples from your own experience.

The framework offers those in practice a clear and useful account of different ways of thinking about health promotion. They can check their ways of working against those in the chart and reflect on how they might want to change. It also draws on practice experience as the basis from which to distil the five approaches and in doing so attempts to illuminate the dilemmas of health promotion. Although some of the language that Ewles and Simnett used has changed – for example, you might now use the term 'empowerment' instead of 'client centred' – the concepts are still very relevant.

It does not tell us much, however, about what might motivate health workers to select one approach rather than another. The 'medical' approach is seen as involving medical intervention but the other approaches are described in terms of particular activities and values which are not occupationally specific. However, the professional training of particular groups in the health and welfare sectors is likely to predispose them to work within one approach rather than another. A 'social change' approach might be seen as appropriate by an environmental health worker, for example, but rejected as irrelevant by an occupational therapist working on a hospital ward.

It could also be argued that the approaches are not discrete. For example, a community health project might include aspects of the educational approach (providing health information) and societal change (lobbying for a local baby clinic or safe play areas), as well as being client-centred. More important, it does not tell us much about how practice changes or how people might modify or transform their own practice. What is described is existing practice that can be observed and reported, not 'what might be'. In contrast to this framework there are models which, while commenting on the appropriate territory for health education and promotion, also make clear which approach is favoured. French and Adams (1986) have argued that health promotion is too complex and diffuse an activity to be neatly plotted, and have drawn attention to the different values which underpin different approaches. They identify three approaches: 'collective action', 'self-empowerment' and 'behaviour change' and comment that collective action is the most effective and desirable approach because of the social bases of health.

Tones and Tilford (1994) identified 'preventive', 'radical-political' and 'empowerment' models and acknowledged that each has its merits, before concluding that they viewed empowerment 'as a central element in health education and health promotion'. Health education is seen as a driving force empowering lay and professional people through raising their consciousness of health issues, policies and choices. Through health education, communities and health professional bodies can become geared up to pressure for change and begin to effect the transformation in public policy that will address social and environmental inequalities and improve health (see Figure 5.1). However, this also works in reverse: environmental and social circumstances exert their own influence on individuals and communities. We might add that they may also, by this means, influence health education messages.

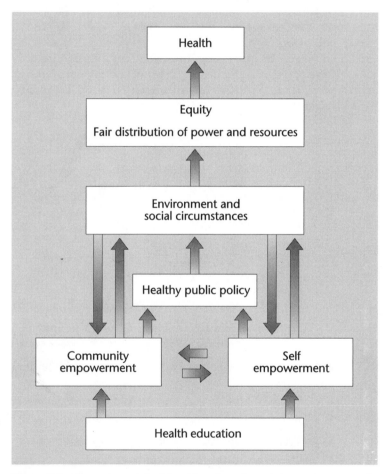

Figure 5.1 **Tones' model of health education, empowerment and health promotion** (Scriven and Orme, 1996)

Downie *et al.* (1990) identified 'traditional', 'transitional' and 'modern' approaches to health education. But it is clear that the first two approaches are found wanting compared with the modern approach which addresses positive health, lifeskills, self-esteem, participation, constraints to freedom of choice and collective dimensions of health and behaviour.

> The modern approach uses a broad information base and sound educational principles, and recognises the importance of socio-political factors in health and health-related behaviour. It is a participatory model.
>
> (Downie *et al.*, 1990: 48)

Having made these claims about health education, the authors endorse a model of health promotion which maps the various domains in an even-handed way (Figure 5.2). The distasteful features of the traditional model, in particular its exclusively individual focus and authoritarian character, do not re-emerge, the transitional model is absent, and all health education is assumed to be empowering. 'Health education seeks to empower by providing necessary information and helping people to develop skills and a healthy level of self-esteem'. Such even-handedness is possible because the model presented is an idealised view from which negative features are excised.

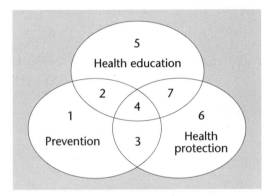

Figure 5.2 **A model of health promotion**
(Tannahill, 1985 reproduced in Downie *et al.*, 1990)

Within these intersecting circles lie seven possible dimensions of health promotion:

1 preventive services, e.g. immunisation, cervical screening;

2 preventive health education, e.g. smoking advice;

3 preventive health protection, e.g. fluoridation of water;

4 health education for preventive health protection, e.g. seat-belt lobbying;

5 positive health education, e.g. building lifeskills with groups;

6 positive health protection, e.g. implementing workplace smoking policy;

7 health education aimed at positive health protection, e.g. campaigning for protective legislation.

Critically review this model in relation to health promoting activities you have been involved in.

The model highlights the potential overlap between prevention and positive action, viewing effective health education as an essential building block for securing change. Contemporary health promotion work, it suggests, does not focus exclusively either on prevention and disease reduction or on structural and social change. A progressive primary health care team, for example, might offer a combination of health education (such as a well woman clinic), preventive services (such as immunisation) and disease management (such as asthma or diabetes education). It might also be involved in outreach work in schools and play a small part in publicising and supporting specialist health promotion campaigns. A specialist health promotion unit might engage in health risk assessment to underpin contract work but also in community-based health promotion work. Community health projects may focus on prevention and disease reduction through their commitment to reducing health inequalities but the targets these use are likely to be derived from the expressed needs of local people.

The model offers many combinations of approach but it does not make explicit the political or social values underlying each approach, or reveal the author's preferences as to methods. Perhaps this offers more freedom of choice to health promoters. Yet different types of health promotion can be in tension with each other and this could create difficulties. Consider a local area where the accident rate is high. The teachers and road safety officers respond with preventive health education about road safety but children and parents pressurise the local authority for health protection in the form of safer crossing places. Where should the main responsibility lie? The different foci reflect not just 'dimensions' of health promotion but quite distinctive ways of conceptualising the issue, with professionals attributing the 'blame' to children and lay people 'blaming' environmental factors. Research on the Corkerhill estate in Glasgow, noted in Chapter 3, did reveal this clash of perceptions about the causes of accidents (Roberts *et al.*, 1995).

5.3 Making sense of models

Models may be exemplars, offering guidance, opening up new possibilities in practice and providing opportunities to review ideas and actions. They may also be constraints, closing down alternatives and requiring conformity. They can provide a potent symbol of an occupational group that has 'arrived' and knows where it is going, yet they can also serve to highlight confusion and disarray. In particular, the descriptive mapping of health education and promotion activities, while useful to highlight issues and even differences, does not provide reliable models of real practice. Such descriptions of practice are not necessarily transferable to other practice settings and they are static snapshots of complex, dynamic approaches.

Explicit in all these models is an acknowledgement of how securing better health is bound up with addressing fundamental questions about social inequality. Yet they are still essentially describing how health promotion happens rather than commenting on the values and conflicts that underpin it. These descriptive models construct health promotion as an eclectic subject drawing upon different disciplines and traditions. A consensus, that all approaches are valid depending on the context and that they are interrelated and work most effectively in combination with each other, is implied. No one approach is seen to take or should take priority.

Whilst this inclusive strategy is reassuring, it may be that recycling descriptions of current practice is ultimately non-productive and does not stimulate practitioners to go much beyond the status quo. Relativism does not encourage clarification of values, whereas the reflective practitioner's task is to go beyond description to analysis (Schon, 1983). To extend representational or iconic maps of health promotion where they do not contextualise or analyse health promotion sufficiently would require a deeper, more analytical and reflective understanding of what health promotion means (Rawson, 1992). This involves moving from models which are primarily descriptive to analytical models which go beyond the present boundaries of health promotion practice and provide a commentary on practice.

The development of analytical models of health promotion is an attempt to aid analysis by being explicit about underlying principles or values, not within the models themselves but within the society in which health promotion is undertaken. Analytical models inevitably involve theory: that is, 'systematically organised knowledge applicable in a relatively wide variety of circumstances devised to analyse, predict, or otherwise explain the nature or behaviour of a specified set of phenomena that could be used as a basis for action' (Van Ryn and Heany, 1992).

Health promotion and social theories

Health promotion has developed within the analytical framework of the social sciences, drawing most evidently on perspectives found in sociology and social policy (Bunton and Macdonald, 1992). It has also been influenced by educational theories. From sociology it has adopted a structural analysis which draws attention to the material and social influences on health and the structured social relationships that help to shape inequalities in health (Townsend *et al.*, 1988). The 'social change' or 'healthy public policy' approach which has recently gained momentum, rhetorically if not generally yet in practice, owes much to a political economy analysis of how ill health is generated by poverty, poor housing and work environments, pollution, discrimination and unemployment (Doyal, 1979). Health promotion has also tentatively adopted a post-modern notion of fragmentation, in the sense that it has attacked the objectivist, monolithic, natural science-driven model of medicine and embraced diversity by celebrating lay accounts of health, subjectivity, social movements, community action and empowerment (Open University, 1992; Kelly and Charlton, 1995).

Social policy has provided an analytical framework for thinking about policy making and policy change. It has also examined the relationships between the shifts in policies for health and wider political ideologies, such as New Right perspectives on the sovereign consumer and on contractualism, which help to explain the shifts in health promotion (Open University, 1992). From social psychology and education, health promotion has adopted a range of theories and models: locus of control, reasoned action, health belief, and behavioural change (Rotter, 1966; Ajzen and Fishbein, 1980; Becker, 1984; Prochaska and DiClemente, 1984).

At the same time, as sociologists have highlighted, health promotion is embedded in contemporary society. It has emerged as a persuasive discourse about 'risk', 'change', 'lifestyle' and 'consumption' not as a matter of chance but because its messages reflect fundamental shifts in ways of seeing and practising health care (Armstrong, 1995; O'Brien, 1995). In particular, the characterisation of health promotion as 'surveillance' carried out by professional health promoters and by people monitoring and policing themselves, offers a powerful critique of what has hitherto in this chapter been claimed to be the 'radical' or 'empowerment' approach.

> Contemporary health promotion techniques that aim to listen more attentively to the views of lay people, by using qualitative interviews, participant observation or health diaries, penetrate into the lives and minds of subjects ... In this respect such techniques can contribute to the creation of a health promoting 'self'. One of the concerns of this critique is to alert us to the possible detrimental or constraining effects of such humanistic and liberal practices within health promotion.
>
> (Nettleton and Bunton, 1995: 47)

This is an important justification for developing analytic models, imperfect and partial though they will be. Analytic models can attempt to represent such tensions and oppositions by demonstrating the ways in which health promotion is embedded in wider social and cultural practices and political struggles. An understanding of the theory underpinning any health promotion practice is important to enable a practitioner to justify a particular programme (Caplan, 1993: 50). However, many of the theories used in health promotion are not highly developed and have not been rigorously tested (Nutbeam and Harris, 1998). The robust evaluation of health promotion programmes and interventions allows the continued development and testing of theories.

5.4 Using analytical models

If health promoters want to acquire a distinctive disciplinary basis, health promotion has to clarify its philosophical (what is the truth?) and epistemological (how do we know the truth?) basis. Analytical models of health promotion provide a possible tool with which to interrogate the basis for practice. By making explicit the links between core values and principles and different kinds of practice, a greater understanding of the philosophy and priorities of health promotion may be derived (Naidoo and Wills, 2000). Analytical models are not bound by current practice and may describe a vision of health promotion practice not yet operationalised. In this sense, theory may drive practice and lead to new insights.

A structural and conceptual map of health promotion can be developed to highlight the assumptions and frameworks underpinning different ways of engaging in practice (Beattie, 1984). It has been adapted (Beattie, 1991) to inspect the theoretical underpinnings of health promotion (see Figure 5.3). Its most important feature is the positioning of various accounts of health promotion within a broader socio-cultural framework. This model is explicitly saying that health promotion is embedded in wider social and cultural practices, in ideologies and political struggles. It is not something apart from the rest of society; indeed, it reflects in its territory struggles about power, control, autonomy and authority.

The typology is generated by means of two axes generated from cultural anthropology: mode of intervention (whether authoritative or negotiated) and focus of intervention in a society (whether individual or collective). In this model social values are seen as driving practice, so that a 'health persuasion' approach to health promotion reflects a paternalist and individual-oriented philosophy. Individualism may not necessarily imply paternalism, however, and the model highlights a 'personal counselling' approach based on negotiation. The 'societal change' approach of Ewles and Simnett assumes a concomitant philosophy of collective action, but Beattie's model demonstrates that collective action could be either participative and community-based or paternalist and state-directed. Such an analysis helps to tease out some of the complexities underlying health action.

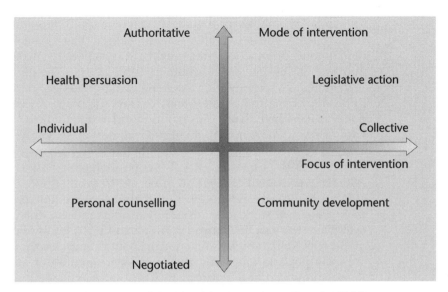

Figure 5.3   **Beattie's Model of Health Promotion**   (Beattie, 1991)

From your experience, note an example of health promotion for each of the four quadrants in Beattie's model.

You might have suggested (going clockwise from the top-left quadrant) anti-smoking advice, seat belt legislation, a community health project, and a psychotherapy session.

Beattie's model enables us to reflect on the social and political perspectives underlying health promotion approaches. Underpinning the 'conservative' model of health persuasion, it is suggested, is a biopathological model of health which sees health promotion as attempting to repair deficits. Underlying a community development approach to health promotion are assumptions about empowerment and equity and the mobilisation of communities to effect change. We noted earlier that prevention and health protection are part of a more traditional, medical approach which focuses on the individual and on the treatment of disease, whereas more radical approaches are linked to Health For All strategies. Health workers, like others, are influenced by socialisation into a family, a social class, a cultural group, and through the values developed in professional training and experience. It is important to try to understand the relationship between values – ways of thinking – and practice – ways of 'doing' (Foucault, 1973).

Assess the strengths and weaknesses of this model compared to those examined earlier.

This approach enables us to understand where health promotion ideas are coming from and what drives them. Rather than being disembodied descriptions of practice, they highlight practice as merely the final outcome of deeper social conflicts and values. The model enables practitioners to identify the values and assumptions underlying different forms of practice and to assess practice from the point of view of others – policy makers and clients. This has its negative side for those who want to know how to take action. If health promotion is firmly locked into competing structures of social values then it is unlikely that one account of 'what health promotion is' will ever be acceptable. Just as health is an essentially contested concept, so too is health promotion.

What can health promoters do if their values are not congruent with their prescribed work role? What about interventions which do not fall neatly into the four quadrants but overlap different forms of practice? The model tells something but not enough about change; are these tendencies the only possible ones? Are they forever in conflict or are there new formulations and new debates which will reflect changing social values? Finally, unlike many of the other models, it is abstract and highly complex and has not been designed to use as a guide to practical action but as a tool for the reflective practitioner.

Other models have also attempted to link health promotion to social and political structures and to frameworks of social knowledge. For example, Caplan and Holland's model of health promotion (Caplan, 1993) plots theories of society (conflict or consensual) against ways of knowing about the social world (subjective or objective) (see Figure 5.4). The resulting quadrants represent different forms of health promotion which are not dissimilar from those set out in the five approaches offered by Ewles and Simnett (1999).

Collins (1993) has attempted to link a micro model of a person's health beliefs, constraints and actions to a macro model which analyses health promotion at a societal level. In both cases the authors argue that health promoters have not made their assumptions explicit and this has resulted in a failure to grapple with the essentially political nature of health promotion practice. Promoting 'healthy public policy' is not a value-free enterprise, nor is public health medicine.

Again, this draws attention to the way in which practice is affected by personal and professional training, beliefs and attitudes, as well as the broader policy environment which regulates its content and boundaries. The two may or may not be compatible. Some practitioners feel uneasy about the kind of health promotion they are engaged in. An example is practice nurses' duties with regard to screening. Their GP practice may be committed to increasing uptake, but nurses might feel they should respect their clients' wishes and not pressurise them to accept screening. Understanding where practice fits into models of health promotion helps practitioners to go beyond a 'common sense' account of their activities. It also clarifies why different parties engaged in health promotion may have very different views as to what it is they should be involved in.

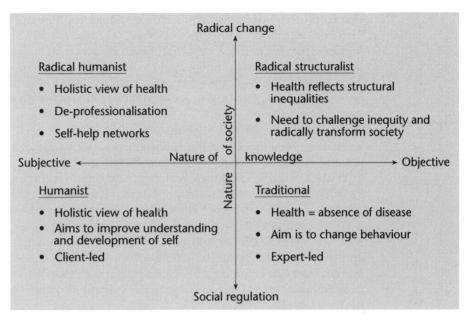

Figure 5.4 **Four paradigms or perspectives of health promotion**
(adapted from Caplan, 1993)

5.5 Conclusion

Health promotion models provide a stimulus to re-examine practice and its underlying assumptions. They challenge those involved in working for health to ask questions and search for plausible answers. Whilst the plethora of models has been criticised as confusing and unhelpful, it could instead be taken as a sign of healthy development. It has also been argued that these models are not mutually exclusive (Rawson, 1992). Although they represent different ways of conceptualising health promotion, and have been reinforced by different ways of training staff and distinctive working arrangements and priorities, in practice health and welfare workers will probably use ideas drawn from a combination of models. Health promoters will undertake tasks associated with a 'health persuasion' model of health promotion and other work which fits more comfortably into a more 'communitarian' model.

Two other issues are important to note at this stage, although they point in opposite directions. One is that, while they have been explained as discrete models, the grouped descriptive and analytical models discussed above do have common features. Both acknowledge diversity and indicate possible conflict. We have also suggested that health promotion is not static and that part of this diversity may be explained by trends and changing ideas over time. Conversely, it will not do to argue that those involved in health promotion should just pick and mix models. There are significant differences between an approach which is based on bottom-up negotiation, one which looks primarily to regulatory frameworks and legislative change, and one which relies on professional dominance. This does not mean that they are absolutely incompatible, only that to bring one into focus inevitably means allowing others to slip into the background. Finally we need to remember that practitioners will use local knowledge and experience, and draw on research data from a wide range of sources to make judgements about community needs and health promotion action (Nutbeam and Harris, 1998).

What is described above are patterns of thought, sets of priorities, styles of working rather than 'tablets of stone'. The type of practice seen as 'professional' and endorsed through training is one factor determining what health and welfare workers will actually spend their time on. People's own sets of professional and personal values and principles constitute another important factor in determining what kind of practice workers feel comfortable engaging in. The next chapter draws on these ideas to explore values and how people's personal value systems interact with their health promotion practice.

Chapter 6
Ethical issues in health promotion

6.1 Introduction

The exploration of health promotion models in Chapter 5 serves to demonstrate the central importance of ethics in health promotion. Ethics is a branch of philosophy and is about studying the basis of moral judgements, principles and values. At its most abstract ethics is concerned with questions such as the meaning of 'right' or 'wrong', but it also has an applied aspect which considers value questions in areas such as health care ethics. As we have seen, working to improve people's health inevitably involves values because judgements are being made about what 'better health' is, and about whether and how to intervene to promote it. This chapter discusses how those working to promote health can become more aware of value conflicts and moral dilemmas and can think clearly through the implications for practice. It explores the way in which health promotion is underpinned by some key ethical principles: respect for autonomy, beneficence (doing good), non-maleficence (doing no harm) and justice. These are discussed in turn and explored through practical examples.

6.2 Values and health promotion

First, however, we need to provide evidence to support the claim that health promotion involves values. Ashton and Seymour (1988) argued that 'the question "What is health and thereby health promotion?" continues to de-energize all those involved in this activity' but it does not follow that the struggle to understand the value conflicts underpinning 'what health is' and 'what health promotion is' is not important. As we have seen, definitions of health are bound up with judgements about values across a broader area of life. For some people health means not being ill, for others it means being fit or at the peak of physical condition, and for yet others it may mean being well adjusted, or content, or well balanced, or full of positive feelings of well-being, or even just happy. The judgements people make about health grow out of their life experiences and influence their attitudes and the actions they take. There is a strong connection between thinking and doing.

This is the case in health promotion as well. The definition of health promotion that you feel comfortable with and the values underpinning it will reflect your life experiences, work, education and professional training. If you have been trained as a doctor then you will most likely feel comfortable with a definition of health promotion which emphasises medical treatment: that is, secondary and tertiary prevention with a strong emphasis on the individual. On the other hand, if you are a health promotion specialist you may well question this approach and see the central thrust of promoting health as influencing healthy public policy, health gain and intersectoral collaboration. You may not be much concerned with health at the level of the individual but with influencing groups and populations through media campaigns, community action or legislative change. For a social worker key values may be promoting client autonomy and non-discriminatory practice.

> **Choose another group of people who work in the health and welfare field and describe what might be their values of health promotion.**

Let us take the example of nurses. For many hospital nurses, health promotion really means health education, which in turn is seen as giving patients advice on health (or often disease) matters. Many hospital and community nurses have received little or no training in health promotion, although health visitors in the UK – as in Denmark and some other continental European countries – have been trained to seek out health needs and to work to improve the health of basically well people. For many hospital and community nurses, therefore, health promotion is an add-on to other activities and may well not be seen as important. Faced with a surgery or a ward full of sick patients it will seem much more vital to treat the presented sickness as swiftly as possible and move onto the next patient. This traditional role of 'nursing the sick' dates back into history and was given a modern, professionalised form by Florence Nightingale.

As Macleod Clark (1993) points, out, although Florence Nightingale discussed two types of nursing, she identified 'nursing the sick' as 'nursing proper' and thereby sidelined health nursing. Professionalised nursing became identified with a model of 'sick nursing' and health education and health promotion were seen as optional extras.

> Health education and health promotion in nursing have been seen until very recently as the specialist territory or province of the health visitor. When health nursing concepts have been taken on board by other nurses they are interpreted almost exclusively in terms of the activities of health education and health promotion. These activities include health advice, information giving and patient teaching and have simply been bolted on to traditional roles. There is no shortage of rhetoric extolling the need for all nurses to develop their role in promoting health. Indeed the whole of the pre-registration curriculum in the UK (Project 2000) has been revised in acknowledgement of the importance of providing a health focus to nursing education. In spite of this, for the vast majority of nurses, the sick model has remained pervasive.
>
> (Macleod Clark, 1993: 257)

The general concept of health promotion, therefore, is one in which nurses spend more time instructing or advising patients. It is not one in which nurses work with patients in new ways. A survey by Gott and O'Brien (1990) indicated that this 'bolt-on' approach to health promotion was widespread, and more recent research by Macleod Clark and her team in acute settings has confirmed this. They illustrate this with descriptions by nurses of what health promotion means to them:

> Health promotion suggests to me someone who is in need of being taught specific things.

> Health promotion is a system of giving health information to individual patients – it's information giving.

> Health promotion means saying to the patient before they go home about smoking, eating a healthy diet and anti-stress techniques.

> Health education – we try to discourage people from smoking.
>
> (Macleod Clark, 1993: 259)

Compared with our earlier discussion of the contribution of health education to health promotion these descriptions appear particularly limited. There is no sense of nurses working to empower patients or even sharing knowledge with them. The words used are about telling, teaching, warning and transmitting information.

What values underpin the type of health education practised by these nurses?

This is a top-down set of values that emphasises professional knowledge and sees health education as being about imparting that specialist knowledge to patients. Ewles and Simnett (1995) call it the 'medical approach' although it may overlap with the 'behaviour change approach'. Beattie (1991) characterised this as 'health persuasion'. It is underpinned by assumptions that professionals know what is in the best interests of their patients. Health education is seen as an unproblematic moral activity of doing good by persuading people to change, perhaps through overriding their own views. As we noted earlier, this has been criticised on the grounds that it imposes a particular set of values on the patient, it assumes a lack of knowledge, and can end up as seeming to blame patients for their own ill health as they 'choose' not to change their behaviour.

6.3 Ethical principles in health promotion

The examples above have begun to tease out how actions are underpinned by value judgements and moral beliefs. We need to take a step back now and ground these observations in a more systematic understanding of ethical principles. The four ethical principles we noted earlier will be discussed briefly here and can be explored in more detail elsewhere (Beauchamp and Childress, 1995). They are:

- Respect for autonomy – that is, respect for the rights of people and their right to determine their own lives. This involves considerations of freedom of choice and whether and when there is any legitimate right to intervene or persuade people to a particular course of action.
- Non-maleficence – not doing harm.
- Beneficence – doing good.
- Justice – being fair and equitable, which is about how to respect everyone and the way harm and good are distributed.

The first question that springs to mind when faced with this list may be 'How am I to know when I am doing good, avoiding harm, respecting autonomy and being fair?' One way of responding is in terms of universal moral duties, which for many people are embodied in a religious or ethical code of valuing other human beings (and in some cases all life) and treating them as you yourself would wish to be treated by others ('do as you would be done by').

A more specific response is to note that most occupations in the health and welfare field have a written or unwritten code of ethics which set guidelines for such decision making. In medicine, for example, the Hippocratic oath requires doctors as a first principle to avoid doing harm (non-maleficence). Inflicting harm through inaction is seen as morally less blameworthy than inflicting it through deliberate action. The Society for Health Education and Health Promotion Specialists (SHEPS) counsels practitioners to avoid engaging in activities for which they are not adequately trained and thus minimise the possibility of doing harm. In the principles of practice there is a strong commitment to equity: for example through countering prejudice and discrimination and working to reduce inequalities in health. It also states that 'the promotion of self-esteem and autonomy amongst client groups/recipients should be an underlying principle of all health education and health promotion practice' (SHEPS, 1993).

Ultimately, while professional and religious codes can guide action, individual professionals have to take responsibility for accepting, interpreting and applying ethical principles.

Utilitarianism

Perhaps the kind of ethical principles most favoured in health promotion are those drawn from utilitarian thinking. Utilitarianism states that people should always act in ways which mean that benefits will outweigh disadvantages. Utilitarianism offers a practical guide to decision making but it also raises some problems if viewed in relation to the ethical principles listed above. For example, smoking bans in hospitals are now widespread and arguably offer the greatest good to the greatest number. But they also breach the principle of autonomy by undermining people's freedom to make their own decisions to smoke or not to smoke.

Another example would be immunisation where the equation is also complex. How far is harm to health offset by positive benefits? The numbers helped, it can be argued, will vastly outweigh the casualties. But we cannot be sure that those who are immunised would otherwise have contracted the disease. Those who are harmed by being immunised may not have been harmed by the disease either (and of course wouldn't have suffered the side effects) if they had not been immunised. Simple utilitarian thinking, by emphasising the overall benefits of actions or policies, can ignore how benefits and harms are distributed between individuals.

A third arena for debate has been screening, which has been projected as ethically justifiable in medical terms. From the viewpoint of a social analysis, however, there are social risks for some women in undergoing screening. Women reported that their male partners associated a cervical smear with sexual pleasure and put pressure on them not to attend and allow the doctor to interfere with them in this way. A positive smear test was interpreted as a sign of the woman having 'slept around' (McKie, 1995).

6.4 Ethical principles and practice dilemmas

Beneficence and non-maleficence

Two central tenets in health promotion are to do good and avoid harm. We shall explore later how 'doing good' is conceptualised. But there is a potential for conflict between the principles of non-maleficence (not doing harm) and beneficence (doing good). Engaging in health promotion which improves the health of people may also do damage to some individuals. As we noted above, encouraging the take-up of immunisation may result in an increase in children suffering convulsions, brain damage and other side effects, even though the total numbers of such cases remains very small.

As well as directly causing harm, a choice of strategy might harm people indirectly. By undertaking one intervention rather than another a health promoter might unintentionally cause harm.

Can you suggest a health promoting intervention which breaches the non-maleficence principle in this indirect way?

Working to improve the health of one group at a community level may involve using up limited resources that could have helped improve the health of other groups and in some cases the health of the groups not targeted may actually suffer. Consider a case where a community health worker has to choose between giving time to get a much needed play group started and counselling sessions for five individuals on their diet. The choice of priorities might have adverse health consequences in either case. The lack of a play group might undermine the mental health of parents and the physical and emotional development of their children. Lack of counselling might have an adverse impact on the health of the clients.

Can the utilitarian principle solve this dilemma by securing the greatest good for the greatest number? On this basis the community worker might decide to support the play group because it helps far more people. On the other hand it would not be easy to determine whether more harm would result from inaction over the play group than over a decision not to run counselling sessions. This highlights a central problem in utilitarianism. It is open to so many interpretations according to what is understood by benefit or harm and how they are weighed together.

Autonomy and rights to intervene

We noted earlier that respect for the rights of people and supporting their right to determine their own lives is an important part of the SHEPS code of practice. The ethical principle of autonomy is very central to western society and is bound up with notions of the 'sovereign individual' who has the ability to reason, understand and therefore make rational choices within their environment. In other societies and among some minority ethnic groups in the UK the sovereign individual has not been seen as of such central importance and the family, the group or the community are more highly valued. Critics have pointed out that, historically, sovereign individualism has been reserved for men and has trampled over the rights of women and children (Dalley, 1988). The particular symbols of autonomy in contemporary society, such as the right to vote or own property, were granted to women only quite recently.

Which groups in society are seen as not capable of being autonomous?

You might have commented that until recently people with learning disabilities were seen as non-autonomous, and this is still a contested area. In relation to health promotion, for example, health workers might argue that enhancing health involves creating opportunities for autonomy in a more active way. On the other hand, parents are often their main carers and may believe that they know 'what is best for them' (Dines and Cribb, 1993). Children and prisoners are also treated as dependent, for different reasons. Prisoners are seen as having forfeited their rights through acting irresponsibly towards others, but children are not yet responsible.

Children are seen as not fully rational and not able to act independently in their environment (Mayall, 1996).

Respecting autonomy raises dilemmas for those involved in promoting health. If the client makes a choice that the professional considers is harmful, the health professional may be torn between respecting the client's autonomy and doing good and avoiding harm. The temptation may be to persuade the client to act differently but if a major principle is freedom of choice it must be questioned whether and when there is any legitimate right to intervene or persuade people to a particular course of action.

In health promotion these dilemmas revolve around the question: 'By what right am I intervening and how do I justify the action I am taking?'. Decisions about the right to intervene involve ethical judgements about the rules and principles that should apply in this area of human conduct. Although we tend to think of dramatic interventions involving life or death decisions about treatment, abortion, sectioning, care orders and so on, there are also dilemmas in more everyday decision-making and action. The most frequently cited conflict is over health protection, with some groups arguing that the government ought to intervene to protect public health and others claiming that legislation and regulation infringe people's freedom of choice.

> **Choose an example in the field of health promotion and assess the type of debate that has taken place.**

You may have mentioned debates about smoking or about control of alcohol. There have been considerable conflicts between pressure groups such as Action on Smoking and Health (ASH) and campaigning groups and libertarians defending the individual's freedom to smoke. Professional bodies such as the British Medical Association have called for high taxation on tobacco, a ban on advertising and stricter controls on smoking in public places. While defenders of the right to smoke deploy arguments about liberty, the freedom of the individual and the dangers of state tyranny, the anti-smoking lobby have highlighted how one person's freedom can undermine that of others – for example through the dangers of passive smoking. Modern states already regulate their citizens in many ways so why should smoking limitation be excluded, it is argued. Moreover, the concept of 'freedom of choice' is essentially undermined by the power of advertising and other media images to shape our tastes and desires and 'hook' the most vulnerable groups (such as children) into habit-forming practices.

Indeed, some health promotion specialists have argued that the best way to counteract media power is not to emphasise the dangers of smoking (seen as boring and irrelevant by teenagers) but to project equally powerful messages about the desirability and advantages of not smoking (Chapman and Eggar, 1993). In its turn, of course, it might be argued that this is as unethical as the undermining of free choice through tobacco advertising! Is the defence of those engaged in health promotion that their action would help to improve people's health a sufficient one? On what ethical basis can such action be justified?

Creating autonomy is also a problem area for health promotion. We noted earlier that enhancing opportunities for people with learning disabilities may be seen as uncalled for interference by their main carers. Seedhouse (1988) suggests that, whereas respecting autonomy involves accepting clients' choices whether or not you agree with them, creating autonomy goes further in actually helping to enlarge those choices. The Ottawa Charter (1986) terms this 'empowerment', which is about raising people's consciousness of issues, developing their skills and understanding of situations and encouraging self-assertiveness. Much of community development work centres on empowerment.

Justice

Avoiding harm and doing good are bound up with the principle of justice. In the extensive territory of health promotion decisions need to be made about dividing time and resources between individuals and communities, high-risk groups and whole populations. Activities such as encouraging people to stop smoking or take more exercise, or attempting to persuade local councils to rehouse people or introduce cycle lanes are underpinned by assumptions about the value that should be placed by individuals or communities on improving health. They reflect on ethical positions adopted by those engaged in promoting health that this is important work and that it is a legitimate activity which can be justified in terms of a vision of what positive health and the 'healthy society' might be. This does not mean that health promotion can be forced on unwilling clients and patients; in fact gaining agreement to act – the so-called 'mandate' – from the client and from the organization or employer is an essential first step.

The principle of justice involves considerations about the degree to which health promotion should be influenced by need, merit and equality. World Health Organisation prerequisites imply that to create the 'healthy society' requires the promotion of equal opportunity and the satisfaction of basic needs. Health promotion emphasises both individual empowerment and healthier public policies which improve people's living conditions. In addition, equity – acting fairly – is a central concern of the Ottawa Charter (WHO, 1986). A high value is put on public participation and liberation – 'enabling people to increase control over, and to improve, their health'. So the 'healthy society' is one in which people are empowered as individuals and where the emphasis in public policy is on meeting needs, equalising opportunities and enhancing equity. This implies that other objectives, such as unbridled economic growth or policies which undermine people's rights or fail to offer them

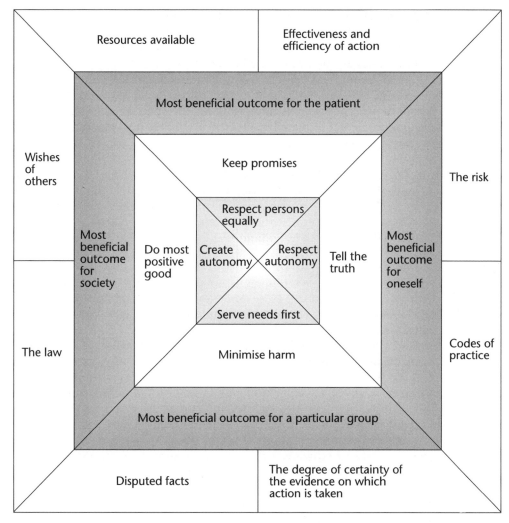

Figure 6.1 **The ethical grid** (Seedhouse, 1988)

protection against disease, are seen as unacceptable – and, indeed, as unethical in health promotion terms.

Seedhouse (1988) developed an ethical grid to enable health practitioners to reflect systematically on situations and to help them to take ethically informed decisions (see Figure 6.1). It is meant to assist rather than to replace personal reflection and individual responsibility. Starting from the premise that each practitioner would answer honestly, the grid offers an opportunity to work through decisions in terms of key principles and potential consequences. It is not, however, morally neutral and Seedhouse signals his values by stating that practitioners should approach the grid with the intention of finding opportunities to enhance the potential of people.

Seedhouse suggests that practitioners should interrogate a proposed action in four main ways. Does it safeguard equity, respect and further the creation of autonomy? Is it doing good and avoiding harm? Will the consequences of the action be good and for whom? How does a proposed course of action measure up against external considerations, such as weight of evidence, legal responsibilities or risks? You will find these questions set out systematically within the four quadrants of the grid, and the questions it raises about health promotion are further explained elsewhere (Seedhouse, 1996).

6.5 Conflicting values in promoting health

Creating an ethical basis for promoting health on the grounds of building a healthier society, empowering people and enlarging their ability to make healthy choices does not do away with the dilemmas involved in health promotion. Whichever set of principles or framework of ideas is adopted there will still be concerns to be raised about the acceptability of different types of action. Let's work through some examples, starting with health education.

Much of health education involves trying to change people's ways of thinking or their behaviour and this may include using techniques of persuasion. You may have asked yourself, as a health or welfare worker, 'What is my justification for trying to persuade Mr X to quit smoking?' or 'What right have I to select information for Ms Y which emphasises the dangers of unsafe sex?'. If you are a parent or carer you may have asked yourself similar sorts of questions about the decisions you make and the advice or guidance that you offer, such as 'Am I justified in not having my child immunised?' or 'What right do I have to try and change the family's diet?'.

> **How do you justify the kinds of advice you give on health matters?**

At one level you might respond by saying that giving advice about health was part of your job (as a professional or as a parent) and that, providing the advice is accurate and appropriate, there's really no problem. People can 'take it or leave it'. If you are a health or welfare professional, however, giving advice on health matters is rarely this straightforward. Professionals may exert considerable pressure on their clients because they are seen as 'experts' and this can undermine people's freedom to choose. Adults exert power over children. There is a difficult balancing act between persuasion and respect for autonomy. In providing people with information and support to make an informed decision it is often quite difficult to avoid putting pressure on them to make the 'right' decision. After all, that is what you want them to make! Recommendations and guidelines alter and there could be conflicts of view. It may be tempting to edit out unwanted ideas to ease the task of decision-making. Yet a real choice is one made when all the options (as far as possible) are known.

There is a real dilemma here, as those engaged in health promotion themselves have recognised. On the one hand we have noted that the ethical basis of health promotion includes a commitment to enhancing autonomy; on the other, the search for the 'healthy society' requires people to value their own health more and to make healthy choices rather than unhealthy ones. How is it to be ensured that people make healthy choices if making up their own minds about health matters is also high on the agenda? The answer given by those advocating healthy public policy is to make healthy choices easier through appropriate policy decisions and frameworks. For example, it might be considerably easier to give up smoking if it were banned in all public places, if advertising were banned, or if taxes on tobacco were higher. This takes us full circle to the discussion about the ethical basis of health protection at the beginning of this section.

There are no easy answers to resolve conflicts of value but it is important not to duck the issues. It has been argued that those who advance the argument that one set of values is as good as another are doing just that.

> If every set of values is as good as every other, then health promoters might as well pack up and go home. It is surely the belief that there are better and worse ways of living one's life that makes the whole practice of health education, promotion, social work, nursing and medicine worthwhile.
>
> (Downie *et al.*, 1990: 144)

In contrast to this, Ewles and Simnett (1995) argue that, in the clash of values between the doctor and the patient over a health problem such as raised blood pressure, the doctor's medical values may be legitimately challenged by the cultural affiliations of the patient. 'Lowering blood pressure may be the most important thing to a doctor, but drinking beer in the pub may be far more important to his overweight, middle-aged, unemployed patient. Who is to say which set of values is 'right' – the doctor or his patient? Whose life is it anyway?' (p. 35).

What would your response be, as a would-be health promoter, in this situation?

You might respond by agreeing that health promoters are committed to putting a high value on health, so taking a doctor's advice about moderating drinking must be the right course of action. There are, however, at least two reasons for doubting this beyond the argument (put forward by Ewles and Simnett) about the dangers of imposing alien, medical 'middle-class' values on people.

First there is the danger of seeing physical health as the only important consideration, whereas for a middle-aged, unemployed man maintaining his mental health and self-esteem through keeping up social contacts and regular habits might be just as important, from a medical viewpoint as well as a health promotion viewpoint. Second, the fact that we may attach value to the medical view does not mean that all other views are wrongheaded. After all, the social model of health emphasises well-being and quality of life as important components of health. If, at the first whiff of medical disapproval, all but people's medically defined physical health is to be seen as unimportant, then health promoters 'may as well pack up and go home'.

What all this demonstrates is that conflicts of value, while they must not be allowed to disempower those who are trying to promote health, cannot be brushed aside. Apart from anything else, there is considerable evidence to suggest that imposed advice which is not internalised and does not relate sensitively to the everyday context of people's lives will be very difficult to follow (Pill and Stott, 1985).

6.6 Ethical dilemmas: some conclusions

Ethical dilemmas lie at the heart of health promotion, not just because it seeks to transform health practice but because there is great scope for uncertainty about how best to achieve health promotion goals. The World Health Organisation produced a report on ethics and health promotion (1989) discussing the principles of social justice, benificence and political and ethical questions of health promotion practice. We have noted that specialists in health promotion, through SHEPS, have a set of principles for practice to guide them but this does not relieve them of the responsibility for thinking carefully through each situation that confronts them. Health promotion is an area in which knowledge is constantly changing and this will have implications for information and advice giving. It is also a 'political' area. Empowering people is not a morally neutral activity; it assumes that raising consciousness and developing advocacy skills are 'good' types of health promotion and that limiting knowledge and choice, imposing solutions and ignoring clients' views are 'bad'.

Market principles are invading health promotion, with increasing sponsorship of research and activities. This results in moral dilemmas as well. Should health be sold as a 'product' and advertised in commercial terms? We noted earlier the support for media advocacy methods, the use of mass marketing techniques and advertising to sell healthy lifestyles (Chapman and Lupton, 1995). The 'marketisation' of health promotion, suggests SHEPS, should avoid dealings with companies whose products undermine health and should not result in outside domination of health promotion agendas. Hence sponsorship of sporting events by a footwear manufacturer might be acceptable but not, for example, by a tobacco company. The concept of partnership with the private sector whose main motivation is profit not health was introduced at the Jakarta Conference (WHO, 1997). Hancock (1998) suggests that health promotion needs to develop ethical criteria to guide health promotion in the selection of partners.

In this chapter we have noted some main types of question to be asked about health promotion decision-making and action. Will I be reflecting the principles of practice in my own occupation? Will I be avoiding harm and doing good? Will I be respecting or helping to create/extend autonomy in my clients? Will I be contributing to a wider social good? Having been raised here, such questions should be kept in mind as you work through the final chapter in this part which looks at developing competence in health promotion.

Chapter 7
Building competence in health promotion

7.1 Introduction

This chapter will apply what has been learned so far about health and its promotion to assess the skills and knowledge required by those working to promote health. The chapter begins by reviewing health promotion in process terms, as adding a new dimension to what in most cases will be a mainly unchanged work role. It asks how priorities can change within work roles so that health promotion becomes more prominent and how relationships with clients can become more supportive and enabling. It then reviews the territory of health promotion: the range of activities, approaches, levels and settings within which it may take place. The chapter ends by identifying key skills for health promotion work, which will be explored in depth in Parts 2, 3 and 4.

7.2 A dynamic process approach

The work of promoting health involves a set of diverse activities at a number of different levels, using a wide range of skills and depending on contributions from varied groups of people, both professional and lay. Chapters 1–6 explored health beliefs, health status, the development and diversity of health promotion and the contested nature of health promotion models and values. The challenge now is to try and organise this knowledge and understanding to enable you to develop your health promotion role.

Health promotion involves adding another dimension to your work. Promoting health is not just a matter of seeking out new opportunities but of working in new ways for health. Acceptance of the underlying values of health promotion, of the ethical principles of beneficence and non-maleficence, respect for autonomy, empowerment of individuals, concern for equity and social justice, acknowledgement and respect for diversity, carries implications about the transformation of the professionals involved as well as their clients. Client-centredness means seeing the world from another viewpoint, starting from 'where the person is at', rather than imposing a professional view. This is difficult for most professionals (whatever their occupation) because professional training and experience moulds them into a professional 'world view' in which their values and views seem both more valid, more rational and 'moral' than those of the lay people with whom they work.

It is a hard lesson to learn that some of that professional certainty and power has to be given up and that it might have to be accepted that the client's priorities rather than your own are what will prevail. But innovative health educators have learned that if health advice is to be of value to their clients it must relate to and build on their lived experience (Ewles and Simnett, 1995; Macleod Clark, 1993). This might need to begin with an acceptance that people will have different priorites for action.

Health promotion work with families, for example, needs to take account of the complexities of family life and of what may be different and conflicting values. For a health promoter health may be the most important social goal but for many parents it would have to compete for attention with financial concerns, work pressures and family dynamics. The financial and social costs of acting on advice about moving to a healthier diet might be too great for poor families to contemplate. Work pressures might lead to increased use of processed foods, even if these were known to be less nutritious than home cooking. Parents might not be prepared to face the conflict involved in resisting children's demands for junk foods, even if these were recognised to be 'unhealthy' (HEA, 1996). Unrealistic or simplistic advice about changing eating patterns, therefore, is likely not only to be impractical but to cause resentment.

Smoking cessation in families is another major objective for many health promoters which parents may not see as a priority. Once again understanding and flexibility are key ingredients of success:

> The complex dynamics behind family smoking behaviours are difficult to unravel ... Effectively tapping into anti-smoking sentiments in the family, and using them in a way that does not increase tensions and pressures, is a challenge for health promotion.
>
> (HEA, 1996: 25)

Power sharing is a crucial factor in health promotion. The objective is not to ensure compliance (although there may be occasions when this is crucial and ethically justifiable) but to enable people to think for themselves about health dilemmas and choices and to support them in their decision-making. Their decisions may not be the ones that you would have made for them, and clearly you will hope that by providing information, talking through issues and debating choices you will guide them to what you see as the 'right' decision for their health. Otherwise, if all outcomes are as good for health as each other, there is little point in promoting health (Downie et al., 1990). But as Kelly and Charlton (1995) have commented, not everyone attaches the same high importance to health. This implies being prepared to accept other people's priorities even if you profoundly disagree with them. On the Corkerhill estate in Glasgow, for example, the professionals' priorities were education of parents and training of children, whereas parents wanted environmental modifications such as traffic calming measures (Roberts et al., 1995). The outcome might need to be a recognition by the experts of the limits to education and the importance of some environmental changes.

Heavy-handed health advice will not be effective unless clients are convinced that the advice is helpful, appropriate and practical for them personally. There are two aspects to this. First, advice, even if well focused, needs to be given within a whole process of enabling the patient to question, challenge and choose. The distinction made by Macleod Clark (1993) between 'sick nursing' and 'health nursing' is pertinent here. Within a sick nurse framework professionals 'cared for' patients and most work was seen with the patient as the object. Hence giving health advice was a largely one-way process of the nurse telling the patient 'what was best'. In health nursing, by contrast, caring was done by both patient and nurse, the nurse enabling and supporting the patient in self-care and personal decision-making and acknowledging the right of the individual patient to make choices, even if they were not what the professional would see as 'healthy' choices.

In addition, we noted in Chapter 2 that making behavioural changes is extremely difficult unless material and social circumstances also changed. Although people unable to stop smoking or change their diet often blamed themselves for their failure it was more often the case that failure was attributable to features of the environment or relationships (Pill, 1990). So health promoters might need to intervene to make changes in the environment which would enable their clients to adopt more healthy behaviour. This process, characterised as trying to make 'healthy choices easier choices' is another of the ways in which professional certainties may be challenged by health promotion values and goals.

Another aspect of working in new ways involves acting collaboratively and in partnership with other agencies and professionals. Professional training and experience is valuable and necessary but it may also be narrowing. Promoting health is not only about empowering clients and the general public; it is also about how interprofessional working, through creating new opportunities for reflection and sharing of experience, can liberate practice.

7.3 Understanding the health promotion role

In Chapter 1 preventive services, health protection and regulation, health education and public policy change were delineated as the four main components of health promotion. But within these areas many different types of activities might take place.

Compare the main health promotion activities of practice nurses and environmental health officers (Box 7.1). How would you account for such a difference of focus?

Box 7.1: Range of activities of practice nurses and environmental health officers

Practice nurse tasks, with per cent of nurses undertaking each:

- immunisations or vaccinations 95.9 per cent

- health promotion clinics 91.9 per cent

- new registration checks 87.3 per cent

- cervical cytology screening 75.6 per cent

- chronic disease management clinics eg. hypertension 69.6 per cent, diabetes 56.9 per cent, asthma 53.2 per cent

- breast examination 66.7 per cent

- minor surgery 51.4 per cent

- counselling/advice, e.g. on anxiety/depression 44.1 per cent, incontinence 33.0 per cent

- health checks, e.g. on elderly people 46.3 per cent, on children 33.3 per cent

- family planning sessions 26.9 per cent

- antenatal clinics 22.6 per cent

      (adapted from Bradford and Winn, 1993:123; Hirst *et al.*, 1995:87)

Environmental health officer tasks:

- food inspection, food hygiene and safety

- housing standards

- health and safety at work and during recreation

- environmental protection, including statutory nuisances

- communicable disease prevention and control

- licensing

- drinking water surveillance

- refuse collection and street cleaning

- pest control.

                              (Allen (1996) in Scriven and Orme, 1996)

A comparison of the duties of practice nurses and environmental health officers highlights the breadth of actual and potential health promotion activity. The core of the practice nurses' workload has a health education or preventive focus. It is mainly face-to-face patient work, such as immunisations and health promotion clinics. Environmental health officers, by contrast, are involved in a considerable amount of regulatory work and, potentially, public policy development. This may be indirect or direct work, in particular checking and enforcing contracts and quality standards. The difference of focus relates most strongly to professional training and legal remit.

In both cases, however, there is a strong health promotion potential. Practice nurses have a 'health promotion' remit arising from the UK national health strategies and the 1990 and 1993 general practitioner contracts which funded health promotion clinics, established health checks and set targets for screening and immunisation. Environmental health officers are now increasingly taking a lead in public policy developmental work, such as recycling and urban conservation projects (Allen, 1993). Many local authorities are undertaking work around Agenda 21 and local authorities are increasingly recognising their health promoting role, particularly in Wales.

> As far as health promotion is concerned the[se] mandatory duties are vital if health is to be advanced. For example, people need sound and adequate housing. It is inappropriate to simply provide a first class primary health care service and new hospitals if adequate and suitable housing is not provided.
>
> (Allen, 1996)

Viewed in these terms primary health care, for example, should involve not just the immunisation and screening services but a range of positive health checks and measures to improve health, such as 'well women' and 'well men' clinics, out-reach advice and support services. In a similar way, health education by health or care professionals, teachers or voluntary sector workers might involve not only working with individuals to effect change but more proactive local campaigns or local health initiatives, working with mass media or supporting community action plans.

Direct and indirect work

Different groups of health and welfare workers make use of different types of approaches and techniques, ranging from an emphasis on information giving or advice work to indirect work with agencies and organisations (see Box 7.2). The critical point here is not to expect to be able to intervene in all these ways yourself but to be aware of them as potential components of health promotion. It may be that there are opportunities to work in different ways within your area of practice. In addition there may be benefits from working more collaboratively with other groups involved in health promotion.

Review which approaches and techniques you would most often use in your health promotion work.

Practice nurses in local health centres or dental nurses might see individual focused support and advice work as the major component, whereas for community workers it might be facilitation of local community action for health. Social services workers already engage in health promoting action, through 'protecting their clients and working to develop their skills for living' (Jones and Bloomfield, 1996). But there may be scope for a broader strategy which focuses on preventive work with families, health education and healthy alliances with the health and voluntary sectors. All of these groups could draw on their national health targets and on the research findings and campaigning initiatives of national health education agencies. Some of the range of approaches to health promotion is given in Box 7.2.

Box 7.2: Types of approaches to health promotion

- Direct work with individuals – treatment, care, listening, information giving, discussion, advice, counselling, empowerment, patient advocacy.

- Direct work with small groups – information giving, discussion, advice demonstrations, experiential learning, training, teaching.

- Indirect work in locality/organisation/system/setting – negotiating, planning, networking, facilitating, organising (people and resources), campaigning, lecturing, representing, training, marketing, publicising/ advertising.

- Indirect work in national and international agencies – epidemiological research, strategic and policy planning, media advocacy, planning national campaigns, funding community and outreach work.

Working at different levels

Identifying the main activities of health promotion work also highlights the diversity of levels at which it might take place. We tend to think about levels in terms of the involvement of different agencies but individual health workers may themselves work at a number of different levels.

Assess the levels at which you currently work by comparing your role with the example given below.

Ms J, a social worker, works in a residential setting, in a children's home. She has responsibility for the teenage girls in the home, who stay there until they leave local authority care at age 16. The girls attend the local school and Ms J liaises with the head and the teachers. She is particularly concerned that the girls receive adequate health and sex education and knows the disproportionately high risks that children leaving care have of being exploited. This involves her in forming links with the local health visitor Ms G who, despite her busy schedule, agrees to run a workshop on offering advice on contraception, HIV/AIDS and venereal disease. The social services department sees this as a positive move and negotiates with the community health trust to introduce these in all its children's homes, offering a small amount of funding to support the work and an evaluation. Ms J evaluates the project over the next three years and she and Ms G write a conference paper which is published in the *Health Education Journal*. They see the focus of their work as empowerment.

Box 7.3: Potential for health promotion at different levels

- Individual level working.

- Focus on small groups.

- Work at neighbourhood, local area level.

- Liaison/networking with local agencies, local authorities, local health services.

- 'Healthy alliances' between individuals and agencies/organisations in a particular locality.

- City/area-wide strategic interventions.

- Mass media and public education campaigns.

- Legislative change/directives/regulatory framework at local and national government level.

- Research, mass media, project and programme work by national health education/promotion agencies (Health Development Agency, Health Promotion Division: National Assembly for Wales, Health Education Board for Scotland, Health Promotion Agency for Northern Ireland Health Promotion Unit, Republic of Ireland).

- 'Healthy public policy' making in government, organisations (e.g. industrial, voluntary, public sector).

- European Community regulations and frameworks.

- World Health Organisation and other international agency frameworks, initiatives and guidelines.

- International agenda setting (e.g. United Nations, world summits, Agenda 21).

Ms J, therefore, works at a number of levels: in individual and small group work with the teenage girls, in linking with the school, developing a small 'healthy alliance' with the community trust and, through her research and publication, helping to influence changes in practice.

Action might take place at a number of levels simultaneously. For example, in HIV/AIDS campaigns in Europe mass media messages about the dangers of unprotected sex were broadcast, large amounts of information were passed out to schools, health centres, hospitals, workplaces and other centres, local HIV/AIDS clinics offered advice to individuals, voluntary groups were given support to care for AIDS sufferers and needle exchange schemes for intravenous drug users were set up. In the UK the four national health education/promotion agencies took a lead in research, mass media campaigns and a range of community interventions and projects. In some countries other measures were used as well. In Thailand, where the government distributed condoms free to sex workers and launched a mass campaign to persuade them not to engage in unprotected sex, the rate of new HIV/AIDS cases among those using brothels fell by 60 per cent between 1990 and 1993 (Tones and Tilford, 1994).

A 'settings' approach

Finally, health promotion involves interventions in a wide range of settings. The settings approach has also been viewed as a potential way of delivering programmes which permeate through a whole organisation and work at a number of different levels (Tannahill, 1994). Such settings include primary health care, hospitals, schools, the workplace, local authority and community settings, and so on (Box 7.4). To demonstrate opportunities for innovation the World Health Organisation has initiated various projects and strategies, such as the Healthy Cities project, health promoting schools and healthy hospitals.

The health promoting hospitals pilot project involves 20 hospitals around Europe, ranging from the Child Health Centre in Warsaw, Poland, to Padua Hospital in Italy, to the James Connolly Memorial Hospital in Dublin, in the Irish Republic. One of the UK initiatives, at Royal Preston and Sharoe Green Hospitals in Preston, has focused on reducing accidents and accident and emergency admissions by a mixture of organisational changes and outreach and educational work. These include work to highlight the causes of accidents, an extended triage system in which people could phone in for immediate advice on self care and first aid, and designing a programme of self care for regular attenders (Harrison and Ashcroft, 1994).

Box 7.4: Some potential settings for health promotion work

- Hospitals.

- Clinics, dental surgeries, GP surgeries/primary health care.

- Primary health care (GP surgery).

- Schools, colleges and universities.

- Workplaces – industrial, commercial, public sector, voluntary etc. (workforce focus).

- Households.

- Day centres, community centres, neighbourhood centres.

- Residential homes, sheltered accommodation and nursing homes.

- Self-help, community and pressure groups.

- Prisons, police stations, legal aid centres, citizens advice bureaux (client focus).

7.4 Identifying skills

This final section outlines the types of skills that may be useful in health promotion work (see Box 7.5). It draws on the previous section where a range of activities, approaches and processes were introduced. In doing this, it encourages you to begin a process of identifying your own skills and exploring where new skills might be of value.

Look through the list in Box 7.5. Identify the skills that you think you already have.

You may have discovered, on close inspection, that you were already familiar with many of the skills listed. One of the issues highlighted here is that health promotion is about using existing skills but giving them a new meaning and dimension. Some of the skills are generic; for example, most people in health and welfare-related work will be involved in some planning, managing, communication and networking. The issue then becomes how to use these abilities and practices in a health promoting way. For example in planning an intervention a health promotion

---

Box 7.5: Identifying useful skills in health promotion

- Planning and research: investigating, defining and identifying needs and priorities, planning interventions.

- Evaluation: assessing the value and cost-effectiveness of actions undertaken, assessing information.

- Communication/counselling: understanding theories and evaluating approaches, client-centredness, listening skills.

- Management of time, people and resources: team building, managing change, managing the implementation of programmes and projects.

- Networking: liasing with people/agencies, facilitating action, negotiating, supporting local groups, fund-raising.

- Teaching: supporting and leading groups, developing teaching/ learning skills, understanding theories, planning, evaluation.

- Marketing: lobbying, using market research, working with mass media, managing publicity, planning a campaign.

- Influencing policy and practice change: brings together skills of networking, marketing, planning and research.

- Writing, research, dissemination, publication.

- Empowerment: understanding concept, developing skills.

- Fundraising: development of project proposals for Single Regeneration Budget, health action zones, healthy living centres, etc.

---

checklist might be added, with questions such as:

> Will this action enhance the health of this client or group and how can I evaluate this?
>
> Has my needs assessment taken into account the needs expressed by the client or group rather than just my professional view of their needs?
>
> How am I going to involve the client or group in the planning of this intervention?
>
> Am I prepared to have my ideas rejected in favour of non-expert ideas coming from my client or the local residents' group?

These are difficult questions to pose and answer and they raise some of the dilemmas that have been discussed throughout Part 1. Most are about sharing power in some way with clients and others, which is a fundamental tenet of contemporary health promotion. All involve putting health – a broad model of health incorporating social and environmental influences and lay ideas – higher up your planning agenda. Such questions may also set you thinking about learning new skills or reviewing old ones.

Many lay people and professionals, for example, engage in some educational work with clients or families, even if they are not teachers. But as we noted in earlier chapters traditional health education was often about telling clients what they should do rather than empowering them to make their own decisions. A health promoting approach to education would be concerned with developing an understanding of education and learning techniques in which the recipient of the education is seen as an active partner and agenda setter.

The skills of managing time, people and resources and team-building are not only needed in health promotion but in a wide range of work roles. Depending on where you work, you may operate as a team or within a more hierarchical line management structure (or the two may be combined). There are particular techniques of management that will aid your health promotion work. Ewles and Simnett (1995) suggest that co-ordination and teamwork are vital because health promotion, at whatever level, often involves working with colleagues from different departments or agencies. They suggest that this puts a premium on building and maintaining good relationships, and where necessary by bargaining, negotiation, joint planning and agreeing policy procedures.

Underpinning health promotion activities are planning, evaluation and research awareness skills. Understanding and assessing the health promotion needs of populations and planning successful interventions depends on being able to interpret health and social statistics. In addition, evaluation, detailed record-keeping and monitoring are increasingly central features of the accountability ethos of the working environment. Evaluation is also about improving our understanding of the processes in which we are engaged in order to improve practice.

Other skills, such as marketing and influencing policy change, may be less familiar, although techniques of lobbying, campaigning and even marketing may well have been used by voluntary sector workers who are trying to raise funding, highlight key issues and keep the organisation afloat. Social marketing is a fairly new technique in health promotion and this and other communication skills will be discussed in Part 2. Part of building healthy alliances for health promotion could involve learning such new skills by networking with workers in voluntary or commercial settings who use them already. So once again it involves power sharing, this time between the health promoters themselves, a process that may be just as difficult in its way as sharing power with lay people. Increasingly health promoters are involved in developing funding proposals for health promotion projects.

One of the strengths of healthy alliances and intersectoral collaboration is that working together enables people to 'play to their strengths'. Not everyone needs to be an expert on everything. Networking has often been seen as a matter of 'keeping up with news' or 'using your contacts' but an intersectoral or alliance approach indicates much more systematic development of teamwork and partnerships for health. The notion of settings and programmes (Tannahill, 1992) also emphasises a team approach to working with a particular group of people in a holistic way.

7.5 Conclusion

This chapter has been about 'taking stock' before 'moving on'. You have been encouraged to apply what has been learned so far about health and its promotion to build up a profile of the skills and knowledge useful to those working to promote health. We began by viewing health promotion as a process and not just a product, as a way of working which added a new dimension to what is probably your usual work role. You were encouraged to review the territory of health promotion: the range of activities, the different approaches, the levels at which action is taken and the settings within which it occurs. Finally the chapter drew together the skills that are central to health promotion work, prompting you to review your own skills and map them onto health promotion work. In Parts 2, 3 and 4 you will be exploring the key issues identified here in much greater depth.

Part 2
Communicating and educating for health

Introduction

The scope of health promotion as described and analysed in Part 1 is broad, encompassing prevention, health protection, health education and public policy change. Although the main focus of this Part is on health education, we begin by exploring communication and counselling skills because they are core skills essential to working in new ways to promote health in the widest sense. These new ways of working discussed in Chapter 7 involve power sharing and the ability to 'enable people to think for themselves about health dilemmas and choices and to support them in their decision making' (p. 109). It was stressed in Chapter 7 how health advice flowing from the health professional to the client will not be of value unless it relates to clients' own priorities and takes into account their particular social or economic circumstances. This client-centredness requires a transformation of the professional who needs to see the world from another viewpoint; communication then has very much to be a two-way process. The development of effective communication to promote health is explored in the first chapter of this Part. However if professionals are to build relationships with clients which are more supportive and enabling, then the communication style has to facilitate such relationships. Here there is much to learn from the world of counselling. Although developed within a therapeutic tradition, the skills of counselling are explicitly concerned with building supportive relationships and so have much to offer those who would promote health. The scope of counselling skills in the promotion of health is the subject of the second chapter in this Part.

Attention in the third and fourth chapters in this Part turns specifically to health education. Education for health is, according to Keith Tones (1983) 'an essential prerequisite in all health promotion programmes'. He identified two distinct functions of health education: one is the traditional function of influencing individual health choices, the other is more radical in that it seeks, through raising public awareness, to influence the adoption of healthy public policies, and is concerned to empower people. In this part we are concerned both with the methods used and the skills required to educate for health in the context of the different approaches and models of health education. Finally we examine the role of mass media in educating for health and explore some of the techniques employed in mass media campaigns.

Chapter 8
Developing effective communication

8.1 Introduction

Communication lies at the heart of all health encounters, both at the one-to-one level and at the groupwork level. It is increasingly being acknowledged (Macleod Clark *et al.*, 1997) that most interactions can in some way be health enhancing, whether in a physical or mental health context. Communication in a way that is health enhancing is not simply a matter of getting the message across; it involves building relationships and empowering people, even in the briefest of encounters, so that they can make choices and decisions about health based on their own priorities and circumstances. Communication is an everyday activity and the skills involved may seem to be deceptively simple. Yet, while the ability to communicate may be taken for granted, there can be considerable variation in the quality of health professionals' communication. Furthermore, poor communication between health professionals and certain groups in the population is a cause for concern. Groups such as older people, disabled people and those from minority ethnic groups, are often disadvantaged by the poor communication skills of professional gate-keepers to health and health care.

There are many types, forms and levels of communication. This chapter analyses our understandings of communication and explores the basic communication skills involved in human interactions. This is done within the broad framework of an understanding that communication should no longer be simply the one-sided conveying of information from the informed to the uninformed but far more an acknowledgement of sharing information between equals. Communication should be seen as a partnership with respect for and understanding of the background, attitudes and agenda of each party. We therefore consider the role of communication in the field of promoting health before looking at the pitfalls that create difficulties in communicating with certain groups and in particular situations.

8.2 What is communication?

This chapter focuses on the characteristics of communication in a fairly specific sense, primarily using the spoken language and non-verbal messages in a face-to-face, usually one-to-one setting. The focus here is on the *communication process*, rather than the *content of the message to be conveyed*.

Communication takes place in many forms, indeed almost every aspect of human behaviour can be a form of communication conveying a message to someone.

When we have something we want to say we formulate our ideas into words which we hope will convey the intended meaning. The more important the ideas are, the more time we spend thinking about how best to communicate them. However, when we talk to someone we do not just communicate with words, we also convey information about ourselves which the listener interprets along with the words we have chosen. When we meet people for the first time we tend to make judgements about them almost immediately. We may do this consciously as part of professional judgement, but whatever the level of conscious assessment, we collect a lot of information about people beyond what they say to us. This information may well change as we get to know people better: our first impressions may have been misleading, or we may find the information serves to confirm or reinforce initial impressions. These judgements are not one way, for the other person is also making an assessment of us to varying degrees of awareness.

There is much more occurring than an exchange of words to express ideas – we are communicating something of ourselves to each other, in other words we are relating to each other. The way we relate is not fixed but is constantly changing as we respond to each other. Recognising that communication takes place within a dynamic relationship is important but we also need to acknowledge the context of relationships. People have different backgrounds and experiences which affect how they experience and interpret the world. Communication is a process but it is one which is bound by structural elements such as age and gender.

What messages about yourself might someone watching you eating alone pick up?

You must have been aware of someone watching you when you've eaten a meal alone in a cafeteria or restaurant and wondered what messages the other person was picking up about you, possibly fantasising about your marital status, your age, what kind of work you do, and why you are eating in this place, alone. Observing someone reveals different forms of communications reflected by body language, facial expressions and gestures.

Communication occurs on several levels because of the perceptions of each person involved in the interaction or conversation. For instance when talking to someone the levels of communication may be seen as becoming increasingly more abstract:

1   This is how I perceive me.
2   This is how I perceive you.
3   This is how I perceive you seeing and hearing me.
4   This is how I think you see me seeing you.

(Murray and Zentner, 1985: 32)

The first level is simply thinking about oneself only whilst talking to someone else. On the second level, the first person is still thinking of him/herself, but also noticing the other person and hearing what he/she is saying. On the third level, the first person is aware of the other person's perceptions as well as understanding what both people are saying and feeling. On this level, the effect the first person has on the second person can be considered and behavioural cues taken into account and responded to. For the fourth level to take place, there must be acute awareness of the dynamics of the interaction because the first person now considers how the other person thinks he/she is perceiving him/her (Murray and Zentner, 1985). This level requires much empathy and perception but will increase the awareness of the other (where the other is coming from) and hence enhance communication.

So what is the purpose of communication? Your answer might include:

- to control, influence or direct others – for example indicating to someone disapproval of their smoking habits. This might include an irritated look, a cough or simply making a noise and moving away
- to express emotion – laughing or giggling, crying, comforting or being angry – expressing enjoyment through play or music
- reflecting – talking through an issue with a colleague, a client or a neighbour and mulling over ideas; asking for feedback from people reading this book, sharing feelings with your partner or children
- providing information – planning the day with your colleagues, teaching students about new developments, explaining findings from research.

Although there is considerable overlap between the four areas described above, they illustrate the form, content and function of communication between people. Although this chapter almost exclusively explores interpersonal communication through speech and physical responses, there are many other forms: such as the media, the internet, written official records, books, music and art. The influences these other forms of communication have on people's lives and indeed on society can be considerable. For example, information stored in computerised documents can lead to changes in people's lives: when different aspects of information stored about one person's medical tests are combined, these may point to major treatment decisions or a decision to change long-standing habits such as alcohol consumption. Even though the person whose results these documents may describe may not knowingly be part of the chain of communication between one test result and another, and all the people who process them in-between, these communications still remain interpersonal at many levels.

> The creation and existence of processes of communication which, as it were, surround rather than target individual people, are an important and powerful part of human experience.
>
> (The Open University, 1992: Workbook 1: 17)

Communication theories exploring interpersonal interactions tend to fall into several categories. Social-psychological approaches address the clarity, openness and effectiveness of the messages. They look at the quality of the interpersonal relationship, whether mutual understanding is achieved, particularly with regard to understanding one another's agendas, attitudes, expectations and goals. In addition they take into account awareness of external social factors, for example the setting in which the interaction takes place and the socio-economic status of the individuals (DiMatteo and DiNicola, 1982). Psychological theories relate to cognition, information processing and interpersonal interactions (for example conflict between the communicating parties). Ley's work (1983, 1986) demonstrates how, if patients do not understand information they receive, they are less likely to be satisfied with their care or adhere to treatment. If understanding is impaired because information is inaccessible (jargon-laden), or recipients are unable to concentrate because of anxiety, illness or are under the effects of drugs, they will have difficulty recalling the information. Mis-communication may be exacerbated by the different perspectives and assumptions of the two parties. However cognition research has revealed that comprehension of both written and oral communications can be enhanced by simple techniques, such as the use of short sentences and uncomplicated words, and by sequencing information – presenting the most important information first and stressing its importance (Joos and Hickam, 1990).

Thus there are a number of factors to bear in mind when communicating about health promotion, one of which is the need to ensure that the communication message is framed in a way that will make the recipient feel valued and respected, and hence will make him or her more receptive. Another is the willingness of the health promoter to relinquish control of the interaction to the other person. In this way, channels of communication will be opened up rather than closed down.

8.3 Forms of communication

As communication links us with other people and helps us understand ourselves and where we belong in society, it is important to examine the impact of these different forms. While for many people the most commonly used means of communication is the spoken, signed or written word, this form of communication is not always the most relevant.

What kinds of communication are there other than verbal?

The following box includes a range of non-verbal communication which is certainly not comprehensive but indicates some of the ways in which communication can be effective without the use of language.

Box 8.1: Forms of non-verbal communication

Speech related

Timing and pauses within verbal behaviour; speech variations and voice; silence and the use of pauses.

Non-verbal behaviour

Posture and position; eye contact; physical contact; proximity to other person; speech variations and voice and facial expressions used to accompany words and indicate listening.

Use of body

Eye contact and direction of gaze; facial expressions, hand gestures; posture and stance.

Aspects of personal appearance

Clothing and hairstyle; smell, including body odour, perfume and cigarette smoke; cosmetics; style and type of dress, for example formal dress or uniform to indicate work, more casual clothes which indicate the cessation of work or an attitude towards dress at work.

Symbols

Colour; uniforms, artefacts such as badges or jewellery; graphic symbols such as Ladies or No Smoking; art and other expressive media; time symbolism such as being late or early, or rushing the encounter.

Sign language

In communication with people who have hearing difficulties; also when communicating with people who are sighted through the use of physical movement, such as gesticulating.

Written word

In letters, and report writing; note-taking; essay and assignment work; sending messages by computer e-mail or fax machines.

Media: newspapers, radio, television

To provide information and entertainment.

This list is far from comprehensive but it illustrates some non-verbal indicators of communication which may occur in health education and health promotion encounters. Indeed, even when we are quiet and on our own, we are still communicating within ourselves – thinking, day-dreaming and reflecting on past activities, encounters and events. All forms of communication affect health promoting activities but non-verbal behaviour needs expanding and exploring further because these messages influence the nature of interactions with individuals and groups.

Non-verbal behaviour, as seen above, includes physical responses such as facial expressions, gestures, movement and eye contact. Whether or not they are used in conjunction with speech, non-verbal signs affect the meaning of what we say and can reveal feelings and attitudes towards others.

Posture is a largely involuntary sign, communicating important information about our attitude to ourselves and to others. For example, a relaxed posture could indicate both a confident self-image and confidence in the person with whom we are interacting. Posture and position may need to be adjusted to promote communication. This involves considering how best to use the physical environment to optimise opportunity for effective interaction. Cues may suggest that a respondent is not comfortable and therefore unable to be receptive or responsive during an interaction.

Buckman with Kason (1992) identified ways of improving an interaction through modifying one's physical position. These include:

- sitting down, keeping one's eyes level with those of the other person
- unfastening or removing an outer coat to emphasise that you are not about to leave
- sitting in a relaxed position with shoulders dropped but looking alert and interested
- removing obstacles to communication, a table, desk or locker, which may form a physical barrier or suggesting the television is turned off for a little while
- ensuring the distance between you and the other person is acceptable, usually 20–36 inches or 50–90 cm. The person will alter position and move to gain attention if this is not appropriate (Matthews, 1983).

Non-verbal cues demonstrate one's intention to establish a good relationship with the other person and a sensitivity or insensitivity to his or her concerns. Keeping people waiting may make them feel devalued, as will being rushed. It is important to appear to have enough time and respond to their individual needs – the person might be feeling ill or have particular cultural concerns which cause discomfort. If the interaction becomes unbalanced, the dominant person will appear more upright and erect whilst the submissive individual will probably have rounded shoulders and the head lowered (Coid, 1991).

Eye contact is important. An interaction with a sighted person usually starts with one person attempting to engage the other in eye contact. If this contact is successful, the other person is under some obligation to return the gaze. Conversely, avoidance of eye contact suggests reluctance to become involved or the intention to break bad news (Buckman, 1993). There is a tendency to look much more when listening than when speaking, and the more difficult the subject being discussed the less eye contact, perhaps because it is too personal, or because of the need to concentrate (Argyle, 1994).

Heath (1986) states that there is a continuing flow of body movement from eye-to-eye and facial expression to changes in body position. Health professionals need to be aware of their own practice and the way it affects interaction: excessive gazing at the other person or at documentation will reduce interaction (Inman, 1996). Different cultural needs should also be considered. People from some different ethnic backgrounds may require *more* eye-to-eye contact (Heath, 1986) or *less*, as in the case of Muslim women when talking to men. The acceptance or avoidance of eye contact can have powerful emotional effects and practice based on knowledge of this will influence the outcome of an encounter. Some facial expressions are so fleeting they are not noticed consciously. The face, however, reflects our emotional state. It is an interesting exercise to watch television with the sound turned off, to see whether emotions can be interpreted from facial expressions.

Touch and body contact communicates a great deal about relationships, status and degrees of friendliness. As some cultures frown on physical contact between different sexes and strangers it is important to be aware of the customs of the other person. Buckman with Kason (1992) states that the most important part of touch is to be sensitive to the recipient's response. If, for example, a light touch on the hand or shoulder helps in reducing emotional distance between you and the other person and fosters the exchange of information, it is beneficial; if they withdraw a little, it is not. It is advisable to limit touch to the arm and shoulder to avoid danger of misinterpretation (Buckman, 1992). If the participant is viewed as particularly vulnerable, care must be taken to prevent misunderstandings and sexual innuendoes.

Non-verbal and verbal behaviour are obviously linked. For example the speed of speech, tone, pitch and volume all contribute towards the voice, and this is readily heard if we make a conscious effort to take notice. For people whose first language is not English, it is important to be aware of meaning that is conveyed by tone and pitch as these may not be understood by people who are unfamiliar with the conventions of tone and pitch in the English language. Initially, one needs to ascertain how the other person usually speaks. If the speech seems very rushed, unclear or if the speaker stammers, it could indicate an unwillingness to participate because of resentment or embarrassment, and the difficulty will need to be explored with sensitivity. We now move on to consider how the use (not content) of language affects interactions.

8.4 The importance of language

For most of us communication primarily means language in some form or another even if we are deaf or blind. Through language people become members of social groups; language transmits values and beliefs which shape development and socialisation into particular ways of thinking and behaving. The use of language serves different functions in a range of settings and speech patterns are regarded as social indicators.

In the 1960s and 1970s many studies focused on practitioner–patient interaction and the power of the medical profession (e.g. Waitzkin and Stoeckle, 1972; Stimson and Webb, 1975). More recently, however, interest has shifted to studying interactions in a range of health-related settings, where language serves a variety of functions (e.g. Silverman, 1987). The list in Box 8.2 relates to functions of language pertinent to health promotion.

Box 8.2: Functions of language

social contact – meeting and exchanging views with others

stimulation – helping to create and maintain interest in others

expression – to give vent to feelings and emotions

alleviation of anxiety – to ease a worry

information – to find out or explain something

persuasion – convince another person to believe

control – to get someone to behave in a particular way

instrumental – to achieve or obtain something

role related – to fulfil a particular role or act in a predictable way

making sense – to order, classify and come to terms with words – to understand the world in which we live.

In a health-focused interview information is *transmitted* or *exchanged*. In addition there may be some interpretation or trying to *make sense* of what was stated or implied. This meeting is *social* and during the interaction some *emotional expression* may emerge. The extent of this will depend on the degree of involvement, personality traits, gender and emotional state. Evidence of the *roles* adopted will vary depending on how the participants relate to the differences in status. Previous learning and experience affect communication patterns.

Everyday language and specialist language

Medical terms are an essential aspect of the vocabulary of health professionals. This is particularly important in diagnostic work and in communicating about health and work-related matters to other health professionals. Specialist vocabulary legitimately evolves as areas of skill and knowledge increase. Think for example of the burgeoning number of terms that have entered the health and lay vocabularies since the beginning of the AIDS epidemic. Essential distinctions need to be made between medical conditions. For example, the term 'myocardial infarction' may seem like a pretentious way of describing a heart attack, but it explains to those versed in physiological processes the precise nature of the problem. See the following extract from a interview between a medical social worker and a cardiac patient:

SW: Have the doctors explained to you the nature of your medical problem?

Mr Morris: Actually it's all rather confusing because the consultant said I had had a myocardial infarction (see I've written it down), my GP told me that I'd had a coronary, and my wife was told in casualty that I'd had a heart attack.

This demonstrates how the use of specialist language can be confusing and indeed may sometimes be employed to 'exclude' people or to emphasise one's own status. Therefore, when communicating with clients/patients, it is useful to introduce specialised language carefully (Maguire, 1993) so recipients are not confused or alienated and, if anything, are well versed in understanding these terms. Awareness of the difficulties caused by 'mystification' is important and efforts should be made to explain any complicated medical terminology.

There are, however, circumstances when appropriate terminology may be particularly welcome to the client/patient. During gynaecological examinations specialist vocabulary and the use of euphemisms may defuse a potentially embarrassing situation. Terms such as micturition, cervix and gynaecological examination may be criticised for being too technical, but the patient may find them a positive aid to depersonalising the situation. In the field of human sexual and excretory functions and malfunctions, medical terminology, by virtue of its formality and detachment, thus may be more acceptable to the lay person than its everyday equivalent. Hence sensitivity to the feelings of others will help to avoid difficulties.

It has often been said that we can only understand the world we live in through language. This embodies two assumptions:

1 that language somehow shapes our thinking and our perceptions of the world (these processes are sometimes referred to as the construction of social reality); and

2 that we can only access this reality through language.

For our purposes here the analysis of verbal exchanges in health-related settings yields insights into the many functions that language may serve; it also highlights ways in which language may be used either to circumvent, bridge or deny social and cultural barriers or even to emphasise them.

Mills (1992) argues that when we acquire language, we are effectively born into a system of logic, a structure of meanings and a set of vocabularies which 'socially canalise thought'. Language is therefore a symbolic system which carries descriptions and interpretations. These 'frames of reference' are grounded in the history and social activity of a particular culture and are used by people to explain and make sense of their world. Mills explains:

Language, socially built and maintained, embodies implicit exhortations and social evaluations. By acquiring the categories of language, we acquire the structured 'ways' of a group and, along with the language, the value-implicates of those 'ways'. Our behaviour and perception, our logic and thought, come within the control of a system of language. Along with language, we acquire a set of social norms and values. A vocabulary is not merely a string of words; implicit within it are social textures.

Moving on from studying the language of a whole culture to studying the languages of sub-cultures, Mills's comments remain valid. A sub-culture can be identified when some members of society experience similar circumstances and problems, attitudes and values which are distinctive to them as a social group (Haralambos and Holborn, 1985). Sub-cultures have a tendency to develop their own distinctive language patterns and vocabulary which may differ from those conventionally used by other social groups. They use the 'everyday' words used by other groups but attach slightly different meanings to the words. They may also utilise their own words that have no immediate meaning for people outside the sub-culture. One example of a group with a culture centred around a specialist communication system is that of deaf people. Different youth cultures also use words in ways that, if anything, are contrary to the dictionary meaning: 'wicked' for example meaning excellent or wonderful. Thus, familiarity with colloquialisms and culture will facilitate better communication.

Those from minority ethnic backgrounds will have particular concepts of health (see Currer and Stacey, 1986) which may be at variance with the white British host society. They may also hold views about health promotion and health promoters. Some people from minority ethnic groups may have only a limited command of English and therefore be unfamiliar with local colloquialisms. Communication problems can, and do, arise as the result of racial prejudice: for example, disapproval of health habits of people from particular ethnic groups may affect a health promoter's attitude towards them. Health promoters need to be aware of and reflect upon attitudes that they may have towards people of different ethnic backgrounds to themselves which may affect effective communication. Clarification of the meaning of asthma in a recently diagnosed asthmatic child for the child and parents from a minority ethnic group might take the form of a description in their own words regarding:

- what tends to trigger an attack and what action to take as prevention
- if an attack develops rapidly what action can be taken.

This will help the health promoter to understand the child and family's perception of the situation. Here a check is made to ensure that the child and family know and understand the relevant information despite differences in language usage.

Health promoters can also be viewed as a sub-cultural group with its own words, language patterns and world view. Esland (1973) suggests:

Every semantic field is serviced by a community of people who participate in organizing the knowledge for which they claim responsibility. This community formulates policy, propagates its essential themes and attempts to persuade the wider public of its value. For its own members, there are often tests of orthodoxy (such as examinations), rules for excluding deviant knowledge and techniques for handling the people who come for treatment, advice or other kinds of service.

The processing and control of knowledge by a particular group, its development of procedures for handling the lay public in those matters, and its power to manage the realities of others are all major questions which emerge from enquiry into the use of language.

The 'power' to which Esland refers should be seen as a form of 'expert power'. He associates two major functions with this 'power':

1 Organising and establishing the importance of certain items of knowledge.
2 Claiming exclusive rights to develop procedures for dealing with the lay public.

He recognises that studying and analysing language will help in the control of knowledge, procedures and people.

Health promotion is associated with developing relationships to enable people to increase their autonomy and ability to make decisions relating to their health. As we have already noted, this is contrary to the conventional view that health information is vested in the control of physicians (e.g. Freidson, 1970). To facilitate self-determination in others, professionals' apparent need to control people (Bopp, 1989) will have to be relinquished and replaced by a participatory decision-making process. It is through the use of language that clear unambiguous messages can be devised and exchanged to facilitate a change in behaviour.

Messages can be conveyed in many different registers: that is, in different forms of language, according to particular circumstances. In health promotion, the language used will be adapted to those with whom you are communicating to reduce the risks of distorting the message. People usually feel comfortable with their own form of words. The health promoter may adopt, to an acceptable degree, a similar style of speech to that of their recipient without appearing patronising. Health promoters who facilitate autonomous decision-making will work hard at ensuring positive communication between themselves and their clients and develop the interpersonal skills necessary for this purpose. Anger and frustration can arise if the language used is not appropriate. Wright (1992) suggests that expressing strong opinions or using patronising language may provoke an angry response.

It is at the interface with the 'lay' public that specialist language can pose problems. It can be confusing and intimidating, leaving people feeling uneasy, anxious, unconfident and embarrassed. It reinforces the power of the professional and undervalues the views of the lay person. It is important to explain technical terms without being patronising. This sharing of language involves the sharing of power and allows the interaction to be more participatory.

8.5 Listening and questioning

Listening is central to all health promotion work and is the most important of all communication skills, but it is a skill that is often assumed and taken for granted. However, for hearing people it may be possible to technically hear what is being said but *physically* hearing another person does not necessarily mean *actively* listening or comprehending. Passive listening is usually non-responsive and may be superficial or selective because the listener is blocking an unpleasant message (Faulkner, 1992). Good listening means active listening and it is a skill which can be learned and improved. Buckman with Kason (1992) suggest that the golden rule is to let the person speak without interruption.

Attentive listening includes

- observing the speaker, if possible
- ensuring eye contact is appropriate and acceptable
- concentrating on both words and non-verbal behaviour
- thinking about what is being said and how it is being stated
- being interested
- indicating your attention with body-language, for example, nodding
- vocalising with occasional 'Hmm' or 'Tell me more'
- being open-minded
- tolerating short silences.

By listening, information is gathered relating to feelings, views and perceptions. Such information can be gathered by noting the way in which information is presented; what is emphasised and what is omitted; whether there are unspoken assumptions; subjects that cause emotional discomfort or topics that cause withdrawal from involvement in interaction. The information gathered is considerable and requires reflection and analysis during or following the encounter.

Non-verbal cues are crucial to demonstrate interest and active involvement in the encounter. An empathetic approach can be signalled through body language – leaning forward, smiling or making appropriate facial expressions which indicate a positive attitude. The other person will quickly ascertain whether the approach is sympathetic, empathetic or judgemental. Non-verbal signs thus also reveal lack of interest, inattention or disapproval. A raised eyebrow, an exclamation of surprise, or too little eye-contact, could give negative feedback. Most non-verbal behavioural signals can usually be controlled. For example, it is possible to avoid appearing very busy by not shuffling papers or looking at the clock. Other positive non-verbal indicators of listening include smiling, being responsive, and keeping channels of communication open in order to increase the effectiveness of the encounter.

Levels of listening

It is possible to identify three purposes or levels when listening to someone speaking, whether one-to-one, or one-to-many. You can listen for *facts*, *feelings or attitudes*, and *intentions*. The importance of each of these levels will vary according to the situation, but usually all three are present to some extent.

Read and reflect on the following transcript from Macleod Clark, *et al*. 1992. Which level of listening is the nurse engaged in in this extract?

Client: I think with lung cancer, I mean if your lungs pack up you have more or less had it, haven't you.

Nurse: Mmm. Yes.

Client: I think that's one that really worries me.

Nurse: Mmm. Women are increasingly getting lung cancer because more women are smoking now. At one time, women used to think it didn't affect them and that more men die. In fact, the statistics are going up for women so it is a definite health risk.

(Macleod Clark *et al.*, 1992: 24)

The nurse agrees that it is a *fact* that if your lungs pack up your life chances are reduced. She then acknowledges the *feeling* expressed by the client and, after encouraging her to continue with a second Mmm, provides additional details relating to the facts. You may have wondered whether this information might lead the client towards expressing her *intentions* regarding smoking. However, you will note that the nurse is generalising and does not pick up on the cues that the client gave as to *why* she is worried. The nurse is effectively blocking the client by providing her with accurate but unrequested information and is closing off avenues for discussion rather than opening them up.

Questioning

The ability to use questions to promote communication is linked closely to listening and is equally important for developing a rapport with the client. To indicate careful listening you might request clarification or amplification of their views. Attentive listening to answers to questions will foster appropriate and sensitive responses. Questions can be framed in a particular way to open channels of communication or reduce interaction: for example, multiple questions! A frequently used strategy is to use questions to reflect back what the person has said as confirmation of understanding, listening and valuing the communication. This is widely used as a counselling technique.

Different types of questions have been used in research and interviewing for many years. The impact of the nature of questions on the recipients in health care settings were identified by Byrne and Long (1976) Macleod Clark *et al.* (1982) and Silverman (1987). Examples of different types of questions are provided below:

Generally speaking, questions are either *closed* or *open*.

A *closed* question usually elicits a yes or no response, and requires the minimum response from clients. This, as you will note in Parts 3 and 4, is a widely used practice in questionnaires. Although they narrow the context they are useful for probing issues in a precise way and for checking that we have understood. For example:

- Are you still living in the damp flat?
- Sleeping well?
- Any breathlessness?
- Have you ever tried to lose weight?

An *open* question has no predetermined answer and encourages people to talk in a way that they choose and to explore new areas. Open questions initiate a flow of information and usually begin with how, when, who, why, what or where (Macleod Clark *et al.*, 1992). Open questioning passes the ownership of the interaction to the client. The following list of different types of questions illustrates how the way in which a question is framed determines the content (and quality) of the answer:

1 Do you smoke? *Closed question*

2 Tell me about your smoking? *Open question*

3 So you haven't been successful in stopping smoking before now? *Rhetorical question*

4 Well, I expect your breathing might be easier if you stopped smoking. *Hidden question*. The hidden question could be: 'Will you consider stopping smoking to make your breathing easier?'

5 The client might ask 'Do you think I need to stop smoking?' The health professional may reflect this with 'How do you feel about stopping smoking?' *Reflecting question*

Consider which of the above questions will promote or inhibit communication.

Only examples 2 and 5 really seem to provide the participant with the opportunity to respond freely.

In health promotion settings, questions may be specifically framed in order to elicit certain types of response.

Directed questions can be used in the following ways:

1 Initially, to assess the needs of a group or an individual. E.g. 'Which of your communication skills need improving?'

2 During a single encounter, or a series of encounters, to monitor progress and test whether objectives are being achieved and needs being met. E.g. 'How have you managed without smoking since I last saw you?'

3 At the end of a health promotion activity or programme, to evaluate what has been achieved and, if appropriate, to improve self-evaluation. E.g. 'So you haven't smoked for a full year now, is that correct?'

Levels of listening, discussed earlier, sought to differentiate facts from feelings. Similarly, when formulating questions, differentiations between *cognitive* and *affective* questioning can be made.

Cognitive questioning is used to discover facts, opinions and ideas, and to provide informative feedback. It is thus useful for:

- gaining attention
- obtaining information
- assessing knowledge levels
- reinforcing facts.

Affective questioning is used to ascertain people's feelings and attitudes to problems or issues, and to help individuals to discover their own feelings. It is thus useful for:

- encouraging
- developing confidence
- exploring feelings and emotions
- exploring problem areas.

As well as being positive and useful, questioning can be either openly or covertly manipulative, communicating various negative attitudes and embedded messages. Our voice, tone and the emphasis on certain words or phrases can imply criticism or reveal hidden assumptions.

Through careful questioning, deliberate pauses, and 'uh-uhs'or 'go on's'(Macleod Clark *et al.*, 1992) reflective responses could be facilitated. In the following quote you will observe a combination of open questioning and encouragement from the nurse (N) when talking to the client (C).

N: What sort of ways have you thought about giving up smoking?

C: I've tried several times, um, and I've always stopped for about a week.

N: Mmm.

C: But I get this really empty feeling inside my stomach.

N: Mmm.

C: I get really moody.

N: Uh-uh.

C: And I've been thinking recently, that instead of just thinking about it, I thought I'm going to set a date.

N:. Mmm.

C: It's best not to think about it.

(Macleod Clark *et al.*,1992: 23)

The client in the quote above has been able to develop her thoughts about stopping smoking without interruption and given permission to control the interaction. Giving cues that you are listening intently may facilitate more free expression of the other person's views and concerns. It also allows more time to consider what, if any, intervention to suggest. At the same time, the other person may provide clues about their worries which can be picked up later by asking for clarification of a particular statement.

Opening and closing

Whatever your area of involvement with health promotion, you have noted that both listening and questioning play a key role. It is important to remember that each of these two activities constitute interrelated skills which can be both learnt and can continue to develop. They are important throughout a meeting but crucial during the opening stage.

The way in which you commence a meeting or interview sets the tone for the occasion. Have the time and composure to make full introductions. Agree on the agenda at the beginning of the interview. Be prepared with relevant documents. Ensure that you use the person's name throughout the interview. Closures are also important as they may help to prepare for future interaction. They also intimate the direction of the relationship: for example, without saying anything you can indicate to the client that the meeting is over, by shuffling papers, looking at your watch or moving away from the desk. Your body language as well as the spoken word will make it clear whether you see this meeting as a one-off occasion or whether you would welcome further contact.

8.6 Barriers to effective listening and communication

Awareness of how well we listen helps us to reflect on our own performance. We can always improve our listening and other communication skills by learning how to recognize and remove the barriers to good listening and good communication. Some of these have already been mentioned such as specialist language, awareness of different cultural concepts and behaviours, and limited or no knowledge of the English language. Acknowledging the existence of the following barriers will help overcome their negative influence and find ways to break them down.

Mechanical barriers can be as basic as the lack of a conducive environment in which to communicate: for example, an interaction might be disturbed by noise and distractions caused by young children, builders or roadworkers or harsh lighting and uncomfortable chairs. Other mechanical barriers include fatigue, the side-effects of medication and impaired sight.

Psychological barriers can emerge because of differing attitudes, beliefs, values and prejudices. Lack of motivation to communicate can be caused by a variety of factors including self-absorption, low self-esteem, uncertainty, fear, embarrassment, hostility, status differences and status conflict, stress and negative past experiences or interactions with health professionals, and low expectations. In addition and less predictable in effect are differences or sameness of gender, age, ethnicity, culture and social class.

Semantics are concerned with the meanings of words. Misinterpretations and misunderstandings can arise because words have different meanings, connotations or associations for different people depending on previous experience.

Having looked at some of the components of effective communication, what do you think are the reasons for faulty listening?

The following table lists some reasons for faulty listening. The listener and the speaker are interchangeable, either could be the client or the health promoter.

This section has explored the importance of listening and asking questions in a way intended to promote positive communication. Developing awareness of the barriers to good interactions which might emerge at any stage of the interaction helps to reduce or eliminate these barriers and facilitate positive communication.

Table 8.1 **Possible reasons for failure to listen**

Location of cause	*Reasons*
The listener	Self-consciousness.
	Negative attitude to the speaker.
	Negative attitude to the subject.
	Impatience to speak oneself.
	Fixed ideas on the subject.
	Not understanding due to difficult concepts or selective information.
	Stress/anxiety about understanding.
	Selective attention, only hearing some parts of the communication.
	Blocking an unpleasant message.
	Not hearing due to a physical problem.
	Limited knowledge of English language.

The speaker	Poor oral presentation.
	Insensitivity to feedback.
	Appearance.
	Preconceived ideas and stereotypes.
The environment	Noise.
	Uncomfortable (heat/cold/pain/hunger).
	Interruptions.
	Lack of privacy.
	Seating and distance.

8.7 Conclusion

An understanding of what constitutes good communication is essential in order to promote health effectively. A range of approaches can be utilised to support individuals and facilitate change. The following chapter explores these different approaches including the use of counselling skills in the context of health promotion.

Chapter 9
Supporting individuals and facilitating change: the role of counselling skills

9.1 Introduction

Much of the work of health promotion with individuals is concerned with providing support and helping people to change behaviours which are either causing them problems, such as drinking too much alcohol, or are potentially harmful, such as smoking.

In this chapter the concern is with the use of counselling skills in providing this support and help. We explore counselling not because those who would promote health need to become counsellors but rather to explore the techniques and understandings that counselling has to offer in the promotion of health.

What is counselling?

Counselling is a diverse activity that increasingly pervades all corners of people's lives. There are many people who call themselves counsellors: educational counsellors, career counsellors, debt counsellors, colour counsellors, sex counsellors and many others, including the more familiar marriage guidance counsellors. It is a burgeoning industry and one where the credentials of practitioners is a matter of some public debate. Although anyone can call themselves a counsellor, there is a distinction to be made between professional counsellors (those who use counselling skills within their work) and others who may call themselves counsellors but have no professional training. Professional counsellors undergo basic training in counselling and have a code of ethics and practice which lays down a framework within which they operate. However there are different schools of counselling and a distinction is sometimes but not always made between counselling and psychotherapy. Anyone claiming to be a psychotherapist should have a recognised qualification.

The aim of counselling, it is claimed, is to help people to help themselves. The British Association of Counselling gives a fairly comprehensive definition:

> Counselling is the skilled and principled use of relationships to facilitate self-knowledge, emotional acceptance and growth, and the optimal development of personal resources ... The counsellor's role is to facilitate the client's work in ways that respect the client's values, personal resources and capacity for self determination.
>
> (British Association of Counselling, 1989)

Counselling is a person-to-person form of communication that is instrumental in character. It is a process designed to help people make choices and take appropriate actions, free from authoritarian judgements or coercive pressures. Much of counselling has developed within a therapeutic tradition but the essential relationship-building skills that are a prerequisite for that therapeutic relationship can inform the relationships that are health promoting.

The dictionary definition of the term counselling is closely connected to the giving of advice. However, counselling has moved away from the notion of advice towards the notion of guidance, and there are those counsellors who see no place at all for the giving of advice or guidance in what they do. A distinction has developed between what is known as 'directive' and 'non-directive' counselling. 'Non-directive' counsellors take a reflective and more passive role, giving clients the time and space to arrive at their own perceptions and solutions to their predicament. 'Directive' counsellors take a more active role, which might involve giving guidance about a behavioural change or intervening to increase the pace of change. Although they represent two broadly different approaches, in practice the difference is often less clear cut. However these different approaches are based on different theories and methods used in counselling as well as the purpose of the counselling. These different approaches are explored later in the chapter. First the scope of counselling within health promotion is examined.

9.2 The scope for using counselling skills in the promotion of health

There is a great deal of scope for using counselling skills to promote health in the everyday encounters health professionals have with their clients. GPs find themselves counselling their patients on a whole range of issues such as smoking or diet. Community nurses may need to counsel someone who is having to deal with incontinence. Health visitors counsel on the immunisation of infants and many other matters. Occupational therapists can find themselves in the role of counsellor when helping someone to come to terms with a chronic illness or disability and when working out how best to cope with the changes that it will involve. Both the directive and non-directive approach can be appropriate.

In the promotion of health the directive approach is likely to be concerned with bringing about a change in health-related behaviour, whereas the non-directive approach is more about supporting someone, perhaps through a difficult or challenging time or for personal development. The two approaches can work in complementary ways. For instance, if the main aim is to help someone to change harmful drinking behaviour, it may be important also to work in a non-directive way to improve that person's morale and self-esteem so that they are more likely to achieve the desired change.

These two approaches also mirror to some extent the preventive and the empowerment models of health education which you were introduced to in Chapter 4. The non-directive personal development approach aims to empower, whereas the directive behavioural change approach is more preventive. But if you think of the three types of prevention discussed in Chapter 4 – primary, secondary and tertiary – then the distinction becomes less clear. Primary prevention (which aims to prevent disorders before they occur) would probably require the techniques of directive counselling to help change behaviour such as smoking. Secondary prevention (which aims to limit the course of an illness or reduce the risk of occurrence) could involve both directive and non-directive counselling techniques. For instance, someone who has just discovered they have diabetes could perhaps benefit from non-directive counselling to help them come to terms with the life-long implications of the condition, but also may need help in changing those aspects of their behaviour which exacerbate the condition.

Non-directive counselling is probably more appropriate in relation to tertiary prevention. The aim is to relieve the symptoms, reduce the burden of disability and achieve optimal health in the circumstances – in other words, to help people to be healthy in spite of chronic illness or disability. For instance, a woman who has had her breast removed due to cancer could benefit from counselling in a non-directive way not only to come to terms with the cancer but also with the threat to her self-image.

As you read through the following accounts where a health professional is engaged in a form of counselling, make a note of how you think the counselling is health promoting and whether you think it is directive or non-directive.

A Well Woman Clinic doctor

When Dr Jenkins decided to do a couple of sessions a week at the Well Woman Clinic she thought she would spend most of her time doing cervical smear tests or dealing with vaginal thrush. In fact what she found herself doing most was what she describes as counselling. Much of this revolves around pre-menstrual tension and menopausal problems. She has felt quite weighed down with some of the complex situations which she has encountered. Take Jenny Burton who came in last week. She looked a cheerful well preserved 52 year old when she walked through the door. Within ten minutes she dissolved in tears saying that she had lost all her self-confidence, was anxious about everything, was sleeping badly had no energy and little interest in life, especially her sex life which was causing some friction between her and her husband. She wondered if Hormone Replacement Therapy (HRT) would help. Dr Jenkins carefully explained to her the pros and cons of HRT, how it was most effective in preventing osteoporosis and also it should stop the hot flushes and night sweats. This might help Jenny's sleeping problems but on further probing Jenny revealed other anxieties. Her husband had been made redundant in the last six months and so was at home all day and was himself very depressed. It was vital for their financial situation that she kept her part-time job as a secretary in a solicitors' office. But they had just changed all their filing system onto computers and she was struggling to keep up, feeling that she would dearly love to be made redundant and a bit resentful at her husband for moping about the house all day. Dr Jenkins suggested that maybe Mr Burton should seek help and got Jenny to think through what may be her options at work. Could she take on more of a receptionist role or should she grasp the nettle and do a training course? Meantime she gave her the reference for two books, one on HRT and the other on 'natural' remedies for the symptoms of the menopause. Jenny would think through her various options and come back in a months time.

A practice nurse

It is practice policy in Heath Road surgery that every new patient should have an initial assessment interview with Gill the practice nurse. Gill uses a computer to feed in the details of these new patients. As well as weight, blood pressure and other physical features, Gill records aspects of the person's lifestyle, for example their average weekly alcohol intake, whether they smoke etc. The computer performs a risk analysis and prints out advice on how to improve or maintain health.

Gary had recently moved into the area and was quite surprised and a little bit annoyed when he went to register as a new patient and was ushered into a room for an interview with the practice nurse. He was in his early twenties and didn't think he needed a health check at his age. He didn't smoke but enjoyed a few beers in the pub, mainly at the weekends. When she started to ask about his diet he felt a bit defensive. His mother was always telling him that he ate too much take-away food and wasn't getting a balanced diet. When Gill started to probe about his eating habits he found himself telling her that since he'd broken up with his girlfriend he hadn't felt like making the effort to cook for himself, there didn't seem to be much point in cooking and eating on your own, and anyway he hated shopping. His girlfriend had always done that and he didn't feel like going round the shops after work. Gill enquired about his cooking and storage facilities and he revealed that he only had two gas rings in his new flat and no fridge. He said that he kept meaning to buy a fridge and his mother had offered to buy him a microwave but he hadn't taken up her offer. Gill suggested that he get a fridge with quite a large freezing compartment which would allow him to shop less often and he agreed to explore microwave cooking. He confessed to Gill that the breakup with his girlfriend had hit him more than he had bargained for but the fact that he had moved into a new area gave him the ideal opportunity to reappraise his way of life.

In the first case Dr Jenkins gave emotional support to Jenny and helped her to explore some choices that she might take. She was also providing information about the prevention of osteoporosis but she was generally non-directive in her approach. The practice nurse was giving more direct guidance to Gary about his eating habits and exploring ways of improving them. However she did create a climate in which Gary was prepared to express his feelings to her and so in a more non-directive way allowed him to re-assess his situation. They were both health promoting in very specific ways in reducing the risk of osteoporosis in the case of Jenny and improving Gary's nutrition, but they were also health promoting in a wider sense of attempting to improve emotional well-being. Neither of the health professionals were specially trained in counselling. These encounters were regular parts of their jobs. But there are trained counsellors working in the health field who have a specialist role and part of that role is health promotion.

Specialist counselling in relation to health

Jot down or make a mental note of the types of specialist counselling that you have encountered which relate to health.

A recent text on counselling and health (Davis and Fallowfield, 1991) included: counselling for diabetes, counselling in renal failure, counselling for disfigurement, counselling in head injury, counselling for spinal cord injured people, counselling people with multiple sclerosis, infertility counselling, pain counselling, genetic counselling, counselling patients with cancer and counselling in heart disease. Others which spring to mind are grief counselling, alcohol counselling, HIV and AIDS counselling, stoma counselling, counselling for incontinence, stress counselling and relationship counselling.

In exploring specialist counselling we will take multiple sclerosis as an example.

Counselling for multiple sclerosis (MS)

There is no known cause or cure for MS and a diagnosis may take years to confirm. MS affects people in very random and unpredictable ways. Some people have it for over 30 years with sometimes quite long relapses, and some deteriorate rapidly and die within ten years. It is characterised, therefore, with a great deal of uncertainty. Temporary or permanent symptoms include fatigue, pain, mobility problems, speech or swallowing problems, clumsiness, loss of sexual responses, disturbance of vision and other sensory problems. Those affected are likely to need a great deal of support at all stages of the disease.

Communicating 'bad news' is always difficult. With MS this difficulty is compounded by the uncertain trajectory of the disease and with the unpredictability of its course. Diagnosis can be a devastating blow and brings many fears and dilemmas. Julia Segal of the ARMS Research Unit (1991:147-61) says that counselling someone with MS requires the giving of emotional support in what can be very distressing circumstances. Health professionals who may be involved in other ways, say as a physiotherapist or doctor, may not be the best person to give this kind of support for two reasons. One is that the depth of emotion which may be revealed can make it hard to maintain the more ordinary therapeutic relationship. And the other is that the health professional who does not have specialist counselling expertise may not be able to cope with the emotions that it could evoke in themselves. This raises the question of whether the health professional *should* be able to cope and what kind of help they need in order to enable them to cope. Segal claims that professional counsellors 'choose and are trained to work with emotions. Their experience, their work setting, their personal supervision and their closely defined task may enable them to work in considerable depth with some of the problems'. Other health professionals, however, are likely to have the opportunity to provide emotional support as they work with a person with MS. A weekly session at a hydrotherapy pool with a physiotherapist provides the ideal opportunity to build up a relationship of trust with someone and may be the person to whom the person with MS will turn. Similarly, an occupational therapist assessing the needs of the person in their own home may find themselves in a counselling role. Clearly they need some of the basic skills of counselling as well as being sympathetic and understanding. They also need to be able to recognise when more emotional support is needed than they can be expected to give and to whom they can refer.

> **How might this type of counselling (which would apply to many other chronic illnesses) be health promoting?**

If we are operating with a wider view of health than just a biomedical one, then helping someone to live with their chronic illness and to relieve some of the anxieties and emotional pain which they may be suffering is in fact a form of tertiary prevention discussed earlier.

Most of the examples discussed so far have been concerned with helping people to make choices which would be health enhancing or which are supportive. Another form of counselling is that which is concerned with personal development.

Personal counselling for health

This type of counselling has emerged from within the context of mental health and the casework method in social work. The focus is on biographical techniques to help people to reflect on their circumstances and review their present dilemmas in the light of their past. A process of self-reflection is set in motion on the scope for personal choice and change, learning from past mistakes and building on positive experiences. The aim is to build self-confidence and improve decision-making skills. An example of this method is the life-skills programme aimed at young people, where it is hoped that they will be enabled to resist unwanted social pressures (Hopson and Scally, 1980).

This non-directive, empowering strand within counselling for health does have some dissenting voices. Beattie (1991) has reviewed a range of criticisms. He draws attention to 'the covert invasion of the private domain' and the 'surveillance of intimate biography' which he sees as a potential infringement of personal rights. Grief counselling is an example which some people find extremely helpful in supporting them through a difficult bereavement, yet to others the idea is anathema. The idea of 'sharing' one's innermost feelings with someone trained to listen can be unacceptable to some people who firmly decline any offers of that kind of help. Some people feel that these are very private feelings or feelings that they would only share with someone close. Some go so far as to express fears of a professionalisation of friendship, neighbourliness or kinship relationships which could have the effect of undervaluing and de-skilling those personal relationships. However grief counsellors would counter that it is precisely because of a lack of those personal relationships that their services are sometimes needed. Family and friends may find it difficult to offer the support needed because they too are involved, whereas counsellors do not have this role conflict.

Part of the problem is the emphasis on self-conscious verbalisation and self-disclosure that lies at the heart of personal counselling for health. As Beattie notes, these are middle-class values and attributes which may be unacceptable to working-class people or to people with different cultural norms. This complaint made by one bereaved person illustrates the point well:

> Many of these counsellors just won't accept that denial can be healthy, that not everyone wants to talk. They don't take into account the cultural background of the people they're dealing with – we Scots are not very forthcoming.
>
> (Bedell, 1991)

There is nothing more frustrating than going to one's family doctor for something very specific only to be treated to invitations to open up and reveal what is 'really' troubling you, like this young woman:

> I went to my GP to change my pill because I thought that it was making me put on weight. I just wanted to try another brand but I was asked

about my sex life, about my self-image, did I see myself as a thin person, why was it important to me to be thin. I thought they were busy. Whenever you do want to talk you always get the one who reaches for their prescription pad as soon as you walk into the room.

(Anon., 1995)

Another criticism of the personal counselling for health approach is that whilst it may be health enhancing in that it aims to help people to learn to cope, it is also encouraging people to be 'self-policing' (Nettleton and Bunton, 1995), to accept their situation, which might be more comfortable for others. However, to counter this, it could be said that improving someone's self-confidence and self-esteem increases the self-determination of people so that they feel better equipped to challenge and change their circumstances. In fact many of the criticisms noted above, it could be argued, are due to irresponsible or inexpert use of counselling techniques. Counselling is based on a range of different theoretical perspectives. Understanding these perspectives can help to clarify the use of counselling techniques to promote health.

9.3 Theoretical perspectives

There are broadly three theoretical perspectives on the types of counselling which we have discussed so far: the psychodynamic, the problem-solving and the person-centred. There are many nuances within these three approaches and counselling does not always espouse one or other approach but may be more eclectic in its methods. These theoretical stances are described only briefly here, but those of you who would like to explore this further should read Dryden (1986).

Psychoanalytic approaches

The founding father of psychoanalysis was Freud but many others have refined and adapted this approach, including Jung, Adler, Klein and, more recently, Bowlby and Winnicott. Although not a unitary movement, the broad central idea is that the past influences the present and that present personal crises result from unresolved developmental conflicts. For instance, if someone has a weight problem, this may well have its origins in early childhood experiences. In order for that person either to be able to come to terms with their weight and feel happy as they are or to set about trying to change their eating habits, he or she needs to understand where the problem originates. Three distinctive features of the psychoanalytical approach have been identified:

1 An assumption that the client's difficulties have their ultimate origins in childhood experiences.

2 An assumption that the client may not be consciously aware of the true motives or impulses behind his or her actions.

3 The use in counselling and therapy of techniques such as dream analysis, interpretation and transference.

(McLeod, 1993: 23)

Perhaps the most important influence of Freud has been his development of the notion of the 'unconscious'. It is not merely the impact of childhood experiences on the present which is at issue. It is the belief that many of these experiences have been repressed and exert their influence on the present through the unconscious mind which is not within the person's direct awareness. Counsellors working within this tradition need to find ways of getting 'beneath the surface' if they are to provide appropriate support and help.

What do you think might be some of the advantages and drawbacks of this type of counselling?

It does provide a framework for increasing the person's self-awareness and for bringing to the surface feelings which have been repressed. But it is an approach which has developed within western culture and may not be appropriate for those who have other cultural traditions. Another criticism of the psychoanalytic approach is that it can leave people with a better understanding of the roots of their problems but no mechanism to change or move on from that position (McLeod, 1993). The problem-solving approach described next is more concerned with the here and now.

A problem-solving approach

Gerard Egan (1982) developed a problem-solving approach, described in Woolfe (1996), which incorporates three stages:

1 The present scenario.

2 The preferred scenario.

3 Getting there.

At the first stage the problem is clarified. Taking again the example of a person with a weight problem, this would be the stage when the person acknowledges that they are overweight. If he or she is unhappy about this then the person would be encouraged to tell his or her story and to acknowledge and confront any blind spots. It also involves the search for what Egan calls 'leverage', which he defines as helping clients to 'identify and work on problems, issues, concerns or opportunities that will make a difference' to their situation. This may involve cutting out snacks or taking more exercise by walking to work.

The second stage involves helping the client to develop a preferred scenario by working out what a better future might look like. This might be a future in which the person was a stone lighter. Having done this the client needs help in translating preferred scenarios into a concrete strategy. This involves setting goals and objectives for making the preferred future a reality. Certain incentives may need to be identified to help clients commit themselves to the objectives set.

The last stage involves developing a strategy for getting there – working out how to achieve the set goals. Egan suggests brainstorming the range of possible strategies and focusing on a particular strategy which is most suitable given the client's personal, emotional and social resources. A brainstorm of strategies for losing weight might include cutting out fatty foods, drinking black and sugar-free coffee and tea, taking up jogging or joining a weight-watchers group. Finally the strategy chosen has to be turned into a step-by-step procedure for action.

Person-centred, non-directive counselling

This type of counselling is sometimes known as Rogerian after Carl Rogers who initially developed this approach. It is very much in the 'humanistic psychology' tradition which takes a very optimistic view of human nature and potential. Person-centred counselling aims to help the client 'to become what he/she is capable of becoming'. In terms of someone who is overweight, this would either be to feel confident as a large person or to have the confidence to tackle the weight problem. As the term 'person-centred' implies, the emphasis is on the client's ability to find solutions to their own problems with the counsellor acting as a source of reflection and encouragement. Thus it is non-directive. The formation of a relationship is central to person-centred therapy. The characteristics of this therapeutic relationship were set out by Rogers as necessary and sufficient conditions for this relationship to take place. McLeod summarises them:

1 Two persons are in psychological contact.
2 The first, whom we shall term the client, is in a state of incongruence, being vulnerable and anxious.
3 The second person, whom we shall term the therapist, is congruent or integrated in the relationship.
4 The therapist experiences unconditional positive regard for the client.
5 The therapist experiences an empathic understanding of the client's internal frame of reference, and endeavours to communicate this to the client.
6 The communication to the client of the therapist's empathic under-standing and unconditional regard is to a minimal extent achieved.

(McLeod, 1993: 70)

These six conditions set up an interpersonal environment in which actualisation and growth can take place. There are three essential ingredients to person-centred counselling; these are: empathy, unconditional positive regard and genuineness. Although the approaches discussed so far have developed within a therapeutic tradition, their importance for health promotion is the emphasis which is put on developing good relationships.

The essential ingredients of a good relationship are identified as follows:

Empathy

Empathy is the ability to see the world from the point of view of another person, through their frame of reference, through their conceptual and emotional spectacles, so to speak. It is not to *be* that person, for that is impossible, but to be 'as if' one was that person and to imagine how it feels to be them. The 'as if' quality should be emphasised. Without this quality, empathy becomes sympathy. Sympathy involves collusion with the other person, taking sides and becoming judgmental. In contrast, empathy involves being detached and dispassionate and remaining non-judgmental and non-evaluative.

Empathy is expressed or communicated by a number of skills; a key skill is reflecting back the emotional content of the message from clients in one's own words. This enables the clients to feel that their message has been understood. In this and similar ways, a working relationship based on trust is gradually built up between counsellor and client.

Unconditional positive regard

This is sometimes referred to as 'warmth' or 'acceptance' and involves a non-judgmental acceptance of clients for what they are, 'warts and all'. People often seek help because they feel bad or unworthy and the very act of asking for help may be seen as an admittance of weakness or failure. If the counsellor is able to convey a sense of warmth and acceptance (to prize the other person) it becomes easier for them to re-evaluate their own worth and to love and prize themselves. This offers the prospect for change. Perhaps the key skill here is to differentiate between the *person* and the *behaviour*. Only by feeling accepted will clients feel safe enough to explore the emotional issues which brought them to a counsellor in the first place ...

Genuineness

Sometimes known as congruence or authenticity, this condition refers to counsellors being honest with themselves about their own feelings and being open in communicating these feelings to clients. The counsellor who is able to be genuine or congruent provides a model for the client and thus facilitates both the development of the relationship and the latter's willingness to take risks in exposing painful or hidden parts of self.

(Woolfe, 1996: 109–10)

Do you see any contradictions or potential difficulties in achieving these qualities?

We tend to associate the attributes of empathy, positive regard and genuineness with spontaneity and naturalness. They are the attributes of someone who cares about another not because it is their job or they are being paid to do so. The idea of learning these attributes and contriving to feel them seems contradictory. Is it possible to feel empathy and positive regard for everyone? If we are able, does this then devalue these feelings? If we manage to convey these feelings regardless of how we actually feel then is there not something inherently hypocritical in that situation?

The term 'emotional labour' has been used to describe the work typically carried out by those who service and care for others. It involves 'formal and ritualised intimacy which is not natural but socially constructed' (Jones, 1994: 466). It was applied by Hochschild (1983) in a study of US airline staff who were well trained in presenting a highly positive emotional atmosphere. The term gives rise to a certain amount of unease because there is an implication that the emotions are managed in order to control the 'other' and avoid conflict. If you look closely at the definitions of 'empathy', genuineness and positive regard given in the quotation from Woolfe you will see that empathy is defined as 'the ability to see the world from the point of view of another person'. Unconditional positive regard is an acceptance of people as they are in a non-judgemental way. To empathise is to try to imagine what it is like to be the other person and to experience his/her world. It is to set aside one's own perspective and to try to think the way the other person thinks. In this way one can avoid making judgements about the other person's situation which are based on one's own views. Of course it is never completely possible to stand in someone else's shoes or exactly experience the world as they do. But it is important to try so that assumptions are not made about what other people think and feel. A good example of where this is particularly important is in understanding cultural difference. It is important to find out the beliefs and customs of people from different faiths and cultures if their perspective is to be understood. Empathy can help to do this by resisting the temptation to interpret the other person's world in terms of our own beliefs and habits. Counsellors also have to confront their own biases if they are to achieve genuineness. The difficulties involved in doing so should not be underestimated as counsellors are not immune from holding deep-seated prejudices, or in the case of health promotion, feeling very strongly about certain behaviours such as alcohol abuse or smoking. The important point is to be able to accept the person even if the behaviour is hard to accept.

9.4 Counselling and supporting skills for promoting health and facilitating change

The Counselling and Career Development Unit (CCDU) at Leeds University categorised the skills of counselling into three groups:

1 Relationship-building skills.
2 Exploring and clarifying skills.
3 Action skills.

Relationship-building skills

Building a relationship based on trust and equality is perhaps the most important skill involved in promoting health. Fundamental to the building of such relationships are the qualities of empathy, genuiness and positive regard which were discussed on p. 143. They involve the ability to understand the other's predicament and point of view without pre-judging the situation. In order to do that it is necessary to clear a space and offer one's full attention so that all aspects of the other person can be absorbed. Clearing a space is not just in the physical environment or in a busy schedule; it is about clearing a space in one's head so that one can listen without the 'distraction' of preconceived ideas or competing issues. The establishment of a good relationship is fundamental to all other counselling skills.

Exploring and clarifying skills

The skills of communication which were discussed in the previous chapter are basic to the skills of exploring and clarifying, particularly the ability to listen. The counsellor aims to explore the clients understanding and feelings, to consider the available options and to examine alternatives. Counsellors tend to use open questions to explore understandings and feelings but they try to get the client to define their problems in a concrete manner using specific examples. They will clarify their understanding with the client to ensure that the facts are as they seem and that half-formed ideas and hidden factors can be identified. Paraphrasing and reflecting back to the client what he or she is saying shows that the counsellor has understood the information that is being given. On occasions a counsellor may need to confront a client, pointing out contradictions which the client may be displaying, or sensitively challenging certain assumptions which the client may hold. The degree to which this can be done will depend on the trust which has been built up in the relationship.

Action skills

The final set of skills are action skills, getting the person to take action which they have decided upon. Often it is useful to set up small actions which can be reviewed at each session and which cumulatively will move the person towards more ambitious actions. The counsellor will help the client to set objectives and form action plans, working out a strategy for carrying out those plans. This will probably need some support from the counsellor.

Facilitating change

So far we have been mainly considering the type of counselling which carefully avoids telling people what to do and which is more concerned with building relationships which enhance the emotional well-being of the individual. But many health promoters and health professionals are being urged to work towards Saving Lives: Our Healthier Nation targets.

Think back to Part 1 where the Saving Lives: Our Healthier Nation targets were introduced. Which type of counselling is appropriate to achieving these targets?

These targets are concerned with disease reduction and prevention, with cutting down the rates of cancers, coronary heart disease and stroke, accidents and mental illness, and other preventable diseases. One of the ways they aim to do so is by getting people to change their unhealthy behaviours for healthy ones. Health professionals are urged at every opportunity to counsel their clients to adopt healthier lifestyles such as taking up exercise or eating less fatty foods. This type of counselling is much more directive as it is trying to advise individuals to change their behaviour. Achieving a reduction in alcohol consumption is a prime target.

Alcohol counselling

Alcohol counselling is more directive and has the specific aim of changing what is considered harmful behaviour. The individual has to make the choice to change but the counsellor gives specific advice on the changes necessary to engage in health promoting rather than health damaging behaviour. Support is forthcoming from the counsellor if the changes or attempts to change are made but without that commitment the counselling relationship will be terminated.

There is a good deal of debate in the alcohol counselling field as to the appropriate use and timing of counselling. A model of behavioural change which is applicable to all addictive behaviours has been very influential in alcohol counselling: that is the Prochaska and DiClemente motivation to change model (1984). The authors describe their model as three dimensional. It integrates changes, processes and levels of change and is made up of four stages of willingness to change:

- *Pre-contemplation.* At this stage the individual is not aware of his or her dependency. This could be due to ambivalence, denial, or selective exposure to information. When the individual becomes aware of a problem, he or she progresses to the next phase.

- *Contemplation.* At this stage the individual admits that something is wrong and starts to think seriously about change. This may last for a few weeks or several years. Some people may never progress past this stage.

- *Action.* A commitment is made to alter the problematic behaviour. This is a much shorter stage; when the decision has been made, the individual progresses to the next phase in the change process.

- *Maintenance.* The new behaviour is strengthened and develops into self-efficiency. The client's feeling of being in control is then maximised. Eventually the exit point to termination of the problem cycle is reached.

(Cooper, 1994: 70)

Individuals do not progress in a linear fashion but in a more cyclical way as indicated in Figure 9.1.

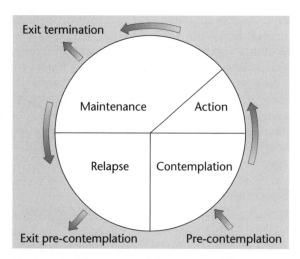

Figure 9.1   **The stages of change model**
(adapted from Prochaska and DiClemente, 1984)

The pre-contemplation stage

One of the main problems in counselling someone to drink less alcohol is to get them to acknowledge that they are drinking too much. People can be very defensive about their drinking habits, and asking people direct questions about their alcohol consumption can be construed as an invasion of privacy (Fennell and Sidell, 1988). However, the Health and Lifestyles survey carried out by the HEA (1995b) reported that a high proportion of people trusted their GP's advice and GPs are probably most likely to be able to inquire about drinking levels when someone comes to surgery for a consultation. If you think back to the practice nurse vignette, many general practices have some mechanism for a health check which usually includes an assessment of drinking behaviour in a non-threatening way. If someone's alcohol consumption is above safe limits for their age, sex, size etc., then this can prompt a discussion about what is a safe limit for them. Providing literature on the subject of safe limits can be helpful as well as giving some guidance on how to cut down. Of course not everyone will be scrupulously honest about their alcohol consumption. This may be because they are aware that it is above limits but are not willing or able to change. It is the degree of willingness to change that is central to the likelihood that someone who is a heavy or dependent drinker will achieve a significant and lasting reduction in their alcohol consumption. Even when such a person does express a willingness to change they are likely to need a lot of help and support in doing so.

The contemplation stage

Specialist alcohol counselling is appropriate at the contemplation stage when there is an awareness by the client that they have a drink problem. They may not have decided to take action but may be seeking information and help with their problem. They may be ready to talk but there may be many barriers to taking action. Gauging their readiness to move from contemplation to action is one of the challenges of counselling. In order to do this the counsellor needs to explore the drink problem thoroughly and recognise that it is likely to be a multi-level problem with related aspects, such as housing, employment and relationships. Counsellors will need to work through the transition stage of contemplation to reach a commitment to change and then help the client to make a plan of action. Together the drinker and counsellor will need to work out ways in which the change can be achieved. They will have to discuss what form the change will take, i.e. a decrease in volume of alcohol or a complete cessation of drinking, who else might be involved or implicated (i.e. partners or friends), and when this change should take place (i.e. the time-scale of change).

The action and maintenance stages

Goal setting and the reviewing of these goals will form much of the subsequent counselling input. However, the counsellor will also need to decide on a treatment plan from a range of possible therapeutic interventions if this is appropriate. Because for many people the maintaining of this changed behaviour is fraught with difficulty, and relapse is always possible, the counselling support is likely to be needed for some time. It is acknowledged that for many who are attempting to alter addictive behaviour relapse is common. This is not considered failure. The relapser can re-enter the change process as a contemplator or may exit back to the pre-contemplation stage.

The stages of change model has been well accepted in health promotion and was the basis for the HEA's course *Helping People Change* (Price and Pry, 1995). However, the Prochaska and DiClemente model is mainly descriptive and does not tell us how or why a person moves from one stage to another. It has also been critisised for presenting a too smooth and unidirectional process of change, whereas change is often much more fluctuating and unpredictable (Bunton *et al.*, 1999).

Helping people to change their behaviour is not just a matter of adopting the right counselling technique and learning the specific skills. Behaviour is firmly rooted in the psychological make-up and located in social and cultural environments. Whether we should try to change people's behaviour in the name of health is an ethical issue, especially if the circumstances of their lives make this difficult. This has already been discussed in Part 1 of this book. Here we are concerned with how to improve the chances of getting people to change their behaviour through counselling, and this entails understanding something of the complex psychological processes involved as well as the socio-economic and cultural context in which the behaviour takes place. Four possible theoretical perspectives have been identified (Naidoo and Wills, 1994; Bennett and Hodgson 1992) which might be of use in counselling aimed at changing behaviour. One of these we have already met – the Stages of Change Model of Prochaska and DiClemente (1984). This model focuses more on the processes of change and the support that people might need to work through that change. The other three, the Health Belief Model (Becker, 1974), the theory of Reasoned Action (Ajzen and Fishbein, 1980) and the Health Action Model (Tones, 1988), are more concerned with the psychological determinants of behaviour change.

All of these psychological models employ certain key terms, such as attitudes, beliefs, values and drives, which need to be understood. Ribeaux and Poppleton (1978) have defined an attitude as a 'learned predisposition to think, feel and act in a particular way towards a given object or class of objects'. There are then three components which make up an attitude: the cognitive, the affective and the behavioural. The cognitive component is made up of a person's knowledge and information, and is the belief aspect. People's beliefs vary enormously and are influenced by religion, culture, class, family background, peer group and education. A person's beliefs may not be in agreement with certain facts or what the majority of people believe but they are the individual's own evaluation of the object or situation. The affective component of attitudes is concerned with emotions, feelings and preferences, and the behavioural aspect – what people actually do – is also determined to some extent by what they *can* do, i.e. the skills they have at their disposal and the circumstances with which they have to contend.

Attitudes are notoriously difficult to change but, theoretically, changing any one of the three components will affect an attitude. For instance providing information which is counter to a person's beliefs may change their attitude to something.

Improving skills can also influence behaviour. A young man may live on take-away junk food because he doesn't know how to cook. Teaching him to cook might change his eating habits but if he really likes junk food and has a distinct preference for it then he may choose to persist in this eating pattern.

Other aspects of behaviour are values and drives. Values are made up of those things which a person cares about and will be influenced by culture, religion, family or peers. We talk of family values which put a strong premium on the institution of the family. Then there are market values which put an economic price on everything. A person may value independence, resilience or flexibility. Drives are the basic instincts we are born with to carry out certain activities necessary for survival. Our perception of hunger and thirst drives us to eat and drink. In general they are thought to be more powerful than attitudes and beliefs as motivating forces for behaviour but there are people in certain situations, for instance hunger strikers, who refuse to eat because of a certain belief. Theoretical models of behavioural change are an attempt to look at the complex interactions of beliefs, attitudes, motives and values in order to understand why people behave as they do and how, if desirable, this might be susceptible to change.

The Health Belief Model (Becker, 1974) suggests that behaviours depend to a great extent on how the person appraises the situation. The individual weighs up the consequences of a particular action in relation to health, taking account of the gains and possible losses that might result from adopting a particular behaviour. This model could explain why parents decide to have their children vaccinated against measles, mumps and rubella. Most people believe that the benefits of vaccination in preventing those diseases far outweigh any slight risk of an adverse reaction. Similarly, it can explain why there was a marked drop in take up of whooping cough vaccine when it was suggested that the vaccine could be as dangerous as the disease. It seems that people were acting rationally. But some would argue that one of the problems with the Health Belief Model is that it assumes a high degree of rationality with people acting like accountants and weighing up the pros and cons of their actions and then modifying their behaviour accordingly. People do not necessarily react in this way and one important intervening variable is the degree to which the individual believes he or she is susceptible to the threat of disease or ill health. 'It won't happen to someone like me' is a common if not entirely rational perception. In the Health Belief Model it is suggested that 'cues' can shock someone out of that complacency.

Take sun bathing behaviour. A woman in her early twenties may persist in baking her body to a golden brown each year in spite of a great deal of evidence which connects sunbathing to skin cancer. She doesn't know much about skin cancer and thinks that it is something that only happens to old people. She also thinks that it is only red-headed people who are susceptible to burning. However, if someone who worked with her had a malignant mole removed from her back which was attributed to too much sun burn, she might begin to think seriously about the messages which make the link between cancer and sun bathing. If that person was a woman in her early thirties who had dark hair and so was not in the category which she regarded as being at risk, this might act as a cue to make her reappraise her views.

The Health Belief Model, however, fails to take account of the influence of family, friends or other role models. The Theory of Reasoned Action (Ajzen and Fishbein, 1980), like the Health Belief Model, is concerned with how people decide to behave in a certain way. But Ajzen and Fishbein put a great deal of emphasis on the influence of significant others. These significant others may be people close, either family or peers, or they may be someone who is looked up to or valued. This might be a celebrity, rock musician or footballer. In this model the urge to conform or be like someone who is valued will influence behaviour. This model has influenced campaigns which use appropriate celebrities to put forward certain health education messages. It is also at the heart of peer health counselling and the use of teenage magazines to convey health messages.

Whether it is 'cues' or significant others who exert an influence, both models place a great deal of faith in the rationality of human behaviour. Certain behaviours, particularly sexual behaviour or addictive behaviours, are not overly reasonable. The pursuit of pleasure and short-term gratification can seem much more attractive than rather vague and longer-term benefits such as 'good health'. The Health Action Model (Tones, 1988) tries to take account of strong motivating forces such as hunger, pain, pleasure or sex in understanding the reasons why people act in certain ways. You will also see from Figure 9.2 that three general systems influence behaviour. The motivation system, the belief system as in the Health Belief Model, is the cognitive element and the normative system which represents the influence of social pressures on behaviour, such as conforming to peer group norms.

The model also emphasises self-concept and self-esteem as important factors which have great significance for health education. It is very much in tune with the non-directive counselling approach which aims to help people understand their predicament and clarify the choices available to the individual in order that he or she can make decisions.

These models serve to alert us to the complexity of people's behaviour and to the difficulty of getting people to change deeply rooted habits. But it always has to be remembered that people's health behaviour is dependent to a large extent on the conditions of their lives, which for many people are outside their control. The work of Roisin Pill (1990: 63-79) with working class women in South Wales discussed in Chapter 3 indicates that although it may be relatively easy to influence attitudes it is very difficult to sustain any behavioural change in the face of adverse social circumstances and the demands of family priorities.

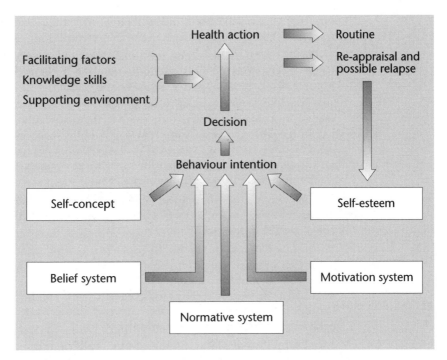

Figure 9.2 **The Health Action Model** (Tones, 1995)

A woman, whose alcohol consumption had reached dangerous levels since her husband had left her, was referred by her GP to an alcohol treatment centre. She made this heartfelt plea:

> What can you do? I'm stuck here on my own in this god forsaken place and I can't afford to move. All I got was, I mean, I know it's basically you that's got to do it, but when you keep getting thrown at you, change your life, change your lifestyle, and you think, well how?
>
> (Fennell and Sidell, 1989: 146)

On the other hand the knowledge that one's behaviour and lifestyle are adversely affecting one's health and that one may have certain choices can be very liberating. Another man in the study of a community alcohol treatment centre referred to above found that the possibility that his harmful drinking behaviour was a matter of choice and change was within his control was a most helpful insight.

> That was magical, no one has said that to me before. From then on I felt on top, you know, I felt that whatever problems I'd got were inside here, and you're the man, you're the man, you can sort them out eventually. But if you talk of the 'demon drink' or whatever, it is something outside yourself – you're not free to influence it.
>
> (Fennell and Sidell, 1989: 143)

Evidence from people who have changed their behaviour indicates that there are certain minimum conditions necessary for change to take place. Naidoo and Wills (1994) have summarised these six conditions:

1 The change must be self-initiated. People will only change if they want to. 'Telling people what to do' will not work.

2 The behaviour must be salient. For a change in behaviour to occur the harmful behaviour must be called into question by some other event in their life so that the advice is timely and relevant.

3 The salience of the behaviour must appear over a period of time. The old harmful behaviour has to be difficult to maintain and the new one has to become part of everyday life. For instance, working in a no-smoking office will make it hard to maintain a smoking habit. Giving up smoking will enable the person to sit in any compartment of a train and go to the theatre or cinema without longing for a cigarette.

4 The behaviour is not part of the individual's coping strategy. Sources of comfort and solace, even if we are convinced of their potential harm, are difficult to resist.

5 The individual's life should not be problematic or uncertain. There is a limit to a person's ability to adapt and change. Someone who has just gone through a difficult divorce, or who has been made redundant, or who is coping single handed with children on a low income will have enough to cope with and changes in their health behaviour will have a very low priority.

6 Social support is available. Changing one's behaviour can be stressful and people need the support of family and friends. Specialist counsellors, such as alcohol counsellors, often provide social support to their clients who are trying to change their harmful drinking behaviour.

9.5 Conclusion

Counselling skills have a place in the promotion of health particularly in helping to facilitate health-enhancing relationships which increase self-esteem and improve self-concept. This is especially important in helping individuals to cope with a particular crisis or problem in their lives or to change a particular type of behaviour which is damaging. Counselling skills are appropriate mainly at the one-to-one level, which is only one aspect of the health promotion endeavour. Many would say that within health promotion there has been too much emphasis on looking inside individuals to find both the roots of and the solutions to their predicament. Perhaps more emphasis should be put on enabling individuals, groups and communities to examine their social, economic and political environment and, if necessary, empowering them to try to change this wider environment. In order to do this they need information about health and an understanding of the impact of the wider environment on their health. Health education, which is the subject of the next chapter, is the mechanism for communicating this information both to individuals and communities.

Chapter 10
Educating for health

10.1 Introduction

Health education is a form of communication which aims to give people the knowledge and skills needed to make choices about their health. This might aim to encourage them to change their own behaviour or to change the wider environment. Health education has been around for much longer than health promotion and has had a chequered history with many lessons having been learnt. The traditional approach of giving advice or providing information through leaflets, lectures or posters is a form of one-way communication where the health educator conveys a message. Current health education practice would avoid the 'telling people what to do to become healthy' approach in favour of self-empowerment which aims to increase the person's autonomy. This approach requires a more two-way form of communication where a dialogue is set up between the health educator and his or her audience.

In this chapter the roots of health education, which can be found in nineteenth century concerns for fitness and hygiene, will be traced as a preliminary to examining the evolution of health education strategies and methods. How these have developed within schools and adult education will contextualise the many themes and issues which emerge.

10.2 The origins of health education

Many would date the origins of health education from the time of the cholera epidemics of the early nineteenth century when handbills aimed at the public at large advised on safeguards against contagion. Blythe (1986) maintains that the main motivating force for nineteenth century attempts to educate the public about health was a combination of fear and philanthropy. Fear was generated around the time of cholera because epidemics were no respecter of class. Later the deterioration of the labouring classes became a cause for concern when three out of every five volunteers for the Boer War were declared unfit for service. It is also claimed that the Temperance Movement had a health educating role. Drunkenness was clearly a health hazard and caused a good deal of misery but the demonisation of drink alienated many who did not like the tactics of the Temperance Movements or share its religious zeal and saw much of this type of health education as blatant propaganda.

Apart from the Temperance Movement's obvious concern with drunkenness what and who do you think would be targeted by the early health educators?

A glance at the titles of some of the publications which came out in the mid-nineteenth century shows that most of the propaganda was directed at the working classes and much of it was concerned with cleanliness and sometimes diet. Typical was *Dirty Dustbins and Sloppy Streets* by H.P. Buenois, published in 1881, W. Bardwell's *Healthy Homes and How to Make Them*, which appeared in 1854 and *A Practical Dietary for Families, Schools and the Working Class* by Edward Smith in 1864. However Hillary Madeleine McBride (1983), in a review of some of this literature, also noted some which would not be out of place in current health promotion literature such as *The Cyclist's Guide to Health and Rational Enjoyment* published in 1886.

Campaigners such as Edwin Chadwick and Thomas Southwood Smith were concerned about the conditions under which the poor lived and worked. Edwin Chadwick's *Report on the Sanatory Conditions of the Labouring Population of England,* published in 1842, was very influential and persuaded the government to pass the 1848 Public Health Act. Jones (1992) notes that although philanthropic to a degree, Chadwick was also concerned with public morality which he equated with cleanliness:

> ...that the removal of noxious physical circumstances, and the promotion of civic, household, and personal cleanliness, are necessary to the improvement of the moral condition of the population; for that sound morality and refinement in manners and health are not long found co-existent with filthy habits amongst any class of the community.
>
> (Chadwick, 1842: 369-72)

It is however important to note that the propaganda coming from the philanthropic element was aimed not only at the poor themselves but also at landlords and the authorities. Just two years after Chadwick's publication, the Health of Towns Association was formed, spearheaded by Dr Southwood Smith. Within a few months fourteen towns belonged. Their stated aim was:

> To diffuse among the people the valuable information elicited by recent enquiries, and the advancement of science as to the physical and moral evils that result from the present defective sewerage, drainage, supply of water, air and light, and the construction of dwelling houses.
>
> (quoted in Frazer, 1950: 33)

Although concerned with the morals of the working class the early campaigners put the onus for the health and well-being of the working classes firmly on the living environment. The Health of Towns Association can be equated with the present day Healthy Cities Initiative described in Part 1. Many Acts were passed and this period marked a leap forward in public health. This goes beyond the scope of this chapter, but it has been well documented elsewhere (for instance R. Woods and J. Woodward

(1984) *Urban Disease and Mortality in Nineteenth Century England* and A. Wohl (1983) *Endangered Lives*).

Another important strand in the history of health education is the emergence of the health visitor which can also be traced to the mid-nineteenth century.

Nineteenth century health visitors

It was from the Ladies' Branch of The Manchester and Salford Sanitary Association, formed in 1852, that the first health visitors emerged. Their brand of health education was a blend of cleanliness and godliness with an emphasis on sanitary and temperance literature. They were closely linked to the Manchester City Mission and employed working-class mission women to deliver their message into the homes of the working-class people who were the target of their endeavours. These working-class mission women were to bridge the gap between the middle-class women of the Ladies' Branch and the 'feckless poor'. They were first known as sanitary visitors and later health visitors. They reported daily to the lady superintendents who were voluntary members of the Ladies' Branch.

> The lady superintendent from her larger knowledge, can direct the health visitor's work, help and encourage her in many ways, and assist her for her special duties... The health visitor is usually a superior woman of the class sought to be helped. She is in touch and sympathetic with the people she visits; she understands them, and they understand her. Each visitor lives in her own district, in a small cottage, or maybe a couple of rooms. She is easy of access at all times, and her home is naturally an object lesson in cleanliness, tidiness, etc., to the neighbours, who of course occupy exactly similar houses. She is regarded as a friend, and proves herself a true one over and over again.
>
> (quoted in Davies, 1988: 43–44)

Their duties were as follows:

> They must carry with them the carbolic powder, explain its use, and leave it where it is accepted; direct the attention of those they visit to the evils of bad smells, want of fresh air, impurities of all kinds; give hints to mothers on feeding and clothing their children – where they find sickness assist in promoting the comfort of the invalid by personal help, and report such cases to their superintendent. They must urge the importance of cleanliness, thrift, and temperance on all possible occasions. They are desired to get as many as possible to join the mothers' meetings of their districts, to use all their influence to induce those they visit to attend regularly at their respective places of worship, and to send their children to school.
>
> (quoted in Davies, 1988: 43)

Celia Davies has described these first health visitors as 'mothers' friends' and their work was seen as particularly important given the growing concern with infant and maternal mortality rates. Areas such as Birmingham, Warwickshire and Glasgow adopted similar schemes with the emphasis on making friends with families and especially mothers. It is interesting that all these schemes were keen to avoid setting up inspectoral work and recognised that if they were to have any influence at all then they had to build up a relationship with the working class mother. Only the Manchester scheme felt that it was important that the health visitor lived in the area in which she worked. But this model could be seen as an early example of community development work with the worker very much in touch with the local community. Another debate which surrounded the role of the health visitor still has resonance for health promotion today. An anonymous male sanitary inspector put it this way:

> It seems to me, Sir, the danger which threatens the public health service is that of looking at things out of perspective – magnifying a feeding bottle, and neglecting insanitary areas... Infants may be badly fed, but landlords still require forcibly reminding their properties must be put in order.
>
> (quoted in Davies, 1988: 50)

Can you think of another debate within health promotion introduced in Part 1 to which this relates?

It recognises the futility of 'blaming the victim' when it was the circumstances which warranted attention. Clearly there was room for both approaches and health visitors were the only people involved in regular one-to-one educational activities.

Health education around the turn of the century was still very much in the hands of voluntary bodies and there was clearly a need for some form of national co-ordinating body. Although the Ministry of Health was established in 1919, suggestions to form a Department of Health Propaganda at the Ministry were not taken up. Blythe (1986) suggests that a possible reason for this was that so much of health education fell foul of a number of vested interests, particularly the alcohol industry, which made governments wary of close involvement. It was the Society of Medical Officers of Health which set up the Central Council for Health Education (CCHE) in 1927. This was initially a committee of medical officers of health, representatives of local authority associations and health insurance committees.

The CCHE published a bi-monthly magazine, *Better Health*, which had a circulation of over a quarter of a million. But health education remained the largely unco-ordinated business of powerful voluntary bodies. The lack of research or feedback on the effects of the health education messages put out by this diverse range of agencies meant that health education advanced little between 1920 and 1940.

The war years

With the advent of the Second World War health education became a part of wartime contingency plans. The threat of epidemics and the possible increase in VD raised the stakes of the CCHE and it moved to a more central role (Welshman, 1997). Between 1940 and 1945 there were massive campaigns to promote diphtheria immunisation. In the space of five years this was very successful, with the percentage of children being brought for immunisation rising from 8 per cent to 62 per cent (Blythe, 1986).

During the Second World War, in response to the government's concern about national fitness and morals, the CCHE mounted a major campaign. This took the form of health talks and the distribution of nearly two million leaflets on four main themes: sex education, the prevention of venereal disease, infectious diseases, and maternal and child health, as well as some more general leaflets.

The messages in the leaflets were aimed mainly at women. As well as those specifically concerned with women's sexual and reproductive development and maternal health, most of the leaflets on infectious diseases were also aimed at women (Amos, 1993). For instance the *Death to Flies* leaflet states 'Housewives in town and country must therefore carry on a never ceasing war against flies' (quoted in Amos, 1993: 142). Those which were concerned with child care, although supposedly aimed at parents, invariably addressed women.

Many of the sex instruction leaflets and those on VD put great emphasis on women's responsibility, duty, self-control and self-sacrifice, making women responsible for male sexual activity:

> Women's Power: Girls know that they are both able to attract and to influence men, but they must always remember that the power of attraction carries with it the responsibility to use this influence in the right way. Many women easily arouse in men the desire for physical contacts and the expression of sex, although they may themselves remain calm and have no difficulty in keeping their self control ... a man whose desires have been excited without being satisfied may be driven to that type of women who merely gratifies the man's sex hunger which has been so unfairly aroused ... often they do give him venereal disease.
> (quoted in Amos, 1993: 143)

The main concern with the sex education leaflets was to direct women away from promiscuity and pre-marital sex into marriage and mother-hood. Sexual development and sexual pleasure were not addressed. Indeed, although most of the leaflets targeted women it was women as wives and mothers who were the focus, not women's own experiences, leaving many childless, lesbian and older women invisible.

The dominant method of health education used was health propaganda and instruction. Instruction on child care was provided by 'experts' on the assumption that women were at best ignorant and at worst lazy or indifferent to their child's welfare. Little or no acknowledgement of the social and economic conditions under which many children were reared was made.

The post war years

With the advent of the NHS there was a broadening of the issues covered by the publications. However, as Amos notes, the home remained the site of potential ill health although there was a perceptible shift from infectious disease prevention to the prevention of accidents. Doctors gave warnings to housewives to 'Be on guard against your children's burns and scalds' and to make sure that their children did not swallow mum's latest and most brightly coloured pills (*Deadly Danger Sweets*, 1957) (Amos, 1993: 146)

During the 1950s a new type of preventive health care appeared, namely screening for cancer. Two leaflets, *A Message for Women – on Cancer* (1952) and *Cancer Can be Treated: A Special Message to Women Over 40* (1956/7), both advised women to consult their doctor if they felt a lump in their breast or had abnormal bleeding from the vagina. However neither leaflet indicated which cancers were being talked about, discussed what cancer was, or what treatments if any were available. Nor did they consider the anxiety that finding a lump might generate.

When the Health Education Council (HEC) replaced the CCHE in 1968 a growing awareness that the purely instructional approaches had little effect on people's behaviour led to attempts at evaluation. The findings from their first major study led them to conclude that attention needed to be focused on middle-aged women, not for their own health and well-being, but in order to influence their middle-aged husbands who were at risk from heart disease. They decided that 'the men surveyed were unlikely to change their behaviour ... there may be some way however of influencing their wives – in relation to the husband's diet' (HEC, 1971).

Women have always been prime targets for health education in terms of reproduction and maternal health and also as gatekeepers of the family's health. By the late 1960s women began to seek out information about their health in their own terms not just as wives and mothers. Educating themselves about health became an important part of the women's health movement and represented a different form of health education which took a much more 'bottom-up' approach than previous forms of health education.

The women's health movement

The pill and the abortion act of 1967 gave women more control over their own fertility, yet pregnancy and childbirth were becoming increasingly medicalised and highly technical. Women were expected to be the passive recipients of health care which still lay to a great extent in the hands of men.

The women's health movement grew out of the reproductive rights campaigns of the early 1970s and the women who had fought to gain control over their own fertility questioned the dominant biomedical model of medical practice which largely ignored their circumstances and experiences. They wanted to play an active role in the decisions which affected their own health, but in order to do that they recognised the need to gain knowledge about their own bodies.

The publication of *Our Bodies, Ourselves*, first in the USA in 1971 and then in the UK in 1978, represented a radically new way for women to educate themselves about their own health. It was information by women for women. The authors tell the story of how it came about:

> We had all experienced frustration and anger towards specific doctors and the medical maze in general, and initially we wanted to do something about this. As we talked we began to realise how little we knew about our own bodies, so we decided to do further research, to prepare papers in groups and then to discuss our findings together. We learned both from professional sources (medical textbooks, journals, doctors, nurses) and from our own experience...

> The results of our findings were used to present courses for other women. We would meet in any available free space, in schools, nurseries, church halls, in our own homes. As we taught, we learned from other women; as they learned, they went on to give courses to others. We saw it as a never-ending process always involving more and more women.
>
> (Phillips and Rakuson, 1978: 11)

The book had a profound effect on many women because it drew on women's own experience, both negative and positive, and emphasised women's rights and responsibilities about their own health. It gave them knowledge about their own bodies and the courage to seek out more information.

Many of the developments of the women's health movement, such as the formation of Well Woman Clinics and Women's Health Information centres, have had greatest impact at the local and community level and are discussed in Jones and Sidell (1997), Chapter 2. But in terms of health education it represented a shift from 'top-down' to truly 'bottom-up' health education. The impetus came from women themselves who wanted to understand their own bodies and take control over their own health. The women's health movement is based on the belief that knowledge is power and without it there can be no freedom of choice. Much of the impetus of the women's health movement came from white and mainly middle-class women, and concern was expressed at how far other groups of women felt excluded (Douglas, 1992). However a survey of attendees at the Norwich Well Woman Clinic and Advisory Service, which was deliberately situated on a council housing estate, indicated that the proportions of working-class women who attended was significant (Sidell, 1985). Black women and women from minority ethnic groups have had to campaign for services which are more appropriate to their needs.

The bottom up method of health education has been a feature of other groups. Many self-help and pressure groups, such as the Arthritis and Rheumatism Society, The National Schizophrenia Fellowship and The Multiple Sclerosis Society, are very well informed about the health issues which affect their members. They also commission research and seek to influence public policy. Recently the self-advocacy movement of people with learning disabilities and disability groups is encouraging people to be better informed about their health.

Can you think of any drawbacks to the bottom-up approach?

The idea that knowledge is control is an attractive one but sometimes the sheer weight of the knowledge is daunting, and sometimes the information is extremely complex and often conflicting.

Between the two extremes of top-down health propaganda and the bottom-up self-help model, a range of models and strategies have developed within contemporary health education. French reminds us that:

> Health education is a practical endeavour focused on improving understanding about the determinants of health and illness and helping people to develop the skills they need to bring about change.
>
> (French, 1990: 8)

10.3 Contemporary health education

It was not until the 1970s that the nature and scope of health education received much theoretical attention with attempts to classify and delineate the different approaches which were in evidence. Tuckett (1979) distinguished between three types of health education: one was concerned with reducing mortality and morbidity by bringing about changes in people's beliefs and behaviours; the second was concerned with the appropriate use of health services; and the third aimed to create a general climate of awareness of health issues. Writing soon after Tuckett, Draper provided a similar three point classification:

- education about the body and how to best care for it
- education on the sensible use of health services and health resources
- education about the wider environment in which health choices are made.

(Draper, 1983)

Think back to Part 1, Chapter 2, where you were introduced to different models of health. Which model of health do you think fits the types of health education identified by Tuckett and Draper?

Reducing mortality and morbidity and educating about the body and use of health services is more concerned with a biomedical model of health which sees health as the absence of disease. The third is open to a wider interpretation of health although this was not entirely clear from Tuckett's work at the time. Draper's third category is more clearly using a social model of health.

Missing from Tuckett and Draper's classification is learning about ourselves and the interactions in which we as social beings engage in our everyday lives. This is taking a life-skills approach. Over the last decade Keith Tones has developed those earlier classifications into a complex typology of health education (introduced in Part 1), which does include this type of 'personal' education. He identifies a 'preventive' approach, a 'radical' approach and a 'self-empowerment' approach.

The preventive model

This approach seeks to 'modify the behaviours which are responsible for disease' (Tones, 1981). Although it falls within the biomedical tradition advocates claim that it is not part of the dominant ideology of medicine which is curative, and although it lends itself to accusations of 'victim blaming', Tones and Tilford (1994) justify its continued use within health education in two ways:

- Curative medicine has a limited capability for managing the major (western) burden of chronic degenerative disease and key infectious diseases such as AIDS. Moreover, its practice is characterised by accelerating costs and it incorporates not insubstantial iatrogenic 'side effects'.

- Prevention is, therefore, better than cure. Since human behaviour plays a significant part in the aetiology and management of all diseases, education is needed to persuade people to behave appropriately.

Tones and Tilford (1994) have set out the functions of health education in relation to the three types of prevention which you met in Chapter 4.

Table 10.1   **Health education and the preventive model**

Level of prevention	Function of health education
Primary	
Concerned to prevent onset of disease; reduce incidence.	Persuade individuals to adopt behaviours believed to reduce the risk of disease; adopt healthy lifestyle.
	Persuade individuals to utilize preventive health services appropriately.
	Concerned with **health behaviour:** those activities undertaken by individuals believing themselves to be healthy in order to prevent future health problems or detect them asymptomatically.
Secondary	
Concerned to prevent development of existing disease, minimize its severity, reverse its progress, reduce prevalence.	Persuade individuals to utilize screening services appropriately; learn appropriate self-care; seek early diagnosis and treatment.
	Persuade individuals to comply with medical treatment and recommendations.
	Concerned with **illness behaviour:** those activities undertaken by individuals experiencing symptoms in order to determine their state of health; subsequent adoption of measures designed to meet perceived needs.
Tertiary	
Concerned to prevent deterioration, relapse and complications; promote rehabilitation; help adjustment to terminal conditions.	Persuade individuals to comply with medical treatment, including palliative measures, and adjust to limitations resulting from disease.
	Persuade patients to resume normal behaviours as appropriate.
	Teach carers to respond appropriately to patient needs.
	Provide terminal care counselling.
	Concerned with adopting and relinquishing **sick role**.

(Tones and Tilford , 1994: 14)

What do you think are the main disadvantages of this approach?

It disregards socio-political factors which were discussed in Chapter 3 such as the context in which a person's health occurs. It also assumes that the individual has free choice and will act rationally when in receipt of the correct information provided by expert educators.

The radical model

This approach 'seeks the roots of health problems and finds them in social, economic and political factors'. Health education is directed at 'critical consciousness raising' to enable people to recognise the factors which are influencing their health and encouraging them to do something about it. Tones and Tilford (1994: 20) see this as a four-step process:

1 Fostering reflection on aspects of personal reality.
2 Encouraging a search for, and collective identification of, the root causes of that reality.
3 Examination of implications.
4 Development of a plan of action to alter reality.

This approach aims to address inequalities in health based on class, ethnicity, gender, and geography by developing organisational policies and fiscal control. The scope for this type of activity may be more limited for most professionals involved in promoting health (Naidoo and Wills, 2000) The skills involved in working in this way include negotiating, lobbying, policy development and implementation. Communication skills will be required at a range of different levels from working with local communities to dealing with key organisations, politicians and policy makers.

The empowerment model

The goal here is to encourage personal growth, by enhancing self-esteem and self-assertiveness. The aim is to teach people the skills to take charge of their own health. Positive health features in this approach as well as the prevention of ill-health. Health has mental and social dimensions as well as physical. The communication process is two way, taking into account the values of the educator and those being educated. The aim is not to coerce or persuade but to foster life skills and increase self-esteem through this participatory process. The rhetoric of autonomy and empowerment has become more prevalent in contemporary health education. To achieve this, a more bottom-up rather than top-down approach is needed. But this approach attracted the criticism that it put the onus back on the individual without addressing the structural changes needed before some people who are in very powerless positions can attempt to take charge of their own health (Rodmell and Watt, 1986). However, those who defend the 'life skills' approach claim that unless individuals have the confidence to challenge the unequal power relationships that maintain structural inequalities they will not increase their control over their own health and achieve any degree of autonomy – which you will remember from Chapter 6 is one of the values which underpins health promotion.

Katherine Weare (1992) maintains that enabling people to be autonomous is a fundamental goal of education. This is to be distinguished from training which aims to encourage people 'to acquire a set of pre-set beliefs, habits and values' (Seedhouse, 1986). However autonomy is not just about the freedom of the individual. Weare maintains that:

> ... it inevitably has a social purpose and a social impact. People cannot be autonomous in isolation: their rights and freedoms depend on how those around them behave and what the social structures within which they live allow them to do. Education for autonomy means shaping a society in which it is possible for people to be free, while ensuring that the freedom of one individual or group is not at the expense of others.
>
> (Weare, 1992: 67)

Accepting the goal of autonomy in health education can leave the health educator in an uncomfortable position. If the individual is to be truly autonomous in relation to his or her own health then they must be free to choose to act in an unhealthy way provided this does not inhibit the freedom of others. If the outcome of health education is autonomy then unhealthy behaviour based on informed choice has to be an acceptable outcome for health education. In practice, health education steers an uneasy course between the goals of education and training. The hope has been that if people have the knowledge and information about what is good for their health and the skills to change unhealthy behaviour then they will choose to change that behaviour. Those who advocate a more radical approach to health education also see a need to change the social environment to 'make healthy choices the easy choices'. In spite of all this, many 'autonomous' people make unhealthy choices, which, whilst frustrating the goals of training, is quite compatible with the goals of education. This clearly has implications for the evaluation of health education programmes which is addressed in Part 4 of this book.

So far we have been concentrating on the aims and functions of health education and the values which underpin them. We now turn to the techniques used to convey the messages of health education. These too can be value laden.

10.4 Styles and strategies

The traditional approach to health education is based on a view of education which sees people as 'empty vessels' into which information is poured in the hope that this will inform that person's behaviour. This view of education assumes that the most important knowledge people can have is rational, scientific and cognitive. It is characterised by a number of features:

- the relationship between teacher and learner is fundamentally unequal; the teacher has a valuable 'commodity' which the learner does not possess
- the teacher is an expert while the learner is basically ignorant
- the relationship between teacher and learner is a hierarchical and stratified one
- it is assumed that the teacher will be the one to initiate action and be the primary agent in making learning take place.

Whilst the communication of rational, cognitive information and thought in verbal form by traditional methods is very important, more modern educational theory emphasises the learning of processes rather than the acquisition of facts. The traditional way of educating people is too narrow for health education which has in many ways pioneered more active democratic and participatory methods of educating people about health.

Modern methods of health education

It has been said that health education aims to start where people are: developmentally, emotionally and socially. What is the significance of this?

This is based on the premise that people are more likely to engage with knowledge which seems relevant to their own situation and experience. A person's stage of development will also determine how he or she will respond to education. People develop cognitively, emotionally and attitudinally right through the life span, and the interests of a person in their teenage years may be very different from the interests which may develop in their middle years. It may be difficult for adolescents to see the relevance of information on the basis of its long-term risks when their pressing concerns are about projecting a particular image in which risk taking is highly prized. Health education must resonate with people's immediate concerns.

The concept of a 'health career' which charts the ways an individual's attitude to health changes over time can be useful in finding ways to make health education relevant to people at different stages of their lives (Weare, 1992). This has been used particularly in relation to health education in schools. The *Health for Life* Primary School Project (HEA, 1989a) and *Exploring Health Education* (HEA, 1989b) emphasise the need to discover where children are developmentally and to adopt pupil-centred learning.

The learner's emotional state and emotional development is also an important issue for health educators and again many school-based health education initiatives have taken a leading role in developing learning materials which emphasise this aspect of learning. There is now an emphasis on child-centred education, focusing on self-esteem and the enhancement of decision-making skills. This approach is featured strongly in some specific projects such as *My Body* (HEC, 1983) and *Health for Life* (HEA, 1989a). But it would be wrong to imply that this method of health education in schools is well established. In her recent study Charlton (1980) asked students and tutors on a teacher training course to rate a list of aims of health education in schools. They consistently rated information-giving the highest, followed by influencing pupil's attitudes and behaviours. Only a few thought that increasing pupils' decision-making skills was a high priority.

Peer health education

You will remember from the discussion of models of behavioural change discussed in the last chapter that one of the main influences on behaviour is the effect of friends and peers. Building on this a range of peer health education initiatives have been developed with young people. Typically a number of key young people are trained as health educators who teach or share health information, values and behaviours with their peers. Kathryn Milburn (1995) has reviewed the rationale for such initiatives. The hope is that peer education avoids the unequal power relationship that exists between pupil and teacher and that through reciprocal interactions young people can help each other and share their knowledge and understandings and empathise with others. Peer education offers the opportunity to participate and promotes acceptance and respect for different views. It is relatively inexpensive, although good peer education depends on trained and committed staff. Milburn also raises some ethical issues concerning peer education asking if adults have the right to manipulate young people's social worlds to promote healthier lifestyles and whether it is not imposing an adultist agenda on young people who are a 'captive audience'. These issues echo some of the ethical issues which have been raised in Chapter 6 about health promotion as a whole. The effectiveness of peer health education remains unanswered, although the HEA in the UK has carried out some investigations (HEA 1993b; Hill, 1993) into the use of peer education about HIV and AIDS . These showed clear benefits to the peer educators themselves although there was less evidence of benefit to the wider target group. One problem they found was that the turnover of students trained as peer educators meant that their commitment could only be short term and that this had resource implications. Overall, Milburn concludes that 'the premise that young people will be more responsive to sexual health education from informed peers should still be treated as yet another working hypothesis' (1995: 415).

The environment for health education

Culturally inappropriate health education, for instance about diet, is likely to be ineffective, whereas health educators who take the trouble to recognise and respect the cultural understandings and values of learners are more likely to be well received (Calnan, 1990; Helman, 1990). The awareness that health education needs to take into account the cultural and social environment in which that education takes place has led to the growth of initiatives which focus on the institutional environment of the school and its relationship to the local community (Young and Williams, 1989). Health promoting schools represent an attempt to pay attention to the social environment of the school (Nutbeam, 1992). This includes the influence of the teachers behaviour so if, for instance, there is a problem with bullying in the school, then it is important that teachers do not provide role models for that type of behaviour. The food available in the school canteen should reflect the health education messages about healthy eating. The concept of the health promoting school is shown diagrammatically below.

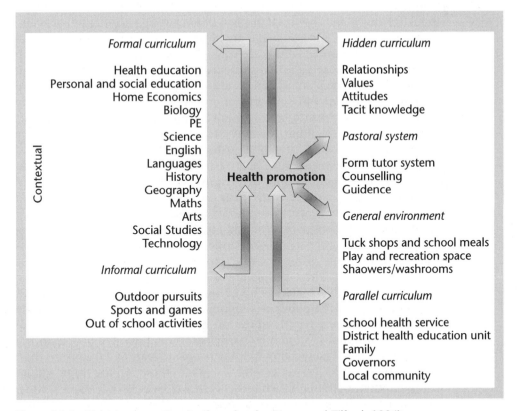

Figure 10.1   **Health promotion in the school**   (Tones and Tilford, 1994)

The European Network of Health Promoting Schools was set up in January 1992 and by January 1996 this involved some 500 schools from almost 40 countries and a practical guide has been provided by Health Promotion Wales (1994). Essentially this initiative is an attempt to make health education an active and integral part of school life rather than a marginalised activity.

Although much education theory and practice has developed within the school situation health education is a life-long activity. In the next section we examine the role of working with groups in health education.

10.5 Working with groups

So far we have focused on one-to-one communication. In this section we want to explore how this can be extended to working with groups as well.

The aim of health education is to provide knowledge and information and to develop the necessary skills so that people can make an informed choice about their health behaviour. Health education can take place through one-to-one advice or one-to-one counselling, the provision of booklets and leaflets or visual displays or increasingly through groups and group discussions. The skills that are important for person-centred work – for example, listening skills – are equally important when working with groups and encouraging active participation of group members. Although the group members may decide the issues for discussion, the group facilitator or leader will support the process of discussion and therefore must be aware of the principles of adult learning and factors which help or hinder this process. Adult learning can involve three aspects: cognitive (information and understanding), affective (attitudes and feelings) and behavioural (skills). All three areas are important in helping people to make informed choices about their health and health behaviour.

Working with groups and using an active workshop style is an appropriate way to engage people in a dialogue about health matters. It allows for the exchange of ideas and provides opportunities for exploring the boundaries of perception, understanding and behaviour. It is important to allow group members to participate on their own terms and to 'start from where people are at'. This recognises that individuals' lives are not simply a matter of his or her own attitudes and behaviour but are influenced by the political, economic and social context in which he or she lives. Because health education needs to start from where people are, it follows that it should be participatory and involve people in the learning process. The secret of helping people to learn is to draw out their own interests and concerns and to relate these to the topic under consideration. Building on what the learner already knows about a topic, and acknowledging the wealth of personal and occupational experience that members of the group bring, is more likely to be effective than bombarding individuals with a multitude of facts.

Small groups may have a number of characteristics that are important issues in relation to group dynamics (Whittington, 1987):

1　They can develop particular moods and atmospheres.

2　Shared themes can build in groups.

3　Groups evolve norms and belief systems.

4　Groups vary in cohesiveness and in the permeability of their boundaries.

5　Groups develop and change their character over a period of time.

6　Persons occupy different positions in groups with respect to power, centrality and being liked and disliked.

7　Individuals in groups sometimes find one or two other persons who are especially important to them because they are similar in some respect to significant persons in the individual's life or to significant aspects of the self.

8　Social comparison can take place in a group.

9　A group is an environment in which persons can observe what others do and say and then observe what happens next.

10　A group is an environment in which persons can receive feedback from others concerning their own behaviour or participation.

The group facilitator or leader must be aware of these characteristics and will also have a number of roles. The first is concerned with setting up the group – who sets the aims and objectives? To enable full participation of group members, the facilitator should allow the group to set its own agenda. The facilitator must be able to develop a 'safe' environment in a group to enable open discussion and debate. This means being aware of the particular experiences and needs of group participants. It can also involve the physical aspects and locations of group meetings and the way in which the room itself is laid out. Other aspects relate to the dynamics within the group, allowing an atmosphere where group members can challenge each other and the facilitator. This means that sometimes conflicts will arise within the group which need to be addressed directly. Sometimes there are hidden agendas or conflicts which sit just below the surface of the group discussions. Group leaders must also be able to confront group members in a sensitive and supportive way and create an atmosphere where members feel able to challenge each other. In this context it is important for the facilitator to establish clear ground rules which ensure that the views of each group member are respected and valued and are challenged in an equally respectful way. The person-centred approaches we have discussed in the earlier sections of this chapter are of particular importance here. The group facilitator must also assist group members in understanding the processes that are taking place within the group. This demands the ability to listen to the perceptions of all the individuals in the group.

In earlier chapters we discussed the diversity, differences and divisions within society generally. These differences will also be apparent in groups.

Groups may have people from a range of backgrounds and experiences; group members may all be from the same ethnic group or from a range of ethnic groups. One aspect of group facilitation will be to enable all group members to contribute and to participate, and to address any discriminatory or oppressive practices which may occur. The use of groups in health education is very effective in involving people from a range of backgrounds and developing participatory approaches to developing health promotion initiatives.

One initiative which has managed to reach older Asian women was set up by a health visitor in Lambeth, South London (Pharoah and Redmond, 1991). The health visitor began to explore avenues into the older Asian community by attending local events and facilities and managed to gain access to Ashram, an Asian day centre for older people with about 300 members. With the enthusiastic support of the centre's co-ordinator she set up a health education programme for the older women with the co-ordinator acting as interpreter. They covered topics such as prevention of heart disease and the problems of diabetes, osteoporosis and osteomalacia, cervical cytology and breast screening. The health visitor noted that, although reluctant to discuss sensitive topics at first, as they relaxed they asked questions and raised personal problems. They discussed incontinence, arthritis, exercise, relaxation and individual health needs.

Between 30 and 35 older Asian women attended regularly. By adopting an outgoing, flexible and responsive approach the health visitor commented that she learnt as much as they did, particularly about traditional remedies and the Asian lifestyle. The health visitor felt that it was essential that a safe environment was created and she identified the following factors which created this safe environment:

- the sessions were held in their own community centre
- a trusted female member of their own community was present
- they were women-only sessions
- a good group atmosphere was created
- a sympathetic non-didactic approach was taken, with a two-way flow of information
- the programme was tailored to the needs of the community.

(Pharoah and Redmond, 1991: 22)

When working with adults, whether from minority ethnic groups, older people, parents or younger adults, group work enables people to participate and to share ideas and experiences and it values those experiences. Health education carried out in this way respects cultural norms and can help and support people to set and achieve their own health priorities.

10.6 Conclusion

Health education remains a key element in the promotion of health. Effective health education promotes autonomy by involving people voluntarily in the process of setting health agendas. In this way health agendas are more likely to be sensitive to the social, economic and environmental influences on people's health choices. This chapter has been concerned with face-to-face health education and the setting of personal health agendas. The mass media present opportunities to communicate with whole populations and influence political agendas. This is the subject of the final chapter in this Part.

Chapter 11

Educating and communicating through the mass media

11.1 Introduction

The use of the mass media represents a powerful agent of communication. News, current affairs and information on a whole range of topics are conveyed to large proportions of the population often straight into their homes. The mass media therefore presents an enticing prospect for health educators to communicate with large numbers of people at the same time. The main way in which educating for health through the means of mass media differs from the other forms of health education discussed in previous chapters is that there is no direct interpersonal contact. The message is communicated through a particular medium. Mass media are often viewed as being newspapers, radio and television, but posters, leaflets and magazines all fit under this heading. In recent years multi-media methods using videos, CD-ROMs, DVD and the World Wide Web have opened up new and exciting prospects for health education.

This chapter will begin by discussing the potential for disseminating health education through various types of media which have a mass circulation before going on to look at some of the techniques used. It will explore some specific ways that the mass media can be used locally by health educators in the course of their work. The chapter will end by taking a look at the future, exploring the multi-media interactive opportunities and the potential of the internet for health education in the rapidly expanding world of information and communications technology.

11.2 The potential of mass media health education

There was a time when health educators were overly optimistic about what could be achieved through the mass media, particularly in relation to individual behaviour change. It was thought that if the message could be conveyed to as many people as possible at one stroke then more people would be persuaded to change their unhealthy behaviour. It was hoped that the mass media could act like a hypodermic syringe injecting the message straight into the mass bloodstream and having maximum and direct effect. This optimism proved to be unfounded and a study which looked at 49 mass media campaigns in the late 1970s (Gatherer *et al.*,

1979) found evidence of only small short-term increases in knowledge, very little attitude shift, and even less actual behavioural change. Nevertheless the mass media still remain an attractive proposition for health educators but the unrealistically high expectations have been revised. Instead of the hoped-for main-lining effect of the health education message the analogy of an aerosol spray is considered more appropriate: 'as you spray it on the surface, some of it hits the target; most of it drifts away; and very little of it penetrates' (Mendelsohn, 1968).

As well as revising expectations for mass media health education there is also a realisation that mass media campaigns alone will have little effect. If used as part of a co-ordinated plan they are more likely to have greater impact. Mass media education is therefore not a substitute for the more interpersonal face-to-face education used in the various settings discussed in previous chapters but should be used in conjunction with face-to-face techniques. The main differences between mass media education and face-to-face channels are summarised in Table 11.1

Table 11.1   **Main characteristics of mass media and face-to-face channels**

Characteristics	*Mass media*	*Face-to-face*
Speed to cover large population	Rapid	Slow
Ability to select particular audience	Difficult to select audience	Can be highly selective
Direction	One way	Two way
Ability to respond to local needs of specific communities	Only provides non-specific information	Can fit to local need
Feedback	Only indirect feedback from surveys	Direct feedback possible
Main effect	Increased/knowledge awareness	Changes in attitudes and behaviour; problem-solving skills

(adapted from Hubley, 1993: 61)

What advantages might the mass media have over other forms of health education?

We have already mentioned that mass media can reach very large numbers of people but they are also able to reach groups of people who may be otherwise difficult to communicate with, for instance young males. Surprisingly it has been claimed that mass media campaigns are relatively cheap compared to the face-to-face and more labour intensive methods. The messages can be put over in very dramatic ways, creating potent images. It has also been argued that because the messages are received simultaneously by large numbers of people they therefore generate social support for the particular behaviour change which is being promoted.

Public health advocacy

Attention is focusing more on the potential for mass media, especially newspapers, TV and radio, as a major tool in public health advocacy which is very much concerned with raising awareness and putting over health agendas. Public health advocacy aims to set and change policy rather than directly change knowledge, attitudes and behaviour. It is concerned with the legislative, fiscal and environmental context in which individual knowledge and attitudes are formed:

> Public health advocacy – sometimes called public health lobbying – is an expression used more often to refer to the process of overcoming major structural (as opposed to individual or behavioural) barriers to public health goals. Numbered among such barriers are some of the most formidable political, economic, and cultural forces imaginable.
>
> (Chapman and Lupton, 1994: 6)

These forces include:

- political philosophies that put economic concerns before health and quality of life
- political and bureaucratic opposition to health promoting policies especially those which try to involve consumers in health care planning
- the marketing of unsafe and unhealthy products often by influential and wealthy corporations
- the persistence of cultural values such as racism and sexism.

(Chapman and Lupton, 1994: 6)

Chapman and Lupton recognise the enormousness of the task and see the use of mass media, especially the news media, as a vital weapon in countering these forces. They quote Allen Otten, a reporter on the *Wall Street Journal* who wrote, 'Well done investigative reporting produces public outrage (or policy maker outrage) that forces new regulations and laws or tougher enforcement of existing ones. Ten-thousand-watt klieg lights turned on a situation focuses the minds of policy makers very fast' (Chapman and Lupton, 1994: 18).

There is much evidence to suggest that the mass media are a leading source of public information about health issues and highly influential in forming public opinion. A study of over 4,000 adults in the US and the UK reported the highest level of interest in medical and health issues in categories of news coverage (Durant *et al.*, 1989). Politicians, senior public servants and policy makers in another American study said that the news media were an important source of information about health and medical issues. Given that television watching and newspaper reading take up a great deal of people's leisure time, the media present an opportunity that health educators cannot ignore. But it is an opportunity which is not without its drawbacks and needs to be handled with care and a great deal of preparation.

The term 'unplanned' is often used to differentiate the use of media to convey health messages which have not been specifically paid for by health promoters as is the case with advertising campaigns. But the art of the public health advocate is to create news about a particular health topic so that it receives media coverage because it is newsworthy, and so it could be argued that media coverage is rarely completely unplanned. Other interest groups may also capture the news with items which impact on health, such as drug companies.

What do you think might make an item newsworthy?

Clearly the item has to be new or unusual or add something significant to an item which is currently in the news, and it has to have impact. An item which is about or includes information from a prominent person is likely to capture the news or a human interest story especially about children. Stories which are highly emotionally charged, dramatic or tragic tend to get into the news. A local event may capture the news in a particular region. Capturing the attention of the media does not mean that they can be controlled and so to some extent they can be seen as 'unplanned'. This raises certain problems. Chapman and Lupton (1994) noted that the news media have a preference for extreme or sensational views which can distort information. Coverage is more likely to focus on dramatic biomedical treatments or health risks which are relatively serious and rare to the exclusion of the more common health issues or ways of preventing illness. Health risks are often not placed in context, little background information is given or the reliability of the source. Sometimes the information is contradictory and confusing which leads to panic. The announcement in the autumn of 1995 that some of the most used brands of the contraceptive pill significantly increased the risk of thrombosis resulted in many women stopping taking their pill in mid cycle with the result that the number of unwanted pregnancies in the subsequent months increased substantially. The mass media are a powerful tool which need careful handling.

11.3 Using the mass media

There are two ways in which the media cover health topics. One is paid-for work through advertising campaigns and specific health education strategies. The other is unpaid-for media coverage, where aspects of health arise in a more general context.

Unpaid-for media coverage of health topics

When are messages about health portrayed in the media which are not overtly 'health education'?

As well as the daily news, current affairs programmes report items such as the latest breakthrough in research into the causes of cancer, or new technologies for dealing with infertility, or new screening techniques. The possible link between BSE and CJD dominated the media for weeks in the spring of 1996 and the findings of a Royal Commission on transport and health created quite a stir in the media and thus generated a good deal of debate about issues which might otherwise not have received much of an airing. Then there are documentary programmes on radio and TV which explore a specific topic. 'Cot deaths' and contraception have frequently been the subject of TV documentaries and they have been accused of causing a good deal of public anxiety. GPs used to be inundated with anxious patients after such programmes but now you might have noticed that invariably after such programmes a telephone help line is offered or a fact sheet on the subject. However the news bulletin about potential dangers of the birth control pill was put out without giving doctors any prior warning, which left them in a very difficult situation.

Even less overtly there are health topics cropping up in the most unlikely places, such as soaps and sitcoms. Problems with alcohol and drug abuse are favourite topics in soaps; teenage pregnancies, domestic violence, HIV and AIDS, depression, unemployment and many other health-related issues are all featured from time to time.

Magazines, particularly those aimed at a young female market, have always had a strong health content and more recently similar magazines have appeared for men and older people. Diet, exercise, sex and reproductive issues, and parenting advice are regularly featured. Clearly there is a market for such features, and books on certain slimming diets have kept major publishing houses in business for some time. Health issues obviously sell media products. This puts editors of magazines, producers of soaps, newscasters, journalists etc. in a powerful position to influence the messages we receive about health. Some of it is for good, some for ill as they may have other interests involved. It is unlikely to be value neutral.

Planned and paid-for use of the media by health educators

So far we have been looking at ways in which health is used by the media. How can those who want to influence health behaviour and put forward their own health messages use the media? There are two separate issues here: one is access the other is objectives. We will return to the issue of access later in the chapter. First we will look at what can be achieved and then explore techniques for reaching specific audiences.

Objectives

Two distinct models of health education via mass media have been identified: the 'direct effect' model and the 'agenda-setting' model (Redman *et al.*, 1990). In the 'direct effect' model, health information is used in much the same way as a health professional might use it. The objective is to change or prevent harmful behaviour and promote health enhancing behaviours. In the 'agenda setting' or advocacy model, the media is used to raise awareness of a health problem or a health opportunity and to influence policy or to gain support for a particular policy. These are not mutually exclusive models and elements of both are evident in most media campaigns.

Think of one of the drink driving campaigns. How far was it agenda setting and how far was it using the direct effect approach?

Drink driving campaigns aim to prevent accidents by changing some people's drinking behaviour. They use a combination of shock tactics and a strong message that makes the link between accidents and alcohol consumption. They are also, and have been very strongly in the past, agenda setting in creating a climate in which it is possible to bring in legislation to breathalyse motorists. You may have noticed that for many years they targeted young people. One year when statistics were showing that there was a hard core of middle-aged men who were not heeding the drink driving message, they targeted them. Again this is setting the agenda by highlighting particular groups in society for attention.

Other examples of public opinion forming and public health advocacy campaigns are the publicising of information on passive smoking which has put pressure on smokers not to smoke in public places. Another example has been the campaign for lead free petrol which has been highly influential in spite of powerful opposition from oil companies. And campaign groups such as Greenpeace have highlighted issues such as the dumping of toxic waste and the sinking of obsolete oil rigs, again taking on very powerful multinational companies.

The national health promotion agencies use the mass media a great deal to convey information on new research or controversial issues. For example 'The Smoking Epidemic' gave statistics by regional health authority on the numbers of deaths and illnesses annually attributable to smoking. This received a great deal of press coverage and a formal request of a briefing from the Prime Minister. They also put out messages related to the Saving Lives – Our Healthier Nation targets which are both agenda setting in terms of the government targets but were also aiming to have a direct effect on these targets.

Can you think of other campaigns which relate to the Saving Lives: Our Healthier Nation targets?

You will be familiar with the anti-smoking and safer sex campaigns. One of the interesting developments in the last few years has been the information given with the television weather forecast. This is related to reducing the incidence of skin cancer and respiratory diseases. In the summer we now get information on the length of time that it is safe to be exposed to the sun and we get information on the air quality. There has also been a national poster campaign alerting people to the symptoms of diabetes in order that people will seek help sooner rather than later and so minimise the damage that diabetes can do.

As well as mounting single issue campaigns, the Health Education Authority collaborated with the BBC to put on the *Health Show.* This was a 90 minute live production, broadcast to viewers in England, Wales, Scotland and Northern Ireland. The show focused on three behavioural topics: physical activity, healthy eating and smoking. It had three main aims. The first was to reinforce the importance of health messages that people might be fairly familiar with already. Second it tried to bring together the three themes of physical activity, healthy eating and smoking as an integrated way of living more healthily. Thirdly it tried to communicate ideas for change which people might find acceptable and suggestions for specific action.

The show was presented by Terry Wogan who was assisted by a Radio 1 disc jockey Jakki Brambles and a TV doctor, Dr Hilary Jones. They used the style and format of the telethon which aims to involve the viewers and get them to participate by inviting them to telephone in at various points. Live audience participation was used, which is another feature of the telethon. Well known celebrities made appearances throughout the show to put over certain messages, often in a light-hearted way.

The show reached an average audience of eight million people during the 90 minutes, rising to nine million at times. It generated 1.6 million telephone calls and 500,000 copies of the *Health Show Guide* were sent out on request. But it is important to discover whether the show had the effect that it was designed to have: that is, to get people to change their behaviour and adopt other forms of behaviour. This information is difficult to get but this show was evaluated ten months afterwards and the methods and findings of that evaluation will be discussed in Part 4 of this book. In television terms it was a success and both the BBC and the HEA were well satisfied.

A criticism levelled at health programmes is that, although they are popular on TV, they are more popular with a middle-class audience. In general there has been a good deal of scepticism voiced about the effectiveness of mass media health campaigns when compared with the effects of advertising 'unhealthy' products. McKinlay has drawn attention to this disparity:

> How embarrassingly ineffective are our mass media efforts in the health field (e.g. alcoholism, obesity, drug abuse, safe driving, pollution, etc.) when compared with many of the tax-exempt promotional efforts on behalf of the illness generating activities of large-scale corporations. It is a fact that we are demonstrably more effective in persuading people to purchase items they never dreamed they would need, or to pursue at-risk courses of action, than we are in preventing or halting such behaviour.
>
> (McKinlay, 1979: 12)

This recognition of the superiority of commercial advertising in persuading people to 'buy' a particular product has led health educators to look at the techniques used in the commercial world to see if anything can be learnt about how to sell health.

11.4 Social marketing for health

Using marketing techniques to sell social and health products was first suggested by Weibe (1951) and developed further by Kotler (1975). They argued that marketing was a universal human activity which could be applied to people, organisations and even ideas. Hastings and Haywood (1991) suggested that there are certain important key elements to social marketing. These are:

- mutually beneficial exchange
- the marketing mix
- consumer orientation
- market segmentation and targeting.

Lefebvre (1992) has further developed the concepts of social marketing and health promotion.

Mutually beneficial exchange

The traditional marketing concept is based on the idea of exchange. The exchange is usually between money and a product. In theory this is mutually beneficial, I have the money you have the product. In social marketing for health the cost to the consumer is in the effort to change a particular behaviour in exchange for improved health and quality of life. The benefits to the health promoter may be altruistic in improving public health. If the promoter is the government then the benefits could lie in lowering expenditure on health care or cutting down on days lost at work.

The marketing mix

It has been said that 'commercial marketing is essentially about getting the right product, at the right price, in the right place at the right time, presented in such a way as to successfully satisfy the needs of the consumer' (Hastings and Haywood, 1991). This involves the four 'p's: product, price, place and promotion. In relation to health promotion the product at a general level would be 'good health'. In marketing terms this would be broken down into the 'core' product, e.g. increased stamina and the tangible product, which might be exercise or smoking cessation. The price is what the consumer must give up or do in order to achieve what is on offer. The price might include money, time, psychological or physical costs. Place concerns the distribution channels used to reach the supermarket or consumer. If the product is healthier eating then the distribution channel might be a fruit and veg co-op. Promotion is the means by which the health promoter communicates the product to the consumer. Other than advertising, this may be a sales promotion such as free condoms.

Consumer orientation

The notion of a consumer is central to all aspects of marketing. Without the consumer marketing has no purpose. The health promoter has to try to understand and ascertain the needs of the consumer if they hope to communicate with them. Haranguing or patronising them is unlikely to be productive. Mendelsohn has expressed some needs that we do not have:

> Among the 'needs' we all have is not to be bombarded with information we already have or do not have any use for (e.g. information asserting that excessive drinking may be bad for us); not to be commanded to do something that is vague and unachievable without explicit simple instructions regarding its achievement (e.g. 'drive carefully'); not to be unreasonably frightened (e.g. any drinking during pregnancy, no matter how moderate, will surely result in the birth of a monster); and not to be insulted by the health communicator who implies that everyone the communicator is trying to address is (1) ignorant ... (2) ... sinfully 'irresponsible' in that they don't give a damn about their own lives/or the lives of others; and (3) they are slothfully 'apathetic' in not immediately doing without question what the communicator commands them to do.
>
> (Mendelsohn, 1968, quoted in Tones and Tilford, 1994)

This also raises the fundamental question which was raised in the first chapter of this book: 'do people want to be healthy?'. You may remember the Australian health promoters view which was expressed there that

people are bombarded with advertising which is health damaging and it
would therefore be irresponsible for this not to be countered.

Market segmentation and targeting

It is a truism that people do not constitute an homogeneous mass. We're
men women, young old, rich poor, fat thin, smokers and non-smokers,
joggers and sloths. We don't all need the same health education messages.
Audience segmentation is the term used in the advertising world to break
down the mixed population into more homogeneous groups. These
'market segments' are thought to share certain characteristics which affect
the beliefs and attitudes of that group of the population. Social scientists
divide us into social classes but marketeers 'segment' us into appropriate
groups or target markets most suitable for their products. Beattie describes
the techniques used:

> A technique of social research known as 'psychographics' has become
> familiar in the market research world, as a method for describing the
> lifestyles and lifecycle positions of segments within these different
> markets. This technique takes analysis away from and beyond the
> demographic categories of age, sex, and income level, and generates an
> astonishing variety of new 'typologies' ... that have little to do with
> traditional perceptions of 'social class differences'.
>
> (Beattie, 1993, Workbook 3, Part 1: 16)

**What might be the significance of dividing people on the basis of social class rather
than lifestyle?**

Many of you, mindful of the Acheson Report and the discussion of the
social determinants of health discussed in Chapter 3 might think that
social class is a very appropriate way of dividing up the health market
given that it is a powerful indicator of health status. This raises the
question about the unequal choices available to the different classes and
therefore the appropriateness of any health messages in the face of, for
instance, poverty and unemployment.

Problems and possibilities with social marketing

Tones and Tilford (1994) have pointed out some of the differences
between commercial marketing and marketing for health. One of the most
obvious differences and one which puts health marketing at a serious
disadvantage is the difference in the nature of the product on offer. As
they say, 'health education is frequently trying to sell a product which
commercial advertisers would consider no one in their right minds would

buy'. Persuading people to stop doing something pleasurable for a rather intangible gain sometime in the future might feel daunting even to the most optimistic advertising professional. In fact Chapman and Eggar (1993: 226) believe that 'future rewards for current deprivations' is the antithesis of the essence of advertising. On the other hand, what people say they want more than anything is good health and a sense of well-being. Perhaps there is sometimes a problem with the credibility of the product. It is getting people to believe that stopping smoking, running two miles everyday, eating fruit and veg etc. will buy them a long and healthy life. Yet commercial advertisers use health unashamedly to sell their own particular products. Supermarkets are full of products with a health promise. There has been a boom in sports clothing which sells a healthy image and the exercise bike manufacturers have done very well out of selling health and fitness. Beattie argues that the problem is that much official health education is dull and negative with an unappetising emphasis on the 'reduction of risk' (1993: 18). He cites the work of Nick Dorn and his colleagues at the Institute for the Study of Drug Dependence in London who have begun to take seriously the importance of pleasure and solace in the health field. Working with youth sub-cultures they recognise the positive elements to many young people of drug and alcohol use and the association of risk with adventure and 'status achievement'. They claim that health promotion has paid insufficient attention to these perceived positive elements. Chapman and Eggar argue that cigarette advertising has successfully created powerful mythological images which have great appeal to adolescents and that the task for health education is to develop an equally appealing mythology around non-smoking.

Tones and Tilford (1994) draw attention to another important distinction between commercial advertising and advertising for health which is a concern with ethical considerations. This must remain high on the health agenda but is less of a constraint on commercial advertising. Rosalind Coward has described food advertising of the 'naughty but nice' variety as a 'pornography of food' (1984: 99) which exploits desire. The portrayal of women as sexual objects in much commercial advertising has long been attacked by feminists. Although we have advertising standards and the Trades Description Act, commercial advertising is, as they say, often 'economical with the truth'.

Another problem with marketing health is that there are very few simple messages. The choice on offer is rarely: stop doing this and you will be healthy, carry on and you will suffer a long and horrible decline. Even if it were, there are ethical problems with creating anxiety and threatening people with a fate worse than death. There is also the issue which we keep coming back to in this book of the context in which you are asking people to make health choices. Persuading them to give up smoking when they live next to a major trunk road might seem pointless. So is urging someone to change their diet when they have very little money or urging old people to wear woolly hats when they need a proper income to afford reasonable heating. However this is precisely why the social marketeers would urge audience segmentation – to make sure that the message does not fall on stony ground because the consumer has very limited choice.

The expectations for health marketing are infinitely more ambitious than most commercial advertising. As Tones and Tilford say in comparing health and commercial advertising:

> The behavioural response is relatively simple – the purchase of a product which in all probability differs from previously purchased products only in its packaging, physical or psychological. Health education seeks to change deeply seated attitudes and even values and sometimes to produce the adoption of often complex behaviours.
>
> (Tones and Tilford, 1994: 189)

One of the ways that social marketing tries to overcome some of the difficulties raised above is through pre-testing. Pre-testing is used in two ways. Firstly to test the characteristics of the audience and their needs. This is part of audience segmentation. Secondly to test the content of the programme and its mode of presentation.

Hastings and Haywood (1991) give some examples. The Forth Valley Health Board in Scotland commissioned the Advertising Research Unit to find out about teenagers' understandings of AIDS and what, if any, information they thought they needed. The research showed that the teenagers had a good theoretical grasp of the transmission of HIV and the risks of unprotected sex but they were unconfident about putting safer sex into practice. They wanted help with the practical problems of actually buying and using condoms and discussing this with a potential sexual partner. The message was that they, the Forth Valley Health Board, should concentrate on promoting safer sexual skills rather than raising awareness.

Pre-testing the actual content of the programme might involve showing a draft, if it is written material, or a preview of a film or TV programme to a group of the target audience for their comments. The Scottish Health Education Group (SHEG), the predecessor of the Health Education Board for Scotland (HEBS), did this when developing a contraceptive campaign aimed at young people. They asked a group of young people to consider two versions of the proposed campaign. One stressed the negative effects of not using contraception, i.e. the threat of unwanted pregnancy. The other presented some positive effects, such as enjoying a more fulfilled relationship because the anxiety was taken out of the activity. The teenage girls were initially more impressed with the negative approach but changed their preference for the more positive approach when presented with the material.

Another important use of testing is of the medium through which the message is being promoted. It was suggested that a popular cartoon character at the time called 'Judge Dredd' would provide a good vehicle for drugs education material. On consulting teenagers this idea was rapidly abandoned as they were scathing of the character: they found him ridiculous and he had no base in reality for them (Hasting and Haywood, 1991: 142). But the right role model can be effective. Jones and Davies

(1996) found that many of the 10 and 11 year old boys interviewed in their study saw Mr Motivator, who appears on breakfast television, as an appropriate role model in relation to physical fitness.

Much of what we have been discussing has been in the context of rather large-scale national campaigns, although the techniques of social marketing apply to all levels of campaigns. However in order to use the techniques one has to have access to the various media and clearly this is less of a problem for the national health education authorities. What about the more local campaign, the ones that health workers may be involved in?

11.5 Access to local media

Although access to national media may be beyond most people's reach, local radio and TV certainly is not and local newspapers, magazines and journals are all accessible. Poster and leafleting campaigns are also methods of reaching a wider audience than are face-to-face contacts. What skills are needed both to gain access to and use these various media to best effect?

Making it on local media

What do you think might be appropriate formats on local radio, TV and in local newspapers which can be used for health education?

News items are regularly put out by most local radio and TV stations. It costs nothing to get a health education item or event mentioned in a news bulletin and it gives widespread coverage. There is usually a spot on local media for public announcements and this can be another source of free exposure. Health is often a favourite topic for discussion programmes on radio or TV or in the features section of a newspaper, especially if it is an issue which is topical. Phone-in programmes on radio and TV and the 'letters to the editor' page present another opportunity to have one's say. A feature or letter should be written simply and not in a literary style, long sentences should be avoided and simple words are better than technical terms or abbreviations.

Interviews and topic-specific documentaries can also focus on a health topic. Journalists and broadcasters in a local area are always looking for interesting issues. The usual way to inform the media of a special event or campaign is to prepare a press release giving the following information:

• what will be happening – a description of the event with the main interest first and details of important people participating

- why it is taking place with background details
- where it is to take place with precise details of how to get there
- when it will take place with date and time of day
- a contact address and telephone number.

If the local media responds with an invitation to do an interview then it is vital to be well prepared, to be clear and concise, and have just a few main points to put across. The language needs to be simple but interesting, with examples and human stories if possible. It is always a good idea to agree the questions beforehand if an interview is live (Hubley, 1993).

11.6 Interactive multi-media health education in the twenty-first century

Today some sophisticated technology is becoming available to health promoters which can be used in exciting and interactive ways. The potential benefit of multi-media applications and packages is that they can facilitate interactivity or two-way communication between the computer and the user. This means that the multi-media applications are under the control of the user. He or she can move through the programme in a non-linear way, stop and start as he or she pleases, skim through some parts yet dig deeper into others, repeat sections and check understandings. Leonard (1995), quoting evidence from the British Audio Visual Society, claims that adding a 'doing' element to hearing, reading and seeing significantly increases what we remember. John Catford (1995) has predicted that the 'couch potato' will become a 'power potato' as consumers gain increasing power over the media with which they wish to engage.

A multi-media package usually contains a mixture of text, sound, graphics, and still and moving pictures controlled through a computer programme. Many people now have the facility to use CD-ROM (Compact Disk Read Only Memory) in the home and increasingly multi-media packages are being developed for this use. No doubt the time will come when every home will have one. The metaphor of a book still dominates the production of multi-media packages. Leonard (1995: 25) maintains that 'we first seek to apply a new medium in terms of an established one' and books are what we know. So multi-media educational packages are often organised into chapters and pages. The metaphor of a menu is used to access these chapters and pages, with menus dividing into sub-menus.

The notion of interactivity needs to be examined and questions asked about whether the new 'power potato' is absorbing the information available. It has been suggested that the encouragement to pick and choose from a menu or click on a topic area actually impedes creative involvement. A recent survey of American teenagers found that the habit of 'grazing' or flicking through the channels resulted in about half never seeing a TV programme through from beginning to end (Leonard 1995: 26). Tony Feldman, a specialist in electronic media publishing warns that multi-media interactivity tends to fragment the user's experience:

> Instead of contributing a spellbinding quality, interactivity interrupts, asks questions or offers choices to which the user must respond. The lack of continuity and the liberty given to the user to choose new directions make it difficult to maintain an underlying coherence. The user's 'freedom' robs multi-media of the storytelling qualities essential to good communication.
>
> Interactivity may be the key to multi-media's future but perhaps we still need to learn how to use it to produce experiences that enrich the hearts as well as the minds of users.
>
> (Feldman, 1992, quoted in Leonard, 1995: 25, 26)

Health information can be communicated and disseminated to the general public in a number of new ways: using stand-alone applications such as computer applications on floppy disks, CD-ROM and video/laser disk; and on-line applications such as the internet (Kolasa and Miller, 1996). Health education materials have been produced on interactive CD-ROMs. For example 'Sex Get Serious', a CD-ROM on sex education produced by a sexual health project in Sandwell, was developed with and for young people. Similar interactive resources have been developed on a range of topics by a number of different agencies and provide materials which young people can access and work through in their own way and at their own pace.

Some health authorities have developed health information kiosks with readily available computer-based systems which provide health informa-tion to the general public. While kiosks facilitate access to health information, they can only be useful to individuals if they are in prominent places. They also need to be seen to be providing a level of confidentiality and privacy to individuals using them to seek/acquire information. Ensuring confidentiality for users, however, prevents any evaluation of the effectiveness of the system for the individual – if you don't know who the users are, there can't be any follow-up.

The internet links up or interconnects computers from all parts of the world. The World Wide Web (WWW, often shortened to Web) is the fastest growing internet service. The Web pulls together vast amounts of information provided by different people in different countries using different computer systems. The Web's main potential is that it offers the capability to disseminate health information.

There are several ways individuals and/or professionals can access a multi-media computer if they do not have their own personal means of access. Internet and cyber cafés are becoming a popular way for members of the public to access the Web and to use interactive health resources.

Although vast amounts of health information are now disseminated through the Web, a difficulty individuals may have when trying to access this information is that the information on the Web varies considerably.

At present it is very easy to publish on the Web; there are no publishing standards, and the information contained in Web pages is not refereed in any way. Therefore any content, brilliant or nonsensical, can be made available. Web page appearance seems to influence readers and Web page design is a burgeoning area of research in its own right. Excellent Web page design can make useless information look attractive, while excellent material in a poorly designed Web page will not stimulate users to stop and read (Dix *et al.*, 1998).

Health information on the internet reflects the broad definitions of health in both its provision and current knowledge. People who use the internet can obtain detailed health information which includes clinical expertise in the tradition of western medicine, the uses of complementary therapies and contact with support networks. Some members of the health professions are critical of the diversity of this information, claiming that it is potentially confusing to lay people. There is, however, contrary evidence, which suggests that users are quite capable of discriminating between conflicting information (Hardey, 1998).

Not only are the users able to discriminate between conflicting information, they appear to welcome information about non-orthodox approaches to health. Some of the people in Hardey's study used information from the internet to renegotiate treatment from their GP.

Each of the health promotion agencies in the UK has its own website: the Health Development Agency has a website which provides a health promotion information service . The Health Education Board for Scotland (HEBS) also has its own health promotion site (HEBSWeb). The site contains more than 25,000 pages of health information; topics covered include information on self-help groups for anything from anorexia to psoriasis, cancer, smoking, stroke, mental health, health statistics, diet, and research (Campbell, 1997). The Health Promotion Division of the National Assembly for Wales has a national health promotion web site for Wales and there is a website for the National Health Promotion Agency for Northern Ireland. These websites provide health information for members of the public and professionals who promote health. In addition, the agencies have also developed specific websites on particular topics. For example, Health Promotion: England, which was established at the same time as the Health Development Agency, has a remit to provide health promotion programmes on drugs, alcohol, sexual health, older people and children and families. It has specific websites on alcohol, drugs and sexual health where members of the public can obtain appropriate health information and advice.

A serious criticism of current users of the internet is that they are mostly educated middle-class people, but in the future digital television will provide much wider and more diverse public access to medical and other health information.

Digital television has been proposed as the next technological innovation to change our lives. Digital television will merge television technology with networked computing capabilities. This will enable information to be delivered directly into people's homes. While this type of technology will widen access, there will still be a cost to individuals in that they will need to replace their current television equipment with digital television equipment, so it may not be available to all members of the public. Also the advent of digital television with the subsequent proliferation of channels means that the appeal of national television to health promoters may lessen with the size of the audiences.

There are a number of health organisations, both statutory and voluntary, which provide telephone helplines on a range of topics from giving up smoking to advice on sexual health and HIV/AIDS. Some of these helplines provide information in a number of different languages. A further initiative developed by the Department of Health, to provide professional advice and information to the population, is NHS Direct, a nurse-led telephone and Internet helpline. This is presently being evaluated to establish which sections of the public use it and the accuracy and consistency of information that is given.

11.7 Conclusion

Catford (1995) notes that we are rapidly becoming a networked society and will be able to communicate anything, anywhere at anytime. Good communication and an ability to develop a rapport and understand the perspective of the 'other' are common elements, whatever the medium.

The appetite for health information and programmes is ever growing. CNN puts a high priority on health news items and a 24-hour health channel is being considered in the US (Catford, 1995). There are tremendous opportunities but also potential dangers. The question of regulation looms, who or what will prevent misinformation on health matters being conveyed by vested interests? The opportunities presented by new technology not only require that attention is paid to the way we communicate health messages, it puts even greater emphasis on the need to be scrupulous about the quality of the information and to evaluate the outcomes. A recent review of research literature on information and communication technology (ICT) in health promotion documented a number of research projects which are trying to evaluate the uses of ICT and reported on projects concerned with the development of codes of conduct for the health/medical domain on the internet (HEBS, 1999). The next two parts of this book explore the issues of information and evaluation.

Part 3
Investigating health information

The road leading to Health For All by the Year 2000 passes through information.

(World Health Organisation)

Introduction

This part explores the nature of health information and its relevance to promoting health. The chapters consider:

- sources of and influences upon health information
- the disciplines whereby information is gathered and made available
- ways in which numerical data is obtained and presented
- the process of planning interventions.

In this part you will explore the different routes to health information and consider the various kinds of available data. Many conflicting interests are at stake. These are explored in Chapter 12 using the example of BSE (mad cow disease) to illustrate the confusion generated by different interest groups presenting contradictory data. This highlights some of the dilemmas faced by those promoting health when providing or deciphering health information. You thus explore the difficulties we all face in interpreting information as relevant, honest or useful.

Many health promotion interventions are based on data generated through the disciplines of demography and epidemiology so it is important to understand the principles which govern them. Both rely on statistics and the presentation of numerical data. Chapter 14 explores the use of statistical data for health promotion and illustrates the importance of presenting information in ways that are accessible to non-experts and minimise the risks of misinterpretation.

Chapter 15 weighs up the considerations to be taken into account when planning interventions. Clearly, accurately assessing need is essential. But this begs the question about whose needs count. The chapter emphasises the importance of consulting as widely as possible before planning any health promotion intervention so that the needs of those likely to be affected are fully represented. The chapter then explores the different stages of the process of planning interventions and some of the likely pitfalls and limitations. It lays the groundwork for Part 4 which examines in detail a crucial component of any health promotion intervention, evaluation.

Chapter 12
What counts as evidence in health information?

12.1 Introduction: the nature of evidence

The modern world may be characterised by an emphasis on rationality and a belief in science and scientific method. Since the Enlightenment people have been concerned about free will and a desire to control the environment and find explanations for all aspects of life through the use of human reason. This desire to understand and therefore control all aspects of life resulted in the elevation of science and the expectation that it would provide answers to all questions. In the late twentieth century, however, there has been a questioning of modernist assumptions both about the role of science and rationality. 'Post-modern' critics have argued that our contemporary society is characterised not by order and reason but by chaos, fragmentation, diversity and irrationality. White suggests that:

> ... our modernity is driven by phenomena that are not easily comprehended within familiar cognitive and social structures.
>
> (White, 1991)

This view replaces one which saw the world as waiting to be discovered and an assumption that one truth would replace another. Whereas modernist science searches for the 'truth', post-modern critics argue that there are pluralist explanations (Williams and Popay, 1995) and that there are ambiguities and uncertainties in our world. According to the post-modern view, truth is not unidimensional, and scientific knowledge as an example can be interpreted with equal justification in a variety of ways by different people and different groups. Aaron Wildavsky, who was concerned to establish the facts about different environmental issues, suggested that:

> It may appear that there is no truth to discover, that there are no clear-cut facts, or that the evidence supports several sides of the question. Perhaps the feeling of uneasiness engendered by the word 'truth' comes from the belief that there is no reconciling the conflicting interpretations of the evidence. Perhaps. But there is no knowing until we try to find the facts that are there.
>
> (Wildavsky, 1995: 5)

This offers a helpful way forward. While it may be impossible to learn the one 'truth' and necessary to accept that there are many different truths, it is equally important to gather and test evidence rather than simply relying on opinion and personal preference.

Why do health promoters require sound and reliable health information?

Reliable health information is essential for health promoters as the basis for multisectoral strategy development and planning services and interventions arising, including health promotion campaigns. If a particular campaign is aimed at the local population to change their lifestyles in some way, for example eat 'healthier food', then this needs to be grounded in information that is reliable and accessible both to the health promoter and the lay public. An example might be a campaign directed at supermarkets to adequately label food: evidence of the dangers of certain frequently-used additives would strengthen the case. The health promoter might be concerned to get the local authority to adopt a transport policy which involves setting up environmental areas, traffic calming schemes or traffic-free roads – to support this case the health promoter would need reliable evidence indicating the local dangers and, for example, might want substantive evidence linking asthma and the atmosphere (Ayres, 1994). Increasingly, health promoters are working in partnership with a range of organisations and evidence is required by all of them before strategies are developed and implemented. Hence, in most aspects of their work, health promoters need to be able to substantiate their arguments with 'indisputable facts'.

But, as noted above, the interpretation of these facts is multi-faceted in the same way as there are many accounts of what constitutes health (Chapter 2). People attribute a variety of meanings to different aspects of health. There are clearly no hard and fast 'truths' and this is a 'slippery' area, one in which health promoters are likely to find themselves grappling with confusing information and possibly contradictory advice. Health promoters will also be concerned to know why the information was produced and who paid for it – the impetus for investigating health issues may come from a number of sources: manufacturers concerned to reassure the public about the safety of their products or the public or pressure groups demanding investigations into the safety of particular food products, or the risks of global warming and the relationship to the incidence of skin cancer.

What constitutes health information, and what counts as reliable evidence?

Health information emanates from a wide range of endeavours and disciplines. These include medical research, the psychological and social sciences, as well as the biological, agricultural and environmental sciences. Health data comes from many different sources including directly or indirectly from major national agencies, for example the Department of Health or the Health Development Agency and other national health promotion agencies. These may be published by The Stationery Office, for example the COMA (Committee on Medical Aspects of Food Policy) reports. The Office for National Statistics and other organisations commissioned by central and local government and health authorities produce reports, surveys and authoritative journal articles describing different accounts of health issues. New Public Health Observatories have been established in each NHS region and are key sources of collated local information on public health. In addition, many lobbying organisations, consumer groups, charities and voluntary organisations also produce material, for example Friends of the Earth. Information available includes details of how one population's health differs from another; perceived health risks from certain activities, for example sunbathing or exposure to pollen, or foods such as contaminated lamb following Chernobyl or salmonella in eggs. It also describes the incidence of certain infectious diseases, or may indicate how people have contracted the current flu epidemic or die of hypothermia.

Those collecting information may have a bias the nature or extent of which may be difficult to ascertain. The information may be interpreted in a number of ways; this may depend on the method of collecting the information and also external as well as internal influences. These influences may determine whether further investigation is warranted or whether the data is neglected or even repressed. Various agencies, government departments, pressure groups, lay people, health professionals and the media will interpret the findings. These agencies have their own agenda which will determine the slant they use and how they present it to others. That is why any agency promoting health or behaviour change from the standpoint of 'independent expert' must maintain its credibility and be seen to be acting independently, providing reliable and trustworthy advice.

The whole population uses current information to make individual and collective choices as well as assess the risk involved in undertaking certain kinds of behaviour, and public interest in assessing risk is growing (Beck, 1992). Two types of risk need to be highlighted: risk perceptions and risk consequences (Wildavsky, 1995). *Risk perception* means that, given the same evidence, two people might view the dangers very differently. In Chapter 9 you looked at models of behaviour change and the perception of risk. This chapter focuses on the difficulties of assessing the *risk consequences*. How can people assess the likely consequences of embarking on a certain behaviour, for example how dangerous is sunbathing? Risk consequences are 'the actual effects of engaging in certain activities or being exposed to certain substances' (Wildavsky, 1995: 5).

Wildavsky sought to understand the relationship between environmental health and safety issues. He recruited a number of students to look at all the accounts of particular episodes when environmental issues posed risks to different populations. These accounts are found in his book entitled *'But is it true?'* He set his students a number of research tasks suggesting a range of particular questions which are equally applicable to investigating health information. Each student was assigned a particular issue and expected to:

> ... read the scientific literature, find as much of the truth as possible, and appraise the relationship between knowledge and action.
>
> (Wildavsky, 1995: 4)

Sorting out what is truth and what is not, and indeed if there is a universal truth, is in itself problematic as we have seen. Large sections of the scientific community have for much of the twentieth century been engaged in investigating truths (Medawar, 1984), which often are superseded by new truths as they are 'discovered'. These claims, whilst often sincere, may conflict with other scientists' standpoints as well as those from people and groups not associated with the scientific community who may feel that they hold equally valid views.

Wildavsky wanted to know the competing views of different claimants. His students were set the following questions:

- What were the original claims?
- What was known about their validity at the time they were made?
- What did the newspapers and news magazines write?
- Did they diminish the force of the claims, present them as received, or increase their seriousness?
- What did the government do?
- What was the claims' scientific rationale and how well did that rationale hold up in the face of existing knowledge?

These questions were to be re-examined as new legislation was passed or regulations suggested, to look at the different permutations of how the knowledge was transmitted and actions taken. Had action and knowledge come closer together or grown further apart? And, finally, as knowledge grows, does it point in the direction of greater or lesser harm than originally envisaged?

When confronted with contradictory evidence from a variety of sources it is hard to know what evidence to believe and which authoritative sources provide reliable and trustworthy evidence. Many people are concerned about the safety of food products. As health promoters you make personal choices about what food is safe as well as having to answer the questions of the people you deal with.

12.2 Influences on health information: a case study

If 'truth' can be interpreted in many ways, one must therefore be vigilant about health messages. Keeping Wildavsky's questions in mind, this will now be illustrated through exploring the sources and nature of the evidence regarding the risks of eating British beef during December 1995.

This case study highlights the problems about knowing the nature of scientific 'truths' and the status of lay information and gut feeling.

In the spring of 1996 British beef was subject to a world-wide ban and international media attention following the deaths of a number of young people in Britain from CJD (Creutzfeldt-Jakob disease – the equivalent of mad cow disease in humans). The BSE/CJD debate neatly illustrates the issues already raised about the nature of truth and the shortcomings of scientific knowledge. It also demonstrates the gap between lay perceptions of what is safe and 'scientific evidence' which in the case of the link between BSE and CJD patently demonstrated the disagreements among scientists.

The debate concerned the 'evidence' that several people died of CJD in the UK and the 'connection' between eating beef and beef products (including beef derivatives) and contracting this disease. Many agencies, organisations and pressure groups all with their own agendas continue to contribute to this debate. Receiving contradictory messages from different sources makes understanding the evidence very complicated.

Since 1986 when BSE (bovine spongiform encephalopathy), also known as 'mad cow disease', was first identified debates have raged over a possible link between eating infected beef and the risk of contracting CJD. The round of discussions that you will follow here began in December 1995, when concern about the safety of British beef was publicised by the media, rekindling the 1986 debate. As you read through a few selective but, as far as possible, representative accounts that appeared in the national and scientific press during that period, recall Wildavsky's instructions to his students. Ask yourself whether it is indeed possible to make sense out of the contradictory evidence. The first article, an editorial in the *Independent*, raises questions about the truth of a range of health advice provided to the public:

To beef or not to beef ...

Ministers tell us that beef products are absolutely safe. There is, says the Health Secretary, Stephen Dorrell, 'no conceivable risk' to the public; he would let his own children eat hamburgers. Dr Kenneth Calman, the Chief Medical Officer, would be happy to join them.

Yet the prospect of bumping into either of them in McDonald's is not wholly reassuring. Despite their advice, more and more people are giving up eating beef products for fear that they might become infected with a human form of BSE, better known as mad cow disease. Some are abstaining quietly and privately. Others are more public, with some parents insisting that beef should be taken off the school dinner menu. A number of eminent scientists have announced that they have given up pies and burgers which might contain offal. We may be on the brink of a panic that could severely damage the beef industry.

The problem is that we do not know whom to believe: the scaremongers, the worried scientists or statements from Whitehall. In the past we would have accepted the word of a health secretary. But respect for politicians has sunk so low that their every utterance is regarded with cynicism.

Governments, after all, have an unreliable record when it comes to protecting public health. Recently, on the positive side, this particular administration was quick to go public on the dangers posed by certain types of contraceptive pill. Thousands of women switched brands in a matter of weeks. But the same government has also refused to order a total ban on the advertising of cigarettes, the only product which, if used according to the makers' specifications, is likely to kill.

Such a ban might damage tax revenue from cigarettes. Likewise, anything less than trenchant backing for the beef industry could lead to a sudden collapse of confidence in its products. No government wants to be held responsible for killing off a major British industry.

In short, there are plenty of reasons for doubting ministers when they express their love for hamburgers. That is why we need an independent assessment of the dangers posed to humans by BSE in cattle.

There is already an advisory group, comprising respectable scientists, which briefs the Government and the public on the threat. It has been more equivocal than Mr Dorrell about the risks, warning that it may be several years until complete reassurance can be given. But however earnest and conscientious this advisory body is, it can never command the trust of the public. It is simply too close to the Government.

A Royal commission, with statutory powers, independent of the Ministry of Agriculture, should be established to give us a trustworthy picture of beef's safety. Its brief could be widened to cover other foods. Such a commission might not be able to provide all the answers. But at least everyone could make as informed a choice as possible before deciding their future eating habits.

(*Independent*, 6 December 1995)

The same day, the *Guardian* reported that a nutritional specialist was warning that small children should not eat beef products for fear of contamination with BSE. This nutritionist (who stopped eating beef six years ago) suggested that 'parents with "niggling doubts" about beef safety [should] buy only certified organic beef'. It continued:

His comments will disconcert the meat industry and the Department of Health, after brain surgeon Sir Bernard Tomlinson's declaration that he would no longer eat beef products such as beefburgers. He called for the sale of beef offal to be banned ... Comments from such authoritative sources have caused a wave of concern among parents, who are pressing local education authorities and schools to drop beefburgers and sausages from school menus. Oldham and Humberside responded yesterday by dropping beef from their schools.

(*Guardian*, 6 December 1995: 5)

The Meat and Livestock Commission responded with full page advertisements in national newspapers quoting reassurances from the Chief Medical Officer. One large multi-national marketing beef products went further, warranting the headline 'Food giant may sue BBC in beef scare' (*Independent*, 7 December 1995).

A BBC radio helpline had advised callers to avoid meat pies, sausages, beefburgers and beef stock. The managing director of a large multinational company (CPC) accused the BBC helpline of 'complete and utter irresponsibility'. CPC said that 'Bovril beef drink and stock do not contain any of the materials that the Ministry of Agriculture, Fisheries and Food has banned'. The same story maintained that the junior health minister, Angela Browning, was disturbed that the BBC was advising consumers to avoid beef. The government's view was consistent throughout the reporting, regardless of the department affiliation – government officials continued to eat beef and maintained that there was no scientific evidence of a link between BSE and CJD. The *Independent* reported that the government was on the offensive to 'bolster beef's public image'. The Meat and Livestock Commission blamed public fears over BSE for the slide in beef sales.

However, the government's position was countered by 'scientific evidence from the nutritional specialist and bolstered up by comments from eminent scientists. One from Leicester University suggested that:

> There is a grand experiment going on in Britain with BSE with us as the laboratory animals.

The broadsheet newspapers, including the *Financial Times*, felt that the BSE situation should be clarified and resolved by reliable authorities and agreed that government statements were not trustworthy. Yet they noted that there were discrepancies in the views of scientists and published conflicting evidence. The eminent neurophysiologist Colin Blakemore proclaimed that recent causes of the human equivalent of BSE in Britain 'most definitely do not support Stephen Dorrell's statement... that there is no conceivable risk of BSE being transmitted from cows to people'. Blakemore claimed:

> This statement revealed ... much about the lamentable ignorance of scientific methods and elementary statistics among British politicians.

However, despite the sparse evidence, Blakemore suggests that:

> Given the quagmire of slim evidence and contradictory opinion, what should the meat-loving public do? Stay calm; do not eat beef pies, burgers or sausages; consider giving up all beef until the picture is clearer; listen to the scientists. And the Government should learn that if it continues to betray its ignorance of the concept of risk by transforming cautious scientific and medical advice into categorical reassurances, which it subsequently has to withdraw, the public will rightly become increasingly distrustful of anything it says.
>
> (*Independent*, 7 December 1995)

This view was challenged the following day by an equally authoritative account from another eminent scientist, Robert Will, the head of the CJD Surveillance Unit at the Western General Hospital in Edinburgh. Will maintained that he and his team continued to consume beef and beef products because their research suggested that the chances of BSE crossing from animals to humans is minimal. He could not explain the occurrence of CJD in four farmers but maintained that no evidence supported the argument that these farmers might have contracted the disease from their animals. There are too few cases to assess the significance of minor changes. However, Robert Will was concerned that the SBO (specified bovine offals) ban, introduced in 1989, is applied rigorously. This ensured that brain and spinal cord, together with other tissues that might theoretically contain significant infestivity, are excluded from the human food chain.

By the third day, the Prime Minister was reported again in the *Independent* to have once more provided reassurances for the public in the House of Commons where he stated:

> There is currently no scientific evidence that BSE can be transmitted to humans or that eating beef causes CJD. That issue is not in question.
> (*Independent*, 8 December 1995).

This article also reported that the government's reassurances were futile with over a thousand schools either cutting beef out of school meals or offering alternatives. At this point the National Consumer Council entered the debate, suggesting that tighter controls be introduced into abattoirs to reduce the risk of infection spreading in meat. The spokesperson from the independent food watchdog, the Food Commission, corroborated Blakemore's argument – that the government seemed more concerned in propping up the beef industry than *admitting that there may be a risk, however small it might be.*

From these extracts you may have noted several different points of view: those of competing scientists, government departments, parents, pressure groups, other media and nutritionists. This example illustrates overtly the conflicts between different interest groups in presenting information about BSE. This problem remains until *universally trusted* scientific conclusions confirm or deny the BSE/CJD link. But in the meantime, the debates rage with the meat industry's interests on the one hand, supported by government sources, and the public health and consumer interests on the other hand with the scientists down the middle.

These debates illustrate the flimsy evidence underpinning assessment of health risks and the difficulty of making informed choice. They also illustrate external pressures on scientific endeavour. Richard Lacey was unable to continue with 'crucial' BSE/CJD research because pressure from the food industry led to withdrawal of his financial support. This raises an important issue regarding general information available to the public – why, since the deregulation of the food industry, have naturally herbivorous cattle been fed with animal offal? Could their change in diet and exposure to new foodstuffs be a contributing factor in contracting BSE?

In the BSE debate, what might count as good information?

The BSE/CJD debacle raised the question of reliable and trustworthy information nationally. Wildavsky's model illustrated the differences between risk perceptions and risk consequences. This raises concern about what is good information and what is bad information. It is apparent that information is controlled and repressed by the government, scientific research institutes and by the media. The Consumer Association goes further:

> The Government's scientific advisers have said the risk from eating beef is *likely* to be extremely small *if* Government controls introduced in 1989 were properly enforced. The problem is, we know that, in the past, government controls *haven't* been enforced. This means that, currently, there is an unquantifiable risk in eating beef: there's no scientific evidence available to us of just how great the risk is.
>
> (*Which?*, May 1996: 58)

Which?, as it has done for years, continues to argue for more accurate labelling to identify food containing beef products, further research to develop a BSE test for live animals, and an *independent* food agency as the Ministry of Agriculture, Fisheries and Food currently represents farmers and manufacturers as well as consumers. A Food Standards Agency was set up in April 2000 to protect the public from risk associated with the consumption of food and to protect the interests of consumers generally in relation to food. However, critics query whether it is truly independent.

Thus the information available is hard to digest – the scientific basis for the opposing contentions, for example *how* scientists differ regarding the link between the bovine disease and its human equivalent, was not clear. If people who enjoy eating beef have to give it up, they then need to have reliable information upon which to assess the risk and the likely consequences. Reading these extracts may make you feel angry or frustrated that the issues about BSE are still unresolved. But this situation of uncertainty applies to concerns about risks of eating other food products, for example food containing raw eggs (for vulnerable people or pregnant women) or non-pasteurised milk products (goats milk's cheese), both of which have been infected with types of salmonella (Rampling, 1996: 67-68). Wildavsky (1995) highlighted the diversity of people's perceptions of risk. These differences may relate to whether the individuals are exposed to lay or professional types of information.

12.3 Lay and professional perspectives

The BSE case study suggests that different accounts can be packaged as authoritative without being regarded as such by the scientific community. In particular, it suggests that scientific truths are only one kind of evidence and that a range of other expert and lay groups – politicians, news reporters, consumer associations – may hold conflicting views and may offer different advice. It is thus important to explore the differences and similarities between the lay and expert views of health information. In Chapter 2 you examined the social model of health. This incorporates lay perspectives on health and moves beyond a 'medical' view of health to encompass the social and environmental causes of ill health. In doing so, it acknowledges the importance of considering lay peoples' views about health and illness.

Give some examples of lay remedies for medical conditions and assess what they have in common.

Lay knowledge includes medical knowledge acquired through life experience or encounters with health practitioners. Lay advice is particularly relevant where medical knowledge is limited or where the health problem is a low priority for the medical establishment. Examples include wearing copper bracelets for 'rheumatic' complaints, eating live yogurt for thrush or drinking lemon barley water for kidney problems. Chapter 2 demonstrated that lay explanations for health conditions and suggestions about remedies abound in most cultures in many forms. Lay knowledge about health has been powerful for centuries in most societies but with increased medicalisation it has lost some of its influence. But not entirely, as lay experts are even today in western societies given access to media airwaves to express their views on a number of health problems such as allergies.

The medical profession may devalue lay knowledge because in many instances it has not been subject to rigorous scientific research, quantified or included in textbooks (for example, Freidson, 1975). However, this includes many current medical procedures which appear to be effective but the scientific explanation is not yet established, for example electro-convulsive therapy (ECT) for depression. Lay knowledge is generally not seen as credible because it is perceived to derive primarily from personal (or someone else's, even over many generations) *experience* and as such does not have the medical imprimatur. Yet lay knowledge is not universally discounted and indeed some lay or complementary medicine remedies have been adopted and adapted by conventional medicine, for example digitalis (from the purple foxglove plant) which is used for heart disease. Indeed, it can be argued that the overlap between lay and expert knowledge is considerable (Cornwell, 1984; Morgan *et al.*, 1985).

Acting on lay knowledge may not find favour with health workers. As Stacey (1994) points out, for many doctors and nurses lay knowledge is seen as leading to non-compliance. This may be seen in the number of people who do not attend outpatient appointments, do not complete their course of prescribed tablets, or do not attend child health clinics. But as Stacey points out:

... not taking your child to the cold and draughty health clinic on a pouring wet day is health-giving rather than health-denying. That's part of the intelligent use of lay knowledge.

(Stacey, 1994: 85)

Lay knowledge is not a monolithic entity, but diverse and shifting. The BSE debate showed the professional authorities speaking with different voices and contradicting one another. Lay people also speak with different voices. In some cases lay views are at odds with health information. For example, thousands of shoppers purchased beef at reduced prices just after the international ban on British beef in 1996, whereas the Consumer Association advice was

... if you want to avoid the risk from BSE-infected beef altogether, there's no choice but to cut out beef from your diet.

(*Which?* May 1996: 58)

Differing perceptions of risk create conflict between lay people and professional bodies. The link between hyperactivity in children and food additives is an example. Parents who associated their children's hyper-activity with artificial food additives such as tartrazine found professionals unsympathetic and even hostile. Medical opposition identified incon-clusive experimental evidence linking behavioural change to food additives whilst many parents claim success using exclusion diets. Personal, lay experience here, as elsewhere, outweighs the conflicting 'official' information (Turney, 1994). This led to the establishment of a self-help group for parents of hyperactive children which publishes reports of supportive research and sponsors its own research findings (Hyperactive Children's Support Group (HCSG), 1992). Although the medical establish-ment is still sceptical of a link, support for the parents has come from individual doctors (disagreeing with their colleagues), complementary therapists and nurses. Like BSE, experimental trials are hard to conduct and consequently lay and professional opinions differ. In this example, health information provides no convincing evidence and each side reports the data that supports their arguments. An interesting by-product of this controversy has been the removal or substitution of food additives by manufacturers because of consumer pressure, without clear scientific evidence of links to ill health. The conflict for nurses (and dietitians) involved in community healthy eating programmes is summed up by the following quote:

Additives and colourings certainly seem to have a link with hyperactivity for some children and there is a lot of evidence to support the influence that diet can have on behaviour, but if nurses do not know enough about this area then they should be given extra training to update them as a part of their continuing professional development.

(Sarah Tooley, senior nurse, Women's Nutritional Advisory Service)

Another example of lay perspectives challenging what is believed to be 'accurate', relates to the evidence produced by the anti-smoking lobby. Some groups of lay people are not convinced that smoking kills and/or causes morbidity. The promoters of the annual No Smoking Day hope to convince smokers to kick the habit. In 1995 the publicity for this was meant to shock. John Cleese starred in a commercial in which he is shown shouting at an armchair about how 'you have ruined my life, tried to strangle me, made me miserable' and so on, and eventually takes out a gun, points it at the armchair and as viewers steel themselves expecting him to shoot his wife, he shoots a packet of cigarettes instead – a very powerful image to convince the viewer that cigarettes ruin lives. Government health warnings about the dangers of smoking are displayed on every packet of cigarettes. Findings published in the *British Medical Journal* and reprinted in the popular press suggest that the dangers of smoking are such that smokers in Britain are now entitled to get legal aid to sue tobacco manufacturers for shortening their lives: 'Claimants suffer from a range of illnesses related to smoking, including circulatory diseases; cardiovascular diseases; cancers, including lung and throat cancer; and chronic respiratory illnesses such as emphysema and chronic bronchitis' (*BMJ*, 11 February 1995).

Yet committed smokers may view the anti-smoking campaign with some suspicion and not be convinced that smoking is all that bad for you, and in any event feel that individuals have the right to decide how to live their lives and run their own risks. You will recall the discussion in Chapter 5 which looked at some of the ethical issues about choice and control This is demonstrated by an encounter which took place in a greengrocer:

> Saleswoman: Derek, you aren't still smoking are you. You know how bad that is for you. My mum smoked for years and now she suffers terribly with her lungs.

> Derek: I don't believe all that stuff – your Mum would have had a problem with her lungs in any case. All the statistics that they put out are rubbish, we all know that. I like my fags, I have no intention of giving them up, I'm not at all convinced that they're bad for me.

For some people their experience of smoking has not corroborated the health warnings of the experts. This experience may be positive and in particular may provide some relief from stress. It is no coincidence that the greatest percentage of quitters is in social classes I and II where health promotion messages seem to be achieving some behavioural change. In social classes IV and V, the prevalence of smoking is linked to the adverse psychosocial conditions of poverty and powerlessness (ASH, 1993; Marsh and McKay, 1994). Just as in the case of diet and health, there is an element of risk analysis in people's responses to particular health risks and health promotion messages. The lack of social support (Graham, 1987), level of stress and feelings of powerlessness are areas for action, all of which might be addressed before any change in smoking behaviour is attempted. As Stacey suggests:

> The aim should be to understand the people's point of view in their terms (not yours) and to work out where they are coming from. Only

then will you be able to convey your own view of the situation in ways salient to them; or alternatively, you may realize that it needs rethinking.

(Stacey, 1994: 96)

Not dissimilar to the conflicts between lay and expert knowledge and professional input in the debate about smoking is that of healthy eating and exercise. Once again there are different strands of expert and lay opinion and the goal posts keep moving. Traditional food habits have been passed down through generations and many people are resistant to change. Despite indications that some sections of the population are concerned about healthy eating, some lay people are unconvinced that they will live longer, healthier lives if they reduce fat intake and increase the amount of exercise they take. Lay voices are sometimes joined by the media. For example, the recommendations of the 1994 COMA (Committee on Medical Aspects of Food Policy) Report on dietary changes needed to reduce the risk of cardiovascular disease were criticised as governmental interference in food choice.

Professional perspectives

So lay knowledge may be seen as derived partly from experience as well as input from experts. Health workers, who also use lay explanations, by and large derive their perspectives on health information from 'official accounts', their professional training and expertise, and publications in professional journals. These journals in turn are picked up by the media who publish newsworthy accounts.

People working to promote health come from a variety of disciplines from within the health and social care fields and their experiences of collecting and processing information will be different. Much of the gathering of information about the health needs of the population as well as current wisdom is done either at a local level or through professional bodies.

All disciplines within the health fields have their own professional journals which provide health information ranging from relatively simple practical advice to debating the complexities of certain issues. The type of health information these provide varies according to the particular focus of the journal. A journal aimed at health visitors might devote considerable space to the advantages of breast feeding whereas a health education journal may be concerned with evaluating particular programmes. *Community Care* and the *British Journal of Social Work* provide information for social, community and residential workers, whilst the *Journal of Epidemiology and Community Health* targets those working in public health.

Many professional bodies send updates to their members which might include details of new drugs or formulae for dealing with particular conditions. Some organisations provide members with specific information about health issues, whilst for many health workers the onus falls upon them themselves to find out current opinion on relevant topics. They may look to, for example, the Health Development Agency which publishes evidence of effective public health practice. Evidence Base 2000 will provide Internet access to a range of public health websites, collated evidence and information on good practice. The professional development newsletter *Network* communicates with an extensive network of over 5,000 practitioners in primary health care.

Health information flows in both directions from the specialist press to the national media, and hence health professionals may be influenced by newspaper articles as much as by their own trade journals. Many topics of general health interest are raised in the national press; for example breast feeding receives frequent coverage. These types of articles published in the quality press, without the hype of tabloid hysteria, may have a considerable influence on busy health practitioners who do not have the time or perhaps the skills to question research papers quoted or the interest to seek out the original papers and keep tabs on the ensuing correspondence which might, indeed, discredit the article. Consider two articles from the quality press which *de facto* are not subject to the potential rigours of academic publishing.

On 7 March 1995, the *Independent's* health page noted that the number of women who breast fed fell from 65 per cent in 1980 to 63 per cent in 1993. Readers were asked to question a mother's motivations for breast feeding a child over eighteen months but were expected to accept the wisdom that it is reasonable to wean a baby between six and twelve months in order to ensure the complete transfer of natural immunity from the mother to the child. An American professor of anthropology was quoted as saying 'There is considerable evidence that breast-fed babies are at less risk than bottle-fed ones for a range of conditions including allergies, obesity, cot death, cancer, diabetes, multiple sclerosis and ear infections.' Professor Dettwyler continues, 'The most recent evidence is that breast feeding is linked to a higher IQ and better graders. And the longer that nursing [breast feeding] continues, the better the results get.'

A second article on the same page of the *Independent* on that day maintained that most brands of formula milk lack a particular component of breast milk called long chain polyunsaturated fatty acids, or LCPs. These are 'thought' to be the 'brain food' which gives breast fed children better eyesight and higher IQs than those who were bottle fed. This information (unlike the article we talk about above which was based on a 'book') is based on an article published in the highly prestigious medical journal, *The Lancet*, widely accepted as publishing the most important medical discoveries in the UK. The research upon which the *Independent* article was based found that children who had been bottle fed in the Netherlands were twice as prone to some degree of brain dysfunction, causing movement abnormalities. The article in the *Independent* carries on to describe the missing ingredient from formula milk, rather than intensively analysing other factors which might have contributed to the findings of the Dutch research team. These accounts illustrate that the general public as well as health professionals may attribute scientific authority to reports in the media that have not been subjected to proper scientific scrutiny.

12.4 Sources of health information

The BSE case indicated some sources of health information – scientific and medical endeavour and government and economic sources. Yet there are other sources of information. If you want to reach people effectively you need to know what these sources are. The Office of Health Economics (OHE) (1994) commissioned two market research companies specialising in consumer population and health care to investigate where and how people obtain health information and to ascertain whether this varies according to age, gender, ethnicity or geographical area. Their remit was to find out:

- what sources of health information people used
- the relative value placed on these sources of information
- how effective health information was in altering behaviour and lifestyle.

In this study 1,194 people were asked to identify and prioritise which sources of health information they used. The data might help health promoters to understand their population and plan interventions. A different survey, *The Survey of the UK Population: Health and Lifestyles* (HEA, 1995), which investigated similar issues, was deliberately planned to provide baseline information on the health of people in England for the Health of the Nation strategy.

Table 12.1 demonstrates that the most important sources of health information identified in the OHE study were television, magazines, newspapers and GPs. Of the respondents, 48 per cent rated the GP as most influential, followed by magazines and newspapers which scored 16 per cent and television with 13 per cent. This is borne out by the *Health and Lifestyles Survey* (1995c) commissioned by the HEA which also suggested that most information, in this case relating to Health of the Nation targets, came from the GP. Men differed from women in relation to ease of talking to doctors and/or nurses, and the topic area (e.g. HIV/AIDS, smoking, weight control) determines the ease with which people raise these issues with doctors or health professionals.

Information received from friends and relatives was relatively lowly rated (8 per cent) except in the under-24 age group (14 per cent) (OHE). Despite the General Household Survey's findings that in any month 99 per cent of the population watch some television, the proportion of those suggesting that they obtained health information from television, despite it being a primary source, was remarkably low.

Table 12.1   Question – from which of these sources, if any, do you obtain your health information?

Response	All	15–20	21–24	25–34	35–44	45–54	55–64	65+
				Age				
MEN								
Number of respondents	**575**	**73**	**34**	**116**	**101**	**85**	**72**	**94**
				Percentages				
Magazines/newspapers	33	36	40	33	36	44	27	21
TV	34	38	28	36	46	29	24	29
Radio	9	4	5	15	8	11	5	11
Leaflets in GP waiting room	12	19	6	14	15	13	7	5
GP	37	19	28	33	29	46	48	49
Practice nurse/health visitor/midwife	4	1	5	5	3	4	7	4
Pharmacist	13	15	3	16	18	11	10	14
Other health professional	5	1	4	8	4	7	3	3
Friends or relatives	19	28	14	23	16	25	21	7
WOMEN								
Number of respondents	**619**	**59**	**44**	**113**	**102**	**85**	**77**	**140**
				Percentages				
Magazines/newspapers	44	53	46	46	57	52	38	29
TV	29	36	34	27	40	22	26	23
Radio	9	2	6	7	13	7	13	10
Leaflets in GP waiting room	16	21	23	18	22	15	11	8
GP	39	43	44	34	38	37	41	45
Practice nurse/health visitor/midwife	10	2	19	18	10	9	7	8
Pharmacist	16	16	23	20	19	15	13	12
Other health professional	7	5	11	7	8	7	11	4
Friends or relatives	19	36	30	22	24	15	15	8

(OHE, 1994 ,Table 1)

Note: Columns do not add up to 100 per cent as respondents were able to select more than one source of information.

The survey identified differences amongst the respondents according to age, gender, social class and the regional health authority of residence.

Age

Although in each age group the GP was seen to be the most important source of information, 45 per cent of the older respondents (over 54) as opposed to 32 per cent of the younger respondents (under 24) relied primarily on this source. The report speculates that the explanations for these differences may include amongst others the respect given to GPs by the older group, or the low consultation rate of the younger group. Another surprising finding related to age was that only 28 per cent of people over 55 thought newspapers and magazines were important sources of health information, as opposed to 44 per cent of the 25–54 group and 43 per cent of the under-24 respondents. The OHE suggests that the lower number of pensioners reading may relate to cost and the fact that few target that age group; other explanations might be problems with literacy or eyesight.

Gender

Women between the ages of 15 and 44 were more likely to use friends and relatives as sources of health information than men of the same ages. This may be because women in these age groups are having and bringing up children and may be more likely to discuss health issues than men. However the finding that men in the older age group (45–64) were more than twice as likely as women to obtain health information from friends and relatives is harder to explain. Perhaps this was due to men's reluctance to consult GPs.

More women than men of all ages regarded newspapers and magazines as sources of health information, which may reflect the health and family focus of women's magazines as opposed to the sport or hobbies focus of men's journals. However the OHE survey indicated that a relatively high proportion of men read women's magazines and nearly 20 per cent of male respondents perceived magazines and newspapers to be important sources of health information.

Practice nurses, midwives and health visitors were also used as sources of health information: 18 per cent of women (5 per cent of men) between the ages of 21–34 used this source, 14 per cent of women aged 25–34 (those most likely to be bearing and rearing children) saw this group as the most important source.

Screening

Men and women differed markedly in the OHE survey in their perceptions of screening. Respondents were asked to what extent media coverage of health problems had affected their attitudes to health screening and whether they would be more or less likely as a result to have some form of screening.

Table 12.2   Question – to what extent do you think media coverage of health problems has affected your attitude towards screening services?

	Age						
Response	15–20	21–24	25–34	35–44	45–54	55–64	65+
MEN							
Made me much more likely to have screening	8	8	8	14	11	7	6
Made me a little more likely to have screening	17	13	22	10	19	25	12
Made no difference	69	72	66	71	64	63	76
Made me less likely to have screening	1	–	1	4	1	–	1
Don't know	6	7	2	2	5	5	5
WOMEN							
Made me much more likely to have screening	33	28	29	26	35	19	18
Made me a little more likely to have screening	18	32	22	34	25	25	16
Made no difference	41	32	46	40	33	52	61
Made me less likely to have screening	4	2	1	–	4	3	1
Don't know	3	6	1	1	3	1	5

(OHE, 1994, Table 4)

What possible explanations could you give for the discrepancy between women and men seeking screening?

The table illustrates the differences between men and women, in that 50 per cent of women as opposed to 25 per cent men say they may seek screening. This finding may be explained by the greater publicity given to screening women for cervical and breast cancer. However, testicular cancer screening was, in the late 1990s, being introduced in some parts of the UK (MORI, 1995). The following is an extract from an interview with a male nurse who was addressing men's health issues in the Welsh Health Promoting Hospital in which he worked:

> We've incorporated within our programme regular opportunities to educate both patients and staff on testicular cancer testing and this is done by nursing staff education and the use of user-friendly leaflets... We think that the males get the short end of the stick really. I got hold of the local Director of Public Health about testicular cancer testing and, as there is no formal screening, its got to be done on an individual basis.

Thus lay people get most health information directly from primary care workers and the media. In addition, leaflets are available in GPs surgeries and hospitals, particularly out-patient departments. These give general information about back and joint pain, genetic diseases, contraception and family planning. For example, leaflets entitled 'Exercise, why bother?' 'A guide to a healthy sex life', 'A whole new ball game' and 'Breast feeding' contain information about preserving function as well as addresses and contact numbers of those involved in research. Obviously people with limited understanding or poor sight are at a disadvantage and will need the leaflets explained.

12.5 What information do health promoters need?

This section will not only introduce you to the kinds of information you may require in order to give advice and run programmes as a health promoter but also enable you to gather data from your own population or other relevant populations. You have already explored the sources and nature of health information. Now you need to ascertain what kinds of information you require about your population and how to go about getting them.

This may range from comparing levels of unemployment, the numbers of single parent families, the incidence of particular illnesses or disabilities or the extent to which your population resembles that of the wider population with regard to particular habits. You may want to know something about the general health status of the population you serve in relation to the general population. This may be important for planning an intervention. For example an assessment of the perceived health of the local as opposed to the national population was carried out in Copenhagen (WHO, 1985).

This demonstrates that those living in Copenhagen rated their health and their prospects lower than those living elsewhere in Denmark. When looking at their health habits the study identified a greater intake of alcohol in Copenhagen than was common in Denmark as a whole as well as a higher proportion of smokers, yet noted that residents of Copenhagen took more exercise. This type of information might be relevant in deciding whether further investigation into lifestyles in large cities was needed.

As a health promoter wanting to acquire health information in your local population, examine the box below and identify which might be the most useful sources.

Box 12.1: Useful sources and types of health information

- *Hospital records* provide information on reasons for admissions, outpatient attendances, operative procedures, accident and emergency attendances and discharges. Information is also available on length of stay in hospital and waiting lists.

- *Notification systems* for births, congenital malformations, infectious diseases, and abortions.

- *Registers* for specific diseases such as cancers, blind and partially sighted people and disabled persons. There are also registers of those 'at risk' of disease or injury.

- *Sentinel recording systems,* such as the National General Practice Morbidity Survey, which provide data on diagnosed disease and symptoms in the community.

- *Surveys* such as the General Household Survey, and other surveys undertaken by the ONS, the Health Survey for England which provide data on self-perceived ill-health and health trends.

- *Department of Health* produces an annual public health report by the Chief Medical Officer, **On the State of the Public Health,** updates Saving Lives: Our Healthier Nation, gives policy guidelines, plus other reports.

- *National Health Service Executive* produces national data on hospital throughput, activity analysis, bed occupancy, admission rates for various causes etc.

- *National health promotion/education agencies* (e.g. HDA) produce national research and survey data on health trends, health targets, projects and programmes.

- *General practitioners/primary care service* practice population health; community nurses may have undertaken surveys.

- *Local health authorities/ health boards* produce local strategy for health promotion based on assessment of population's health promotion needs; may have carried out local studies of health behaviour, local population statistics.

- *Regional offices of the NHSE* produce regional statistics on hospital admissions, activity analysis, five year health plan etc.

- *Community Health Councils* report on service monitoring, particular issues, patient groups.

- *Voluntary agencies* produce national or local surveys.

- *Local authorities* produce data on environmental health, social services, employment, population profiles by electoral ward.

- *Public Health Observatories* collate local information on public health.

- *Directors of Public Health* produce annual reports.

(adapted from HEA, Morbidity Slide 31)

Box 12. 2 Information from new technologies

CD-ROM –   **reference sources** e.g. the British National Formulary

databases e.g. MEDLINE, CINAHL, PsychLIT, ERIC

newspapers e.g. *Times, Sunday Times, Financial Times*

Internet –   **e-mail discussion groups**

electronic conferencing

news groups e.g. Usenet

websites Health Development Agency and Health Promotion: England; Health Education Board for Scotland; Health Promotion Division of the National Assembly for Wales; National Health Promotion Agency for Northern Ireland; UK Dept of Health; Centre for Health Information Quality (CHIQ); NHS Direct; National Institute for Clinical Excellence (NICE); UK Stationery Office; Centre for Disease Control and Prevention in the United States; World Health Organisation; Libraries e.g. National Library of Medicine (including MEDLINE); Library of Congress

electronic journals including the *Internet Journal of Health Promotion* (IJHP); the *Health Education Journal; Health Promotion International; Health Education Research; Nursing Times; Nursing Standard On-line; American Journal of Nursing;* the *Australian Electronic Journal of Nursing Education; JAMIA,* the official *Journal of the American Medical Informatics.*

Although none of these sources is likely to yield information that is fully reliable, comprehensive and appropriate to your needs, they may provide some guidelines. Through obtaining data from different sources about the same problem you may be able to compare local and national trends (as in Copenhagen). Some sources may not be accessible to non-medical people, but may be obtainable through the office of the local Director of Public Health. It should be noted, though, that in many instances the importance of a particular disease or condition in a population can be assessed only by means of specific studies of incidence or prevalence. Such studies can be quite complex and would normally require the help of a statistician or epidemiologist.

Information from new technologies

As the amount of information about health has escalated sharply in recent years, new methods have been devised to help people access, evaluate and utilise this wealth of material. It would be impossible for any individual to continue to practice in a health-related profession and keep abreast with all the recent and relevant advances in their field. However there is pressure for the practice of all health professionals to be research based. Nurses who have studied in the Project 2000 pre-registration education system are required to have a considerable knowledge of the research studies relevant to their nursing practice. Doctors and surgeons are also being targeted in an effort to increase their access to research findings so that these can be incorporated into their patient care – what is known as 'evidence-based medicine'.

According to an editorial in the *British Medical Journal:*

Evidence-based medicine is the conscientious, explicit, and judicious use of current best evidence in making decisions about the care of individual patients. The practice of evidence-based medicine means integrating individual clinical expertise with the best available external clinical evidence from systematic research... By best available external clinical evidence we mean clinically relevant research, often from the basic sciences of medicine, but especially from patient-centred clinical research into the accuracy and precision of diagnostic tests (including the clinical examinations), the power of prognostic markers, and the efficacy and safety of therapeutic, rehabilitative and preventive regimens ...

Evidence-based medicine is not 'cookbook' medicine. Because it requires a bottom up approach that integrates the best external evidence with individual clinical expertise and patients' choice, it cannot result in slavish, cookbook approaches to individual patient care ... Evidence-based medicine is not restricted to randomised trials and meta-analyses ...

(Sackett *et al.*, 1996: 71-72)

There is now a Centre for Evidence-Based Medicine, a *Journal of Evidence-based Medicine*, a *Journal of Evidence-based Nursing*, the NHS Centre for Reviews and Dissemination and the UK Cochrane Centre (dedicated to providing clinicians with up-to-date information on randomised clinical trials) as well as national and local initiatives to help make health care research based. Health promotion is also developing a research base and requires as much research information as other health areas. The EPI centre at the Institute of Education of the University of London seeks to provide information on evidence-based practice in health promotion. Health information changes rapidly. Computer data handling and access technologies are addressing these issues, and health promoters are now able to access CD databases, for example Medline and CINAHL (Cumulative Index of Nursing and Allied Health Literature) which enable readers to scan a comprehensive literature. There is also access to electronic journals online for many individuals. Some sources of information from the new technologies are listed in Box 12.2.

The Internet has facilitated rapid access to health information and amongst many other health-related facilities there are health promotion e-mail networks which enable health promoters to exchange data, experiences and good practice. These advances in communication can bring together people at a local, national and international level and enable them to co-ordinate their efforts more effectively as well as process the ever increasing amounts of health information.

With the emphasis on evidence-based health promotion and clinical governance in health services, a number of national organisations have been established. NICE – The National Institute for Clinical Excellence – was set up as a Special Health Authority for England and Wales in April 1999. It is part of the National Health Service and its role is to provide patients, health professionals and the public with authoratitive, robust and reliable guidance on current 'best practice', although its remit is much wider than health promotion. Similarly the Centre for Health Information Quality, established in 1997, aims to bring together skills in consumer health information, evidence-based healthcare, public involvement and research.

Finally whenever looking at the information you have gathered together it is important to recall the questions that were posed at the beginning of this chapter. Is the information unidimensional or could there be a number of explanations for contradictory evidence or findings that are difficult to explain? We now move on to explore the ways in which information about health is collected.

Chapter 13
Studying populations

13.1 Introduction

Chapter 12 explored *sources of health information.* This chapter investigates *what kinds of information* are collected about health. People involved in promoting health need to understand the principles underpinning the disciplines whereby information about health matters is obtained, as well as the ways in which such information is assessed and evaluated (to be explored in Chapter 16). Two major disciplines collecting information about health are *demography* (the study of human populations, focusing in particular on numbers of people) and *epidemiology* (the study of the occurrence and spread of ill health and disease).

If as a health promoter you are proposing a particular intervention, there are several questions requiring answers before you can ascertain the most effective methods to reach your target group. You will need to know certain features of your population and its geographical distribution. You may require certain demographic facts, for example how many people are homeless, or the distribution of very old people.

13.2 Demography

Chapter 2 noted that since 1801 demographers have conducted a census to ascertain the number of people residing in the UK. Demographers count people according to certain social characteristics such as age, gender, marital status and housing conditions. Demographers want to know how many people live and/or work in a particular geographical area, what kind of work they do, and the age and gender distribution of that population. They are concerned with change resulting from births, marriages, deaths, movement of people and alterations in population characteristics. Demography provides information on the number of divorces compared with the number of marriages. It identifies whether employed people move away whilst unemployed people stay in the area. Demographers calculate unemployment statistics showing numbers of long-term unemployed people as well as the temporarily unemployed, such as school leavers.

Demographic data can be divided into two discrete forms.

1 Data collected through *registration systems,* giving information on events during a particular time period, often a year. This is dynamic in nature as it illustrates flows, for example births, deaths, house moves and so forth. This data facilitates comparing levels of mortality and

fertility, rather than just births or deaths. Demographers count and compare birth and death *rates* in different places and at different times. These rates are calculated on the basis of returns to the registrar following a birth or death. Birth and death rates are usually expressed per thousand, rather than a percentage (per hundred). (These will be discussed later when you explore epidemiological concepts.)

2 Data gathered through population *censuses and surveys,* which gives a snapshot view of individuals at a particular moment in time. The information it yields is about the size and structure of a particular population as it was on census night. Comparisons between or within censuses involves absolute numbers or the calculation of proportions.

Many questions in censuses and surveys relate to people's health directly or indirectly and therefore are of interest to health promoters. The kind of information obtained in censuses or surveys often reflects the concerns of those commissioning them and the results may influence decisions about provision of services and priorities. Criticism has been directed at certain surveys conducted by the Office for National Statistics, on the grounds that the questions asked may determine the answer, for example that surveys may not adequately reflect the diversity of the population or levels of disability (Oliver, 1993).

The national census

The concept of counting people originated in biblical times. Moses was instructed to 'take the sum of all the congregation of the children of Israel, by their families, by their fathers' houses, according to the number of names', hence the book 'Numbers' in the Old Testament. In ancient Rome, census (meaning to tax) takers prepared lists of people and property, chiefly for purposes of taxation and enforcement of military requirements. During the Anglo-Saxon period in England a tax known as Danegeld was collected by conducting a census. After William the Conqueror invaded England his officials organised a count of the country's land, people and property. Records were collected from every parish and the details sent to London where a central register was compiled – the Domesday Book. Parish-based censuses took place occasionally thereafter but not necessarily in the same places. However, only summary information was sent to London for central collation. The first modern periodic, direct and complete census took place in the United States in 1790. The first UK census followed shortly in 1801 and has been repeated decenially on a regular basis, except in 1941 during the Second World War. The 1840 Population Act appointed a Registrar General responsible for a complete census of the population of England and Wales.

Questions asked in censuses have changed reflecting contemporary concerns and since 1891 data has increasingly been collected providing information about aspects of health and lifestyles. In the 1891 census, questions were asked about types of dwelling and the number of rooms each household occupied, reflecting concern about overcrowding. From

1911 details were asked about family size, to be considered alongside mortality and morbidity data. The 1921 census contained questions about place of work and methods of transport to work, reflecting growing concern with traffic density. By this time questions were included about educational level as well as information about the ages and numbers of children in the population (for educational planning purposes).

Social classes were identified in Chapter 2 as a major indicator of health. The 1921 census redefined occupational classification and introduced the five social class groups which have recently been modified as illustrated in Table 13.1.

Many scales have been devised to give a precise definition of socio-economic grouping for research. Classification is by current or former occupation of head of household in the two most widely-used systems – the Registrar-General's social class system, used in the Census, and the National Readership Survey system used by most UK market research.

What are the main differences between the current classification and the original classification of social class groups?

Table 13.1 **Social grading systems**

NRS system	Registrar-General (OPCS)	Description	Examples
A	I	Professional/upper middle class	Professor, doctor, bank manager
B	II	Intermediate/middle class	Journalist, nurse, teacher
C1	IIIN	Skilled non-manual/lower middle class	Clerical worker, shop assistant
C2	IIIM	Skilled manual/skilled working class	Bus driver, miner, carpenter
D	IV/V	Partly skilled/unskilled working class	Agricultural worker, hospital porter, labourer, cleaner, dock worker
E		Those at lowest levels of subsistence	Old-age pensioners, widows, and those totally dependent on social security through long-term unemployment or sickness

As the table shows, the two systems are roughly comparable. However, the Registrar-General's system classifies the retired and unemployed by their last significant period of employment, whereas the ABC system merges groups IV and V into D and creates an additional category E for those dependent on social security and state pensions. The scales are unsatisfactory for several reasons: married women are classified by their husbands' occupations rather than their own; there can be quite marked lifestyle differences within occupational groups; and grading systems can vary slightly between different market research agencies.

(HEA, 1993a)

The notes surrounding this table describe some of the changes that have occurred over the years and also the inadequacies of the scales.

Since 1911 census data has been analysed mechanically. Initially data was entered on punch cards and sorted by electrical machines. Computers were used for the first time in 1961. Now the Data Protection Act 1984 ensures that personal and identifiable census information stored on computer files remains confidential. The censuses of 1971 and 1981 saw the introduction of a 'cohort study' on a sample section of the population. Babies born on four days in 1971 were identified and followed up in subsequent censuses. This data was used for medical research as well as demographic purposes.

Census data forms the basis of a great deal of statistical information at the national, regional and district level. Indeed, since contemporary censuses extend over some 100,000 separate enumeration districts, accurate statistical information about each and every one of them is available. This facilitates accessing information about, for example, one-parent families, employment, housing, education and other health-related issues for small areas of the country.

The 1991 census requested the following information:
1   Name
2   Sex
3   Date of birth
4   Marital status
5   Relationship in household
6   Whereabouts on census night 21/22 April 1991
7   Usual address
8   Term time address of students and school children
9   Usual address one year ago
10 Country of birth
11 Ethnic group
12 Long-term illness
13 Whether working, retired, looking after the home etc. last week
14 Hours worked per week
15 Occupation
16 Name and business of employer (if self-employed give the name and nature of the person's business)
17 Address of place of work
18 Daily journey to work
19 Degrees, professional and vocational qualifications
20 Number of rooms
21 Accommodation
22 Housing tenure

23 Floor level of household's living accommodation
24 Amenities (bathroom, WC, etc.)
25 Whether living in a shared household
26 Cars and vans (available for use)

Which census questions are of most interest to those involved in promoting health?

The range of questions is quite comprehensive and data gathered from questions 11, 12, 13, 18, 23 and 24 might be useful for those involved in promoting health. These can reflect information about poverty, disability, long-term illness and housing conditions. The questions asked in the census are not without controversy: for example, considerable debate was generated following the 1991 census regarding the categories imposed for ethnic identity (Raleigh and Balarajan, 1994) and the 2001 census contains different categories for ethnic identity. Evaluating census data and providing the information required by interested parties is an extensive task and takes much of the subsequent decade to produce. The publication of reports for the 1981 census took place in 1987, and despite the computerisation of the data evaluation process a similar time was required for the 1991 census.

A range of health-related surveys have been carried out regularly by the Office for National Statistics (ONS, formerly OPCS) since the Second World War when the Social Survey Division monitored population morale as well as diet during food rationing and sickness absences from work. In addition, in contrast to the census, government agencies commission other studies to elicit opinion or attitude, for example those undertaken by the Social and Community Planning Research Organisation. The General Household Survey (undertaken by the ONS) collects information annually from 12,500 households on five topics: population and family, housing, employment, education and health. The annual National Food Survey reports on expenditure on food and dietary patterns for a representative sample of the population. Since very close links exist between diet and health, this is a particularly useful source of information about the types of food that make up a typical British diet and also looks at the relationship between income and diet. In addition the Health Survey for England (HSE) provides baseline data from which to monitor health trends.

Counting births and deaths

Since 1836 registration of births, marriages and deaths has been compulsory. Prompt registration was encouraged by instituting a fee payable if the birth was not registered within six weeks. Local registrars were responsible for registering deaths and births and entitled to perform civil marriages. This, combined with other kinds of local registration, has facilitated recording movement within different localities and computations of local populations.

So how are the numbers calculated? The population of an area at time t + 1 is just the population at time t plus the number of births between t and t + 1, less the number of deaths, plus the number of migrants entering the area, less the number of emigrants.

The equation can be written as:

population change = natural increase + net immigration

Thus it is important to record deaths as well as births. Through compulsory recording of deaths (without a death certificate, for example, it is illegal to dispose of a body) the ONS is able to publish detailed mortality statistics. This data includes deaths classified by age and sex, and also by cause and area of residence. In addition, through the evaluation of census data, information about mortality in relation to cause of death and occupation is obtained, and this is published every ten years. The combination of mortality and census data facilitates the study of trends and changes in mortality over time.

13.3 Epidemiology

Epidemiologists are concerned with the health status of a population and compare groups within a specific population. They then analyse the results and provide explanations for any differences. Epidemiology is dependent on demographic details (Majeed *et al.*, 1995) to provide total population numbers so that it is possible to count the people with a particular condition or illness as a fraction of that number. The kinds of events that might interest epidemiologists may be morbidity (disease), disability, mortality (death), recovery, or the use of health services. Although many people assume that epidemiology is only the 'science of epidemics', it actually has a much broader remit and explains why and how epidemics occur, spread, what causes them, and how they can be contained. It can be defined as

> ... the science concerned with the occurrence, distribution and determinants of states of health and disease in human groups and populations. Epidemiological studies may deal with the distribution of diseases or health-relevant characteristics in groups (descriptive surveys) and with the factors influencing this distribution (analytic surveys experiments, and quasi-experiments).
>
> (Abramson, 1990)

Epidemiology can be seen as the scientific foundation for health promotion which assists in identifying the health problems in particular communities, assessing the relevance of prevention and evaluating the effectiveness of preventive interventions (Tannahill, 1992: 97). Thus health promoters rely to a large extent on epidemiological data to provide them with valuable information about the health of their population. It is therefore useful to understand the principles behind epidemiological methods and techniques. These have impinged upon almost every area of medical science, yet epidemiology is not purely a medical discipline; its concern is with *groups* of people, not individuals as such (which is the primary focus of concern in clinical medicine). Public health physicians are generally trained epidemiologists, but people from other disciplines such as statisticians, sociologists, scientists, economists and geographers, may also be involved in epidemiological study. Thus, epidemiology is multidisciplinary in nature and, although its concerns are with issues of health and disease, its methodology and techniques can be applied in many other areas, including the social sciences and economics (for example, market research). You may want to refer back to Chapters 1 and 2 where you explored the different perspectives and questions posed by 'lay' and 'expert' epidemiologists – it is important to keep these perspectives in mind as you explore who, when and what epidemiologists study.

Early studies in epidemiology

The first important epidemiological map illustrated a health problem which today would interest environmental health officers. In the mid-nineteenth century Dr John Snow suspected that drinking water might have caused the spread of cholera in Soho, London. He found that people who had drunk water provided by a particular water company were more likely to have developed cholera than those who had not. He plotted all the cholera cases in Soho on a local map and noted that they clustered around Broad Street.

Figure 13.1 identifies the water pump on Broad Street used by many local residents. Dr Snow suggested that the pump's water caused the cholera outbreak. On removal of this source of water, the cases of cholera began to decline. Snow's interest was not so much in treating the individuals with cholera as in the *patterns* of where the victims lived and got their water supply so that he could prevent further spread of the disease. Thus the link between the water and cholera was established before it was understood precisely what was in the water which caused the illness. Hence the epidemiological explanation preceded the biological explanation and was able to halt the rapid spread of the disease. There are two twentieth century parallels – the link between smoking and increased incidence of lung cancer (Doll and Hill, 1950) and AIDS, where understanding of the biology of the disease is far behind epidemiological explanations. Epidemiology can thus help highlight populations or certain groups with an above average death rate, or high disease rates, and that information is essential to all those involved in working towards equality in health. Epidemiology thus provides two types of information

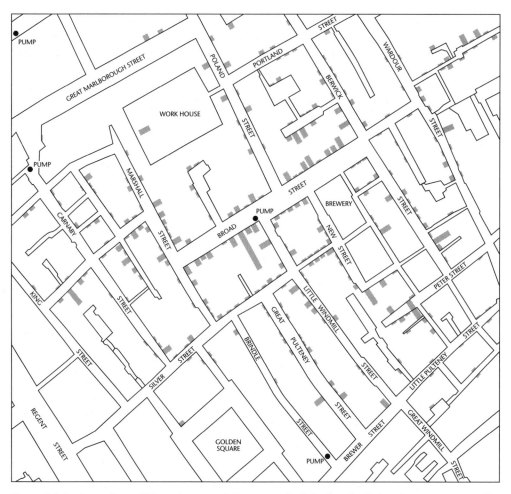

Figure 13.1   **A portion of Snow's map of the spread of cholera in Soho. Bars represent the number of fatal cases in each house. The position of the Broad Street pump from which all the victims had obtained water is also marked.**   (HEA, 1993a)

useful for health promoters: it identifies structural problems such as poverty and poor housing and points out aspects of behaviour that might be amenable to interventions, such as the links between heart disease and exercise or lung cancer and smoking.

Epidemiological concepts and terms

It is helpful at this point to understand what epidemiological data is collected routinely.

Routine data

This is collected on a regular basis and kept accessible in an index or database for epidemiological use. This includes denominator (the population at risk) data from Census and Population Registers, Death Certificates, Birth Certificates and Congenital Malformation registrations, Registrations of Notifiable Diseases, e.g. infectious diseases and Cancer Registration, Health Service Data on consultations, treatments and diagnoses, and data about potential risk factors from the census and surveys.

Routine data is used in two particular ways by epidemiologists, on the one hand for providing descriptive statistics and surveillances and on the other as a resource for analytic epidemiological studies. For example, routine mortality and cancer incidence data can generate aetiological (causation) hypotheses by comparing rates of disease between places where lifestyles clearly differ or between different subgroups of the data set.

Rates

'Death rates' are one of a number of different rates showing the numbers of a population at risk. A *rate* expresses the frequency of a characteristic per 100 (or per 1,000, per million etc.). To calculate a death rate the number of deaths (numerator) is divided by the number of persons in the population (denominator) and multiplied by 100, 1,000, or another convenient figure (Abramson, 1990: 99). Rates can be useful indicators of changes in health patterns in any given population and consideration of these may lead directly to a health promotion intervention. When looking at disease indicators, rates are a measure of the frequency of the appearance of new cases. Rates are usually measured per thousand.

Standardised and other *adjusted rates* estimate what the rate might be in particular circumstances, for example if the groups being compared were similar according to defined independent variables. For example, *age-specific rates* are a rate for a specific age group. The numerator and denominator refer to the same age group. Rates that are not age specific are called the *crude rates,* in other words they have not been adjusted.

Thus *crude death rates* show the number of deaths in the total population, and to make the numbers more manageable the crude rate is quoted per thousand. In 1993 the crude death rate in England was 11.1 per 1,000. Crude rates, however, do not show the burden of deaths in particular groups of the population, which is an important aspect for those involved in health promotion programmes. For example, one might assume that a town on the south coast of England is an unhealthy place to live as it has a high crude death rate. However, when you look at the population distribution you realise that the average age is higher here as a popular place for retired people to live than many other places in England, and hence the higher number of deaths.

Perinatal Mortality Rates refer to the number of deaths after the 24th week of pregnancy plus deaths under one week of age. The *Infant Mortality*

Rate (IMR) is the number of deaths per 1,000 of infants under one year old compared to the total number of live births. IMR is used as an indicator of the overall health of a nation or community as this rate correlates well with adult mortality and is more sensitive to improvements in the health care than other health measures. IMRs are often used to compare nations with very different health care systems. Such data can be valuable for promoting health. For example, health workers are able to use the IMR to identify certain groups at risk from Sudden Infant Death Syndrome (SIDS or 'cot death') (Gilman *et al.*, 1995). These high risk groups included some ethnic minorities, those living in crowded conditions, very low birth-weight babies and babies in families where a parent or both parents were unemployed. Although the cause(s) of SIDS is still unresolved, as are the influences of these various factors, it has been found that if babies slept on their backs the incidence of SIDS is reduced. The dramatic drop in IMR confirmed the effectiveness of the campaign to change babies' sleeping positions (Hiley and Morley, 1994).

The *Fertility Rate* is the number of births per 1,000 women in certain age groups. The Department of Health document *On the State of the Public Health 1993* used fertility rates within certain age groups (15-19, 35-39 etc.) to show changes in the patterns of childbirth that may have ramifications for health promotion programmes aimed at pregnant women and those considering parenthood.

Chapter 2 defined the *Standardised Mortality Ratio (SMR)* as the rate measuring the relative chances of death at a stated age. Death rates from many diseases differ between the sexes and between age groups within each sex. Therefore, the death rate for a specific condition in a particular area may be higher than the national average, simply because the area contains relatively more residents in a susceptible sex/age group than the national population. The SMR is thus a means of compensating for the effects of differing age and sex distribution (how this is calculated will be addressed in the next chapter). Using this method, fairer comparisons of death rates in populations can be made than are possible on the basis of crude death rates alone. The south coast resorts have a preponderance of older people and consequently a high death rate, while a population with a high proportion of young people, as in a new town, is likely to have a low death rate. A direct comparison of crude mortality rates for the two localities would obviously produce a distorted picture. Hence, standardised mortality ratios have to be used. Despite the very different age structures of the populations involved, regional comparisons in the UK can be made. Calculations such as this have shown up regional variations, the so-called north-south divide (with higher SMRs in the north) as Figure 13.2 demonstrates.

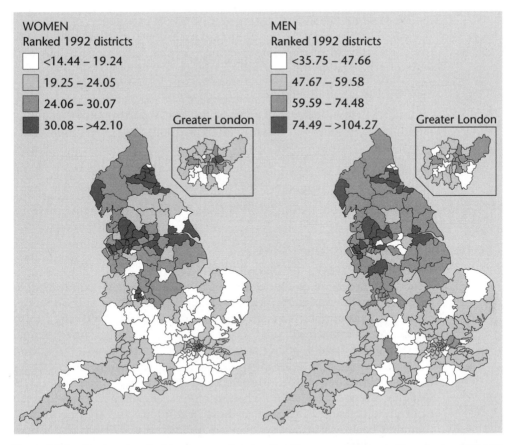

WOMEN
Ranked 1992 districts

- [ ] <14.44 – 19.24
- [ ] 19.25 – 24.05
- [ ] 24.06 – 30.07
- [ ] 30.08 – >42.10

Greater London

MEN
Ranked 1992 districts

- [ ] <35.75 – 47.66
- [ ] 47.67 – 59.58
- [ ] 59.59 – 74.48
- [ ] 74.49 – >104.27

Greater London

Figure 13.2   **Regional variations in age-standardised lung cancer mortality rate per 100,000 in men and women aged under 75, average for the year 1990-1992**   (HEA, 1991, Figure 12)

Incidence and prevalence

Epidemiology involves estimating the frequency and distribution of diseases in populations and comparing the effect of suspected risk factors on the frequency of diseases. Measures of disease frequency are tools to describe how common an illness (or another outcome event) is in relation to the size of the population (the population at risk). These measures count the number of cases in a population and a measure in time. The two main types of measures of disease frequency are incidence and prevalence.

Incidence is the number of new cases of a disease or disorder that arise over a set period of time. *Prevalence* is the total number of people suffering from a specific condition or exhibiting a particular characteristic at a certain point in time. Prevalence studies are commonly used to survey characteristics such as smoking habits or alcohol use.

The *incidence rate* of a disease over a period of time is:

$$\frac{\text{number of new cases over the period}}{\text{population at risk}}$$

Whereas the *prevalence rate* is:

$$\frac{\text{total number of cases of the disease at that time}}{\text{population at risk}}$$

Both these rates are expressed as percentages or as rates per thousand or per hundred thousand people in the population. It can be useful to think of prevalence as a 'snap-shot' of a health problem whilst incidence charts the progress of the disease/disorder over time.

The health status of a population

Why is it necessary to know the health status of the population to promote health? Mortality (death) and morbidity (illness and disability) statistics are essential information when planning and evaluating health promotion programmes, whether at a local, national or international level. You only have to glance at any document on the health promotion needs of a population to see the use made of these indicators of health, for example the Black Report, the Acheson Report and *Saving Lives: Our Healthier Nation* or local health strategy reports. However, as you will recall from the discussion in Chapter 2 these health measures are not without their drawbacks, particularly as they are indicators of *ill* health rather than of health. Finding adequate measures of health is as difficult as defining health. However, these two key statistics are important because of the influence they and other epidemiological measures have had on health promotion activity in the past. In looking at mortality and morbidity you can see the patterns of disease in different populations which reflect, for example, differing social circumstances. Comparing mortality rates within populations by social class enables researchers to expose inequalities in health.

Epidemiologists, in investigating the health status of a population, look in particular at which people develop health problems, when they contract illness and in which locations a problem is particularly prevalent. The information regarding who develops health problems is partly collected, as you have noted, through morbidity and mortality statistics. But epidemiologists are particularly interested in patterns of disease spread.

What are the health problems and which groups have them?

We need to know the breakdown of the population, the age groups, proportions of men and women and occupational groups. Other population variables that should be considered are the social circumstances and conditions in which people live, as well as religion, culture and ethnic origin. This is important since there may be associations between these variables and the health status of individuals.

Look at Figure 13.3 which illustrates the prevalence of obesity by age and sex. What age groups would you deem to be most at risk?

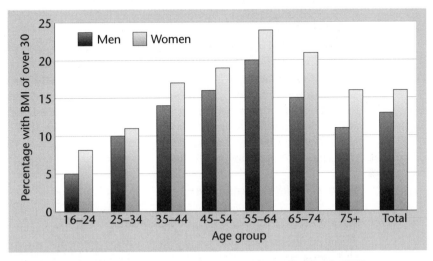

Figure 13.3   **Prevalence of obesity by age and sex: England, 1993** (Bennett *et al.*, 1995, Figure 2.2)

You will note that there is a sharp rise in obesity following young adulthood which is where the greatest jump occurs in prevalence.

Where do the problems occur?

The cholera epidemic in the 1850s described earlier demonstrated the influence of geographical and environmental factors on the occurrence of disease. Disease patterns vary internationally, for example 'tropical diseases' such as bilharzia, malaria and leprosy. Within countries, regional variations in the occurrence of diseases are not uncommon (for example, there are regional variations in the occurrence of heart disease and different types of cancer, see Figure 13.2). In addition, differences in disease patterns between urban and rural communities are frequently observed. Even within one health district, mortality rates due to particular diseases may vary from one electoral ward to another.

Studies of immigrant populations can separate groups within geographical areas. One such population was that which migrated from Japan to the United States between 1890 and 1924. It was found that heart disease in Japan was only one quarter the rate in the United States, whereas stroke and cerebral haemorrhage were two or three times more common

(Marmot *et al.*, 1975). Stomach cancer was five times more common in Japan, but cancer of the breast and prostate were very uncommon there. Cancer of the cervix was twice as common in Japan as in the United States. As the Japanese population settled in the USA some of their disease patterns changed, and conditions such as stroke, cerebral haemorrhage and cancer of the cervix approached the rates of the community to which they had migrated. This suggests that environmental factors played a considerable part in the causation of these particular diseases. Cancer of the stomach also declined, but not to a very great extent (Hirayana, 1980). Cancer of the breast, however, did not alter significantly when the population had settled in the United States.

Caution must be exercised when making international comparisons of ill-health. In developing countries access to health services and the availability of facilities for investigation tend to be rather restricted. This means that there may be problems with the accuracy and completeness of diagnosis. The age structure of the population in developing countries, with a greater proportion of young people than in the industrialised world, also makes comparisons of disease frequency difficult. The recording of data may be limited.

When do health problems occur?

The question of when (in time) diseases occur or peak is of considerable interest to the epidemiologist. For example, it is well established that a range of well-known infectious diseases (for example, measles, influenza and whooping cough) show cyclical variations in occurrence, which results in epidemics every few years.

Look at Figure 13.4 and identify in which years notifications about pertussis (whooping cough) cases peaked.

You will note that in 1978 over 60,000 cases were reported and this fell dramatically in 1981 only to rise again in 1982. The rises may be explained by media coverage of the dangers of the vaccine in the mid 1970s and then again in the early 1980s.

When considering time in relation to the occurrence of diseases, we have to bear in mind that time can be measured in a variety of ways: as secular time (referring to centuries), as cyclical time or time intervals, as seasonal time (i.e. summer, autumn, winter and spring), or by specifying particular times of the week or times of the day. In relation to 'secular time' in this country and elsewhere, infectious diseases constituted a major health problem throughout the nineteenth century. Fortunately, most of these diseases have declined and even been eliminated altogether (like smallpox). However, at the end of the twentieth century, AIDS, heart disease and cancer have become the major health problems.

Seasonal variations in the incidence of disease are most common for respiratory tract infections (during winter months). Salmonella food poisoning also frequently shows seasonal variations, with peaks during the

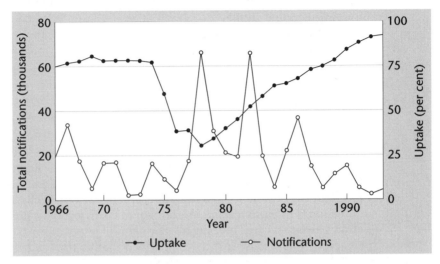

Figure 13.4 **Pertussis notifications and immunisation uptake 1966 to 1993 (England and Wales)** (HEA, 1995d)

summer and in the Christmas period. Hayfever and other allergies occur primarily in the early summer.

Outbreaks of diseases can also be related to specific points in time, locations or events. For example, the sudden occurrence of infection such as typhoid or salmonella food poisoning is usually due to the simultaneous (or near simultaneous) exposure of groups of susceptible people to a certain micro-organism, as might happen at a wedding reception or a hotel.

Thus, despite considerable evidence about the influence various factors have on people's health, epidemiologists cannot infer that the link between a factor and ill-health is necessarily a causal one. Causation of ill-health is difficult to determine. Other than infectious diseases most evidence relates to the risk associated with particular factors, rather than the direct causes of ill-health. Even in the case of infectious diseases, it is not known why certain people succumb to them, whilst other, seemingly similar people do not.

Occasionally, descriptive studies give an indication of the cause of a disease, but normally special epidemiological studies are needed to determine the positive causation of a disease. Only certain types of causative mechanism are amenable to investigation by epidemiological methods and no disease can be said to have a single cause. Epidemiological evidence regarding disease causation is mainly circumstantial.

13.4 Types of epidemiological studies

Epidemiological studies generally fall into three broad categories:

- cross-sectional studies
- case control and cohort studies
- intervention studies.

Cross-sectional studies

Cross-sectional studies are used to determine the prevalence of conditions or characteristics of people in a population. These are essentially descriptive studies, although their results can often suggest causative factors associated with particular illness or behaviour. They may be used to ascertain the prevalence of a health-related behaviour, such as the wearing of seat-belts or participation in exercise. In cross-sectional studies, it is not always necessary to investigate the whole population: a sample (see Chapter 14) is usually sufficient, provided that its size is adequate and the individuals in the sample are representative of the total group under consideration.

A population or group can be studied in a variety of ways: by questionnaire, by taking measurements (such as blood pressure), by analysing blood specimens (for example, for blood cholesterol levels), or by examining health-care records. Questionnaires are often used to obtain data and information about populations and groups. They allow information to be gathered from relatively large groups, whereas other techniques (such as interviews) usually have to be confined to small population samples. Questionnaire design will be discussed in Part 4. Many health districts have undertaken health and lifestyle surveys at regular intervals of 4–5 years to examine changes.

Case control and cohort studies

These focus on determining disease causation. *Case control studies* tend to be relatively quick and cheap whereas cohort studies are time-consuming and expensive. A case control study is often undertaken to test a particular hypothesis or theory, and may if appropriate be followed by a cohort study. The 'case' is a person who has a particular symptom or medical condition. Thus, the focus is on a group of cases which is then compared with a 'control group' consisting of persons not having the symptom or the medical condition. Investigations are then carried out into the previous exposure of the two groups to particular factors that are suspected of causing the symptom or condition. If the two groups differ regarding their exposure to such factors, a causal link between the symptom/condition and the factor is inferred.

A good example of a case-control study was the important study reported by Herbst *et al.*, (1971) and Herbst and Scully (1980) in which a clinician noticed a cluster of unusual cancers in adolescent girls. On investigation, it was found that the mothers of these girls had been treated with a hormone during pregnancy, whilst the mothers of the adolescent girls in the control group had not. (The particular hormone had been prescribed to prevent miscarriages in the girls' mothers, but no one had suspected that their children might develop cancer.)

Cohort studies focus on groups of people who show certain attributes or characteristics (for example, with respect to their health behaviour). The groups are then observed over a period of time in order to discover what happens to their members and to check whether there are any associations between behaviour and disease (see Chapter 14). To test this theory, the famous epidemiologist, Sir Richard Doll, and colleagues investigated doctors' smoking habits and *prospectively* followed the sample over 40 years, by which time two-thirds of the sample had died. The finding obtained during the first 20 years was that doctors who were heavy cigarette smokers were 32 times more likely to die of lung cancer than doctors who were non-smokers (Doll and Hill, 1964). Mortality associated with smoking doubled during the second half of the study (Doll *et al.*, 1994).

Cohort studies may also be *longitudinal studies* (studies over time), as well as prospective or retrospective studies. Longitudinal studies can be very costly in time and money and require following up subjects which may prove difficult. They have the advantage of being able to accumulate very useful information in determining the long-term effects of biological, environmental and social factors on health. Comparing cohorts born in 1946, 1958 and 1970 could throw light on the effects of changes in social and health policy and education on beliefs about diet, smoking, exercise and other issues of interest to those engaged in promoting health.

Intervention studies

Whereas the types of study described so far are purely observational in nature, intervention studies involve intervening with a group of people, with another equivalent group acting as a 'reference'. The most popular study of this kind is the *randomised control trial*. These divide the population to be studied into the groups on a random basis, one group is then subjected to a treatment, procedure or intervention, the other not. If the two groups are exactly similar in their characteristics, then any measurable differences between them should be due to the intervention. Statistical tests are used to assess whether the difference between the two groups is significant (a 'real' difference rather than as a result of some error in the trial or through chance). Ideally the randomised control trial should be carried out using a double-blind method: that is, neither the researcher nor the subject knows who is in the study. An ongoing longitudinal study using this method is a large study of twin women over the ages of 40 which is looking at a range of similarities and differences and testing, amongst other variables, the effectiveness of hormone replacement therapies (Spector, ongoing). Designing these studies can be quite complex and the advice of a statistician or epidemiologist should be sought in the planning stages.

Intervention studies are conducted in the following way: initially, observations (or measurements) are made on a population which is then divided (by random sampling) into two equivalent groups. Of these, one is subjected to the intervention. After some predetermined period following the intervention, the observations are repeated and the results for the two groups compared to establish whether or not the intervention had any effect. Objections to trials such as these are often on ethical grounds (see Chapter 6) and relate in part to whether the participants are fully informed about the potential effects of participating.

Drug trials are by far the most common type of epidemiological intervention studies. Their purpose is to discover the effects and effectiveness of new drugs developed by the pharmaceutical industry (for example, propranolol, a cardiac betablocker). Intervention studies may be useful for health promotion. The effect of a 'stop-smoking' campaign could be investigated this way. This might take the form of initially investigating the smoking behaviour of a group of people and subsequently exposing one half of this group to an appropriate health education programme. After a predetermined time interval the smoking habits of the two groups could be compared to see if the campaign had had any significant effect. However, there are many problems associated with the use of randomised control trials in health promotion (Speller *et al.*, 1997). This will be discussed further in Part 4.

Intervention studies can also be used in order to determine the relative effectiveness of different health promotion techniques, or for finding out how different population groups react and respond to particular techniques.

13.5 Conclusion

The nature and methods of demographic enquiry and research are of considerable importance to those engaged in promoting health. And even more important to health promoters is the data generated through epidemiological study which is concerned primarily with understanding the distribution of disease and ill-health in populations and population groups. However, as you noted in Chapter 12 when considering the sources of health information, the usefulness of epidemiological evidence will obviously depend on whether the 'right' questions were asked and for which people and which groups these questions were indeed appropriate. In order to gauge the questions epidemiologists have attempted to answer it is important to understand how they analyse and present information collected in numerical form. This is explored in Chapter 14. This chapter has considered quantitative approaches to studying populations. We consider some qualitative approaches in Chapter 15.

Chapter 14
Analysing numerical data

14.1 Introduction

Health promoters may be called upon to explain and contextualise health information. In addition, they may be expected to collect data as well as interpret it. Information requirements about health issues go in both directions: epidemiologists, public health physicians and other information specialists have, as part of their work, the responsibility for interpreting data for various bodies, including health authorities. They do, however, often need the guidance of health workers and others who have a thorough knowledge of an area of practice and who may have collected some of the data themselves. It is therefore essential for those involved in promoting health to understand the ways in which information about health matters is obtained, as well as how to evaluate and assess such information.

There are various terms that are used in everyday language but which also have a specialist meaning for researchers (including, for example, the social sciences) when describing data. You will be familiar with the terms validity, reliability, sample and population in a variety of contexts. We shall now explore how such terms are used more narrowly when describing research findings.

Instruments are measuring devices which are used in particular studies. These might include devices such as questionnaires, inventories, observation schedules and interview schedules.

The *population* under study is the number of individuals or items from which the samples are drawn, for example all those resident in a specific locality or all mothers with children under the age of five living in a particular village. As it is only rarely possible to study the whole population, it is necessary to *sample* that population. The *sample* is thus a set of individuals or items selected from a population and analysed to test hypotheses about that population. There are different ways of selecting samples depending on the size and nature of the population and also the purpose of the study but usually the researcher aims to get as *representative* a sample as possible. It is important that the sample reflects the characteristics of the particular population under study. *Random sampling* is a technique whereby each member of the population has an equal possibility of being selected. *Systematic sampling* occurs when a predetermined system is used, for example choosing every tenth pregnant woman attending antenatal classes to enter the study. *Stratified sampling* means that the population is divided into subgroups according to particular characteristics (e.g. age and sex) which then have random or systematic sampling performed on them. A *purposive* sample is one where people, organisations or objects exhibiting particular characteristics are chosen for study, for example pregnant women over the age of 40 with diabetes

Validity is the degree to which a research instrument measures what it is intended to measure. There are several kinds of validity: *content validity* looks at whether the research instrument measures all aspects which it hopes to measure, in other words is the content of a complex concept like health adequately measured by the proposed indicators? For example, could you measure health by the number of aspirins someone takes? This would be nonsensical because some people don't take aspirins for headaches, and others take them as a preventive measure against cardiovascular disease. Another type of validity is *criterion validity,* where one looks to see whether another measure would give the same result. An example would be to see whether you get the same results when measuring a particular health status using two different questionnaires. To establish both kinds of validity you might approach experts in the specific field to enlist their help in evaluating the instrument. *External validity* reflects how well the research results can be generalised to the wider population of interest (Bowling, 1997: 162). The sampling methodology is important for enhancing this.

'*Reliability*' can be illustrated by the following case studies:

In a study in rural India, in which the incidence of accidental injuries was studied by paying periodic home visits and asking about injuries occurring since the last home visit, the incidence was doubled when inquiries were made at intervals of two weeks instead of a month.

A number of studies have shown that if children are measured during the morning they are on average taller, by half a centimetre or more, than if they are measured in the afternoon

(Abramson, 1990: 137-8)

These examples clearly illustrate inconsistent or unstable information. Reliability refers to the stability or consistency of information (Abramson, 1990) and means that similar answers would be obtained if the instrument was used repeatedly on an unchanging object or person. 'The reliability of a procedure of measurement is equivalent to a marksman's capacity to hit the same spot each time he fires, irrespective of how close he comes to the bull's eye.' To assess reliability, the same scale is usually administered at different times to the same population (test-retest). Within reliability there are a number of additional measures to test. Internal consistency is tested by measuring the same concept by different scale items; inter- and intra-rater reliability is tested by looking at the consistency of the measure when administered by a different interviewer or the same interviewer at different times. A measure can theoretically be reliable without being valid.

When collecting data, it is important to appraise critically your own data-collection skills. Developing valid, reliable data collection instruments (be they questionnaires, interview schedules or observation schedules) is time-consuming. As health promoters may not necessarily have time or money available to develop these instruments you will find yourself modifying instruments developed by others (for example existing health and lifestyle surveys) for specific purposes. However, this may mean testing the instruments carefully in the new context.

14.2 Introduction to statistics

This section is not designed to teach you statistics but to introduce you to statistical concepts so that when you are confronted with statistical data you can ask yourself the following questions before deciding whether you should invest the time interpreting it:

- Is the source reputable?
- Was the context in which the statistics were collected similar enough to the situation you want to understand that the figures are applicable?
- Was the data collected relatively recently (or in the last census)?
- If sampling was involved, was the sample representative, and was it large enough?

Data available from records and published sources is often secondary data: that is, originally collected and presented for a different purpose. When making use of such data, it is important that you have satisfactory answers to the questions summarised above. One measure which is used frequently and which may seem uncontentious is mortality data; however, this depends on the consistency with which death certificates are completed.

Mortality statistics

In Chapter 2 you noted that the two key statistical measures used to understand patterns in health are mortality and morbidity data which are used as proxies for health. Mortality statistics are based on death certificates which list the cause of death, the date and place of death, and the name, age and sex of the deceased.

The doctor completes the cause of death box and a relative or friend delivers it to the local registrar of births, deaths and marriages who sends it to the Office for National Statistics (ONS). This information is transformed by codifiers into a number which is given to a particular cause of death on a list called the International Classification of Diseases, Injuries and Causes of Death (ICD). For example, cancer of the lung is ICD 162. The accuracy of death certification may be questioned which obviously presents those who have to analyse such data with a number of problems. It is important to note here that routine mortality statistics are based on the underlying cause of death. However, the ONS also now codes additional causes mentioned on the death certificate.

The usefulness and validity of mortality statistics depends on the accuracy with which death certificates are completed. Variations in diagnostic decisions between countries, between physicians and over

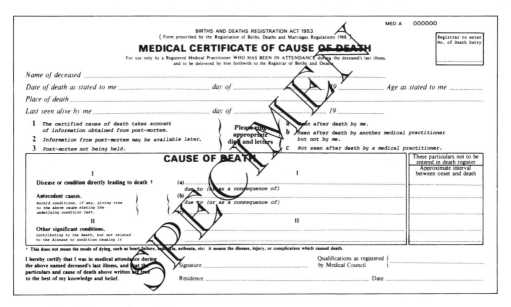

Figure 14.1   **Death certificate**

time can influence the mortality rates derived from these certificates. In addition the cause of death or underlying disease or diseases mentioned on the death certificate might mask a serious disease problem which is not identified either because the person completing the death certificate is unaware of underlying causes, or because the dying person or his or her family put pressure on the doctor certifying the death to withhold this information (for example people with AIDS). This misrepresentation could occur following a fatal road traffic accident. The deceased may have had a CVA or a heart attack before or during the accident. Alternatively the deceased may have suffered from a number of conditions that would not be explored during a post-mortem.

In the past 'old age' was a perfectly acceptable cause of death. Even nowadays registrars vary in their willingness to accept this as a cause of death. When my 94-year-old grandfather died in 1982, the doctor certified his death as due to carcinoma of the liver. On enquiring what the GP had written on the death certificate, the consultant physician informed me that this was indeed inaccurate – my grandfather had secondaries (spread of the cancer, not the primary tumour) in his liver, but had died of bowel cancer. So the ONS would have added one case of liver cancer instead of the 'accurate' diagnosis, bowel cancer. Has this inaccurate information on my grandfather's death certificate contributed to a belief that liver cancer was more common than previously thought? There may be discrepancies in up to 30–50 per cent of cases (Peto, 1994) and this is likely to be more common in older people where there is multiple pathology.

Mortality statistics measure outcome at a point which may be remote from the disease itself. What of the miners who were exposed to asbestos but died of lung cancer? Does the information from death certificates that we get about lung cancer differentiate between the initial causes of the disease – was it due to industrial exposure or to smoking, or is the diagnosis inaccurate? What about someone whose death is attributed to pneumonia but a post-mortem, had it been carried out, would have revealed that that person had lung cancer, or possibly at the end of the twentieth century, AIDS?

Autopsies are sometimes requested if there is some doubt about the actual cause of death. These cases may have been 'difficult' to certify, in which case these findings may exaggerate the inaccuracy of death certification in general. The implications of this are costly – doctors should be more careful when certifying deaths, or maybe more autopsies should be performed to enable us to have more accurate information. More properly performed autopsies would document changes that follow on lifestyle changes and would therefore provide useful information about disease patterns.

Chapter 2 explained that the statistical measure SMR (standardised mortality ratio) measures the relative chances of death at a stated age – the death rate. To calculate the SMR for a particular cause of death, in a particular area, age-specific death rates are first calculated for contiguous age ranges in the national population. These rates are then multiplied by the corresponding age-specific populations for the area to give the number of deaths from the particular cause that would be expected if mortality in the area varied with age in the same way as in the nation as a whole. Finally, the observed number of deaths in the area, due to the particular cause, is divided by the expected deaths and expressed as a percentage. The resultant figure is the SMR. A value significantly higher or lower than 100 (see 'confidence interval' below) indicates that mortality in the area differs from the national mortality for some reason other than the age/sex distribution of the population of the area.

Look at Figure 14.2 which shows lung cancer death rates.

What does Figure 14.2 show you about SMRs by social class in Great Britain?

You will note that SMRs are greatest among those in social classes IV and V. How might this be explained? Smoking prevalence is three times greater in men who work in unskilled manual occupations compared to professional men (Townsend *et al.*, 1994). This has been sustained over 20 years. The figure demonstrates that lung cancer mortality in men in unskilled manual occupations aged 20-64 is four times greater than in professional men. The social class gradient is present but not as steep in women.

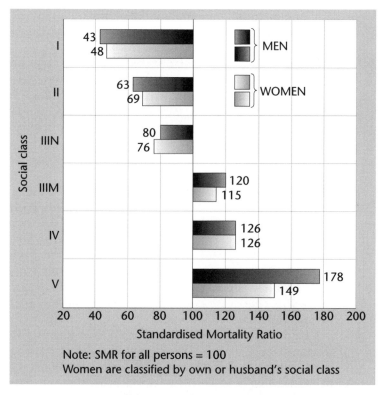

Figure 14.2 **Standardised mortality ratios for lung cancer by social class in Great Britain: men aged 20–64 and women aged 20–59.** (HEA, 1991)

Confidence interval

Even if an area has the same underlying mortality rate as England and Wales, its SMR (calculated as above) is unlikely to be exactly 100 because the number of deaths observed is subject to random fluctuations. It is possible to calculate the range within which the true SMR lies, with 95 per cent *probability* (could a certain pattern of numbers, a situation or event have arisen by chance?). This range is called the '95 per cent confidence interval'. If this interval does not include the value 100, then the SMR can be said to be significantly different from 100. This suggests that the death rate in the area is significantly higher or lower than the national average, even when adjusted for differences between the age distributions of the national and area populations.

Figure 14.3 shows SMRs and their confidence limits for acute myocardial infarction for each district health authority (DHA) of the Yorkshire region. The confidence interval for each DHA is shown as a horizontal bar, against a horizontal scale of values, with the calculated SMR marked as illustrated.

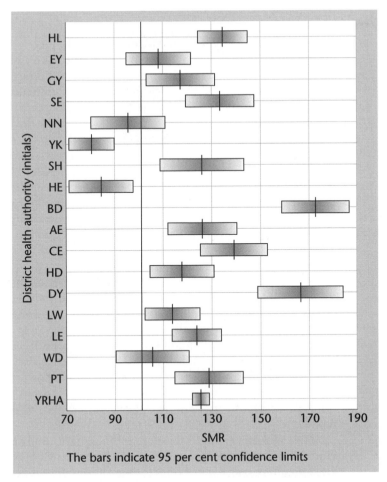

Figure 14.3 **Standardised mortality ratio (SMR) for acute myocardial infarction, ages 35 – 64 (males, 1985–89, Yorkshire DHAs)** (HEA, 1993a: 29)

The vertical line indicates the SMR for England and Wales which, by definition, is always 100. The top bar (Hull) does not overlap the vertical line; therefore mortality in Hull is significantly higher than that in England and Wales. Conversely, the second bar (East Yorkshire) does overlap the vertical line; therefore, mortality in East Yorkshire is not significantly different from that in England and Wales.

Before looking at how data can be represented and misrepresented it is important to look at some additional terms which apply to data interpretation.

Morbidity statistics

Morbidity statistics, as you will recall from Chapter 2, are indicators of ill health and collected by clinicians, hospitals and primary care teams using certain outcome measures. These may entail biochemical tests, observed symptom rates (pain, exercise testing) or role performance (Bowling, 1991). Looking at return-to-work statistics can be misleading as other factors such as age and economic and social opportunities need to be taken into account. There are a number of physician-assessed morbidity scales but many have severe limitations as their definitions of health or what being healthy entails are not necessarily consistent. Morbidity data may be more successfully collected from self-reported health status questionnaires focusing in particular on functional ability and status, and broader concepts of positive health and quality of life (Bowling, 1991).

Morbidity data collected by epidemiologists provides information about the incidence of diseases which are non-fatal. It is relatively easy to collect some data, such as the incidence and prevalence of infectious disease, as cases can be easily recognised and reported by health professionals. Outbreaks of Legionnaires disease (an acute respiratory infection) and Salmonella food poisoning are quickly noted by organisations such as the Public Health Laboratory Service and are immediately taken up by the media (Entwistle, 1995). These reports, as we said earlier, influence and sometimes drive public policy. However, even with easily noticeable conditions such as infectious diseases, there can be under reporting.

Many chronic conditions such as back pain and arthritis are under reported and do not appear in official statistics. Mental health problems are difficult to assess as not only is there an unwillingness to report mental problems but also the diagnostic categories into which those suffering mental health problems are placed are subject to debate and redefinition. The *Health and Lifestyles Survey* (1987) documented many incidents of illness that went unreported to the medical profession and therefore did not appear in morbidity statistics. Morbidity statistics are even more prone to inaccuracy and incompleteness than mortality statistics.

With conditions such as HIV/AIDS, there are many confounding factors which make accurate estimations of those affected difficult, if not impossible, to obtain. AIDS is now the fifth leading cause of death among American men aged 35-44, following accidents, heart disease, cancer and suicide. AIDS is the fifth highest cause of death in the USA among women after cancer, accidents, heart disease and suicide. Nearly 600,000 cases of AIDS have been reported by the Centers for Disease Control and Prevention since the disease was first recognised in 1981.

Look at Figure 14.4 and try to answer the question on the next page.

Consider why it might be difficult to judge accurately the number of likely cases of AIDS through morbidity statistics.

Only those having an HIV test will appear in official morbidity statistics. Anonymous testing of women attending antenatal clinics has given some prevalence data but this has only been undertaken in small studies and cannot be extrapolated to the general population. The continual redefinition of AIDS diagnostic characteristics also affects the morbidity data. Of course, being HIV-positive does not mean having any overt symptoms and again medical diagnosis can come at a very late stage in the disease.

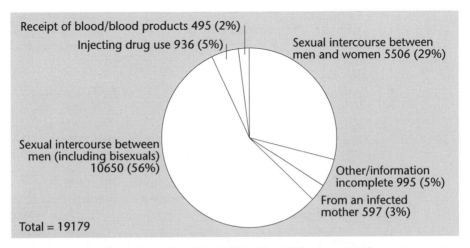

Receipt of blood/blood products 495 (2%)
Injecting drug use 936 (5%)
Sexual intercourse between men and women 5506 (29%)
Sexual intercourse between men (including bisexuals) 10650 (56%)
Other/information incomplete 995 (5%)
From an infected mother 597 (3%)
Total = 19179

Figure 14.4 **Number of people with AIDS in the UK by transmission category to the end of 1999**

14.3 Interpreting data

In this section we will explore the meaning of some commonly used statistical terminology.

Mean, mode and median

Many terms, such as average, median and mode, used when interpreting data are found in everyday life. Let's look at the term 'mean' (or 'average') first.

If the numbers of HIV-positive adults in seven districts are:

40   50   60   60   60   70   220

respectively, what is the average number of HIV-positive cases per district across the seven districts? The answer can be obtained by dividing the total number of HIV cases by the number of districts, in other words 560 divided by 7. Thus, the average, or mean, is 80.

The number that occurs most often is known as the 'mode', in this case 60. If, instead, we look for the number of HIV-positive adults for the district that appears in the middle when the districts are placed in order from the lowest to highest number of HIV cases, then the figure we get is 60. This is known as the 'median'.

As this example shows, the definitions of mode, median and mean are clear-cut. However, what is not clear is *when* each of them should be used. Here are some general guidelines. If the prime concern is the *total* (in this case, the total number of cases in all seven areas), then the mean is usually most appropriate. If the aim is to obtain a figure that is representative of all the districts, then the median is usually the appropriate measure. If, however, we wish to identify the largest subgroup of districts with a similar number of cases, then the modal group would seem to be the most appropriate.

In many small groups, the pattern of ages of the group members will not reflect anything more than that particular group. For example, a group of pregnant women is likely to be concentrated in the 20–35 age band with a number of outliers. Suppose you are meeting with ten pregnant women who get together because they are all diabetic. Their ages are as follows:

    18   19   23   26   28   32   37   38   39   43

Thus we have two teenagers, three women in their twenties, four in their thirties, and one in her forties.

How would you calculate the mean (average) age?

The mean = total size / sample number, i.e. $303/10 = 30.3$, which in fact is the actual age of none of the pregnant women. The median being the middle of this range would co-incidentally also be around 30, but might not have been had there more pregnancies in the middle band (25–35). The median age is also around the 30 mark so would be an appropriate average to quote. An average is meant to be a 'typical' value. When summarising data, make sure you choose a form of average that has this quality of 'typicalness'.

Percentages of different groups are also important. Surveys relating to staff eating habits were conducted by several of the Health Promoting Hospitals in Wales (Cefn Coed Hospital, 1995) One staff cafeteria offered a free vegetable with any meal for a period of time to encourage staff to eat 'greens'. If this was used as an indicator of lifestyle change and the survey found that 43 out of 50 people attending the staff cafeteria continued to order the green vegetable, they might conclude that 86 per cent of the staff modified their eating habits as a result of the intervention. However, only with a large group of people are percentages relevant.

Correlation

Data collection often involves taking one single measure from each person or item in a sample to provide a picture of the variables in question, for example the height of eleven-year-old girls in a class. However, sometimes data can be collected in pairs. As well as looking at single variables and which statistics summarise them (for example, averages and percentages), using paired data we can look at the relationship between the two things being measured. It is often useful to draw a scattergram to illustrate the way in which two variables are associated with each other. The regression line, or 'best fit' line, is the best line which can be made to fit the line point it passes through.

The degree of scatter of the points, or the correlation, is a measure of the strength of the association between two variables (Graham, 1994). The correlation coefficient (r) measures the extent to which two variables move together in a straight line. The correlation coefficient can take values between minus one and plus one:

$r = -1$ means perfect negative correlation

$r = 1$ means perfect positive correlation

$r = 0$ means zero correlation

$r = -0.84$ means strong negative correlation

$r = 0.15$ means weak positive correlation

(adapted from Graham, 1994)

However, the number of points on the scattergram is relevant. The smaller the number of points, the larger must be the value of r to provide evidence of significant correlation. With too few points, high values of r can occur by chance alone. So we must always ask how many points a value of r was based on.

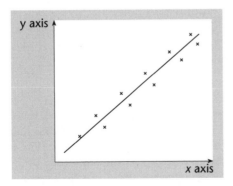 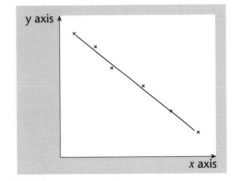

Figure 14.5   **(a) Positive correlation; (b) Negative correlation**

Secondly, we need to be aware that 'correlation does not imply causation'. Just because two variables are highly correlated, this does not necessarily mean that a cause-and-effect relationship exists between them. All tall children do not necessarily weigh more, there are many factors which influence weight, for example genetics and food intake.

To exemplify this point, think of the association between lung cancer and smoking.

Look back to **Figure 14.2** which demonstrated lung cancer SMRs by class and compare it with **Table 14.1** which shows the percentages of people who smoke by social class. Do they tell you anything about the possible connection between smoking and lung cancer?

Table 14.1 **Cigarette smoking prevalence (per cent) adults, 1992**

	Males	*Females*
Professional (SCI)	14	13
Employers and Managers (SCII)	23	21
Intermediate and junior non-manual (SCIIIN)	25	27
Skilled manual and own account non-professional (SCIIIM)	34	31
Semi-skilled manual and personal service(SCIV)	39	35
Unskilled manual (SCV)	42	35

(DoH, 1995)

Many experts and lay people argue that smoking is a risk factor for lung cancer and that social classes IV and V are more likely to contract lung cancer (See Chapter 2). But it is impossible to establish that any particular case of lung cancer is directly attributable to smoking. Indeed some people develop lung cancer without ever having smoked. Thus, a *causal* connection between lung cancer and smoking cannot be established. All that can be stated on the basis of the statistical evidence is that lung cancer and smoking are statistically correlated.

Tests of significance

In this sub-section we explore some terminology used when looking at statistical information in health research papers and articles: hypothesis, null hypothesis, statistical significance level or p-value. The terms 'test of significance' and 'hypothesis test' both refer to more or less the same statistical process of deciding whether there is a difference between two values or two sets of results.

To ensure that experiments are conducted with the issue of random chance kept in mind, every experimental hypothesis has a null hypothesis. The null hypothesis in most cases states:

the results of the experiment will simply be the product of random chance.

The null hypothesis is *not* the opposite of your hypothesis, *nor* is it an alternative hypothesis. If we can *disprove* the null hypothesis we gain *support* for our hypothesis. It simply states that your results will be due to chance.

(Open University, 1998: 28)

In scientific research it is a convention to accept odds of either 1 in 100 (i.e. 1%) or 5 in 100 (i.e. 5%) as grounds for rejecting the null hypothesis and accepting that the research hypothesis has been supported. This is expressed by stating that the probability of a result being random is less than 1% or less than 5%, that is, that findings were significant ($p < 0.01$) or ($p < 0.05$).

(Open University, 1998: 40)

The p-value may be attached to some conclusions that have been drawn from research data, as in 'the mean amount of spinach eaten by men is greater than that eaten by women ($p < 0.05$)'. In general, p-values indicate the probability that a conclusion drawn from data collected from a sample and extrapolated to the population at large could be the result of an unrepresentative sample. The smaller the p-value, the lower is that probability. Here a p-value of 0.05 denotes that this probability is 0.05 in 1 or, expressed differently, 5 in 100, or 5 per cent. In other words, a conclusion for which the p-value (or 'statistical significance level') is 0.05 would only in five out of 100 cases be the result of an unrepresentative experimental sample. Thus, p-values help judge the confidence in the correctness of the results. The value of p can lie between 0 and 1, but an upper limit of 0.05 is usually imposed if the findings are to be accepted as reasonably dependable.

14.4 Ways of representing data: graphic presentations

Data can be represented graphically in a number of ways. Some of the most useful are graphs, disease maps, pyramids, histograms, scattergrams and pie charts. We'll look briefly at the value of each in turn.

As a practitioner you may well have used *graphs* and *tables* in building a case for a particular health action or social intervention. Many parents plot their children's height on a wall or a door to measure their growth patterns. Consider an example where a particular child (Gary) seems not to be growing according to the normal percentiles and another child (Graham) is. You could plot Graham's age/years on one axis and his height on another and represent this on a graph. On the same graph Gary's growth patterns could be done as a comparison using a slightly different colour or a broken line:

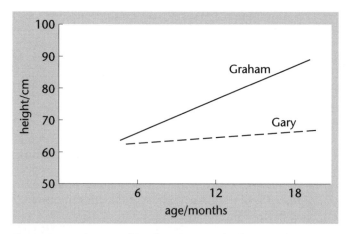

Figure 14.6   **Gary and Graham's growth chart**

What problems might be encountered in the creation and interpretation of this graph?

It is very important when drawing graphs to decide at the outset the range of numbers on each axis, as these figures will determine the shape of a graph and could be misleading. For example, if there were very large intervals for the height as opposed to the age, Graham's increase in height might look fairly normal. To practitioners reading the graph this could make a difference as to what conclusions they drew about Gary's growth patterns, and the need for health advice or social work intervention. The Radical Statistics Health Group have sometimes been critical of official statistics on precisely these grounds, that the range of axes can serve to misrepresent health trends quite significantly (RSHG, 1983).

Another way of presenting complex data is through maps, for example those showing the geographical distribution of diseases. Look back at Figure 13.2 which shows the regional variations in the age-standardised lung cancer mortality rate. This illustrates that the further north you go, the greater is the incidence of death from lung cancer. Small pockets of lung cancer deaths are also reported in the Midlands and in certain areas of London.

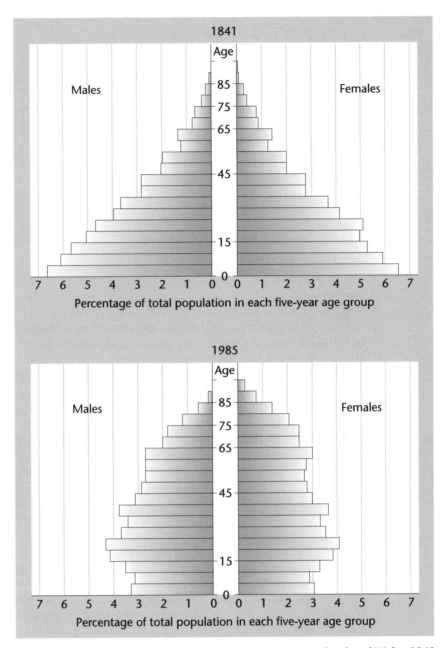

Figure 14.7 **Sex and age structure of the population, England and Wales 1841 and 1985** (HEA, 1993)

An effective way of demonstrating age distribution is through population pyramids. Figure 14.7 shows two population pyramids comparing 1841 and 1985 for England and Wales. Each bar represents the proportion of the total population in that particular age/sex group.

Compare the general shapes of the two population pyramids – what changes do they indicate?

- In 1841, 6.5 per cent of the population consisted of males aged under five years, whilst in 1985 the percentage of males in this age group was only 3.2 per cent. (The figures for the equivalent population of females are practically the same.)
- In 1985, the number of women over 65 was greater than the number of men of similar age.
- In 1841, 35 per cent of the population was under 15, and 5 per cent was aged 65 and above. In 1985, only 19 per cent of the population was under 15, whilst the percentage of the 65+ age group had risen to 15 per cent. (These figures are obtained by adding the lengths of the appropriate columns.)

The broad-based pyramid shape for 1841 indicates a combination of high fertility rates and high mortality rates. The more rectangular shape for 1985 shows a low fertility and low mortality pattern.

Population pyramids express the age distributions within populations in terms of percentages, not in terms of numbers. Therefore, if we are interested in showing *how* the number of people in different age categories has changed with time, another type of graphical representation is required. One such type is a 'stacked' bar chart or histogram which you have met several times before (e.g. Figure 13.3). If you look at Figure 14.2, you will note that histograms present bars of equal width to illustrate changes of data. This is very effective for illustrating comparative information. For example, as part of the Liverpool Healthy Cities Research Consortium, Croxteth Health Action Area (CHAA) produces information about various health issues and uses histograms to illustrate, for example, levels of disability in Croxteth.

Finally, a number of pie charts have appeared already in this book. Figure 2.1 looked at major causes of death from 1931–91 in England and Wales and Figure 14.4 illustrated the number of likely cases of AIDS by transmission category. Pie charts are a convenient way of representing the relative importance of causes or events since it does not matter whether in interpreting such charts, you focus on the angles at the centre, or on the areas of the various sectors, or on the arcs round the outside: they are all proportional to one another.

Liverpool's city health plan uses the pie chart in Figure 14.8 to describe the water quality in Merseyside. If translated into percentages this chart shows that 33 per cent of water sources are class 3 (poor), whilst 11 per cent are Class 4 (bad). That leaves only 56 per cent of Mersey water as falling into the Good or Fair (Classes 1a, 1b and Class 2) categories. Another form of representation might have been more useful for demonstrating the different classes, as pie charts are not suitable if there are a number of small categories (or slices).

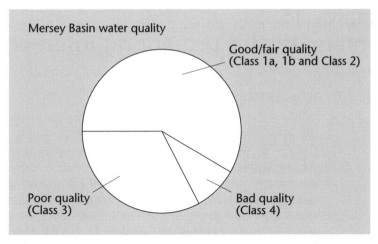

Figure 14.8   **Water quality in Merseyside**   (Liverpool Healthy City 2000, 1995)

Using visual aids such as graphs, histograms and pie charts enables us to read data easily and explain it in relatively simple fashion to those not familiar with the presentation of statistical data. There are many software packages, such as Excel, to assist with presenting statistical data.

14.5 Conclusion

In this chapter you have looked at the different ways numerical data is analysed and presented. You will recognise that statistical data needs to be interpreted in a cautious manner. When looking at the results and conclusions of any study it is necessary to examine the sources of the data before ascertaining whether it is reasonable to apply the conclusions drawn from one sample or context to another. In addition, it is important to remember that statistical inferences should not be accepted at face value, without some indication of confidence levels. The principles covered in this chapter and Chapter 13 form the foundation for Chapter 15 in which you will examine the conditions required for planning health interventions.

Chapter 15
Planning health promoting interventions

15.1 Introduction

In most health, welfare and education work people undertake some planning. In initial training, and possibly in subsequent professional updating, you will probably have been involved in reviewing how to plan interventions. The nursing process offers a useful starting point, for example, since it directs nurses to investigate, assess, plan, implement and evaluate their care giving. This draws attention to the fact that planning is one of a number of stages and needs to be preceded by investigation and assessment and followed, after implementation, by evaluation.

This chapter concentrates on both the pre-planning stage of investigating and assessing needs and the steps towards implementation of the plan. Planning can be seen as part of a cyclical process ending with evaluation and this chapter forms the bridge between health information (the last three chapters) and Part 4 of this book which will investigate the process of evaluation.

Why plan?

There are many opportunities for health promoting encounters which occur spontaneously, such as during a GP consultation. The consultation may ostensibly be about a painful knee but if the person is overweight then the GP can discuss weight reduction as well as investigating the knee problem. We have also stressed throughout this book the importance of communicating in such a way as to make all relationships between health workers and their clients health promoting. However, health promotion takes place at many levels and all health promoting interventions need to be given some forethought. Making plans can be an end in itself and a substitute for doing. On the other hand doing without planning can lead to disappointment and frustration and can be a waste of time and resources. Planning can help to make sure that resources are used well and are most effective. Without planning, health promoting interventions run the risk of being marginalised and not having priority in resource distribution. Perhaps most important of all, planning is a reflective activity: it focuses the mind on the job in hand and forces people to prioritise and justify their activities. For many people, planning is a taken-for-granted activity and something that they embark on many times a day in the course of their life and work. Plans can be made for small-scale activities such as planning a talk to give to a parent and toddler group, to big events such as planning a national no smoking day. Increasingly health, local authority and community workers are involved in developing health improvement programmes. This requires planning across health services, local authorities and the voluntary sector. Although the scale is different the planning process is fairly similar. Ewles and Simnett (1999) suggest that all plans should provide answers to three basic questions:

- what are my objectives?

- what do I need to do in order to achieve these objectives?

- how can I establish whether I have met my objectives?

15.2 What is planning?

The term 'planning' is used in a variety of ways and often other words are used instead to describe an aspect of planning. The terminology can be ambiguous and Box 15.1 differentiates between some of these different meanings:

Box 15.1

Plan – how to get from your starting point to your end point and what you want to achieve

Policy – guidelines for practice which set broad goals and the framework for action

Programme – overall outline of action. A package of services, or information, in planned sequence that is intended to produce a particular result

Strategy – the methods to be used in achieving goals

Priority – the first claim for consideration

Aim – broad goal

Objective – specific goal to be achieved

(adapted from Dignan and Carr, 1992, and Naidoo and Wills, 2000: 347)

Effective planning requires anticipation of what will be needed along the way toward reaching a goal. This statement implies that the goal is defined, as are the necessary steps involved in reaching the goal. Perhaps, most importantly, it requires an understanding of the steps and how they interrelate.

(Dignan and Carr, 1992: 4)

This implies that planning is a rational activity which involves noting and examining a range of options from which to choose before deciding on a programme. Figure 15.1 sets out a rational planning model which highlights various stages and their interconnections (McCarthy, 1982).

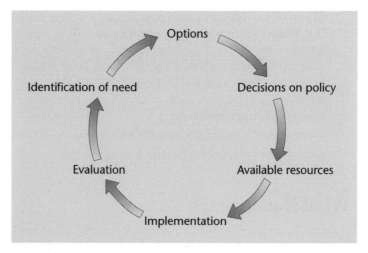

Figure 15.1 **Model of rational planning** (McCarthy, 1982)

Study McCarthy's model of 'rational planning'. What messages does it contain about how planning should be undertaken?

The McCarthy model suggests that the planning process is complex and cyclical. Identification of need, influenced by previous evaluation, is seen as feeding into a stage at which a whole range of options is considered. Only after this process are policy decisions made and resources committed to enable implementation to get underway. You may be rather sceptical about this view of the process and it is clear that in practice policy decisions are often made, and may have to be made, without knowing all the options. However, the early history of health education demonstrated that mass media campaigns or community development projects which lacked real insights into the audiences at which they were aimed were singularly ineffective (Rodmell and Watt, 1986; Sutherland, 1987). This suggests that evaluation of previous interventions and identification of needs are crucial stages in planning.

There are a range of different types of planning. This would depend to a large extent on the nature of the intervention to be undertaken. Some interventions, such as a local breast feeding awareness campaign, might need only a few people to be involved to set it up. On the other hand it might be more effective if representatives from local neighbourhood groups, the practice nurses from the local surgeries, and a representative from the National Childbirth Trust were involved. Some interventions might require a whole population approach. Some of the AIDS awareness campaigns have targeted whole sections of the population, for example young single people, with regard to condom use.

Planning an intervention may take place only with colleagues who share your perspective and your goals. However, if you are trying to reach a wide target audience you are more likely to want to plan this intervention with a variety of interested individuals or agencies, each of whom will have their own agenda to promote, as well as with funding officials or those representing local statutory or health services.

Figure 15.1 looks at rational planning and this suggests that being rational implies noting and examining a range of options from which to choose before deciding on a programme (McCarthy, 1982) But limited financial and human resources mean that it is not always possible to have a range of options. Certainly it would seem foolish to embark on large national campaigns without a rational and organised plan. Indeed, Tannahill (1990) argues for an overarching integrated planning framework for health promotion which goes beyond the narrow disease-oriented and risk factor approach:

> An integrated approach to health promotion planning involves dove-tailing comprehensive programmes of health education, in key settings and with key groups, with specific preventive services and with health protection measures appropriate to the places and people concerned.
>
> (Tannahill, 1990: 197)

Often, however, there is not a 'grand design' and planning ends up being piecemeal or incremental, each stage being added as deemed useful or appropriate (Naidoo and Wills, 2000; Jones and Sidell, 1997, Part 2). The rational model may be ideal but not always manageable in practice. Constraints on time, energy, budgets and uncertain futures can make planning an *ad hoc* activity often dictated by circumstances. Any planning then takes on an incremental nature moving forward towards only small but perhaps realistic goals. French and Milner (1993) suggest that the incremental approach is more flexible and enables collaborative working practices. This is particularly suited to working with individuals or small groups. For instance you will remember from Chapter 9 how one of the goals of counselling is to help people to make action plans. If this plan was to take action to change harmful drinking behaviour it would be very unwise of any counsellor to encourage the making of a grand plan with ambitious aims. Small manageable goals which are achievable and which can be built on incrementally would be much more realistic.

> **Go back to the three questions which Ewles and Simnett suggest are basic to any plan and ask yourself if they are appropriate to rational or incremental planning.**

The first two questions are appropriate to all forms of planning. In addressing the first question 'What are my objectives?' it would be necessary to identify needs, set priorities and specific aims and objectives. Underlying the question 'What do I need to do in order to achieve these objectives?' are decisions on the best way to achieve those aims and objectives, identifying resources and setting action plans. It is the third question which is perhaps more a feature of rational planning. Addressing the question 'How can I establish whether I have met these objectives?' involves building plans for evaluation into the overall plan so that evaluation becomes an integral part. Incremental planning is characterised more by trial and error building on successes and rejecting ways which do not work. Figure 15.2 provides a useful flowchart which works through the three questions. Although the chart is laid out in a linear fashion the arrows lead round in a circle with the evaluation feeding back into the whole process.

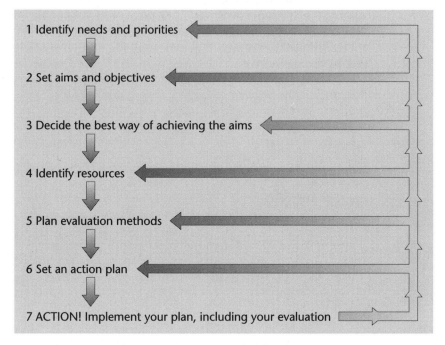

Figure 15.2   **A flowchart for planning and evaluating health promotion** (Ewles and Simnett, 1999)

Hawe *et al.* (1995) argue that rational programme planning is important for devising a health promotion programme that is appropriate to the health problem and the identified target group, within the resource available, and which will have the best chance of bringing about the desired change.

In the rest of this chapter we concentrate on the first four and the sixth element in the model, taking up the question of evaluation in Part 4.

15.3 Identifying needs

This section explores concepts of need and the different interpretations of need that may be made by lay people and professionals. It evaluates a range of needs assessment approaches and discusses how such assessment can inform planning for health promotion interventions. It builds on the previous chapters by demonstrating the central importance of having reliable and relevant health information in the planning stage of any health promoting activity.

An essential starting point for any health promoting intervention is identification of needs, yet the process of identifying and prioritising needs is complex and resource intensive. Systematic analyses of national health status are undertaken by the Chief Medical Officers, the national health promotion bodies, directors of public health medicine and health authorities/ health boards, and they provide much of the data on which health purchasing decisions and priority setting are based. They rely on epidemiological enquiry and are framed within scientific discourse (Bunton and Burrows, 1995). In contrast to this, health promoters are increasingly attempting to incorporate the ideas and reflect the needs of lay people who otherwise merely figure as the 'objects' of professional health promotion. While the national health strategy targets of the early 1990s, such as those to reduce the incidence of suicide or reduce smoking levels, were generally welcomed they were also seen very much as 'top-down' and expert assessments of health needs. A parallel development, it was argued, should be systematic participation by local people in priority and target setting for health gain (DoH, 1993). This has been reinforced in recent government policy (DoH, 1999).

A central problem in identifying needs is determining what needs themselves are and, in particular, what types of needs should be regarded as legitimate. At one level there are 'normative' or 'criteria referenced' needs: that is, needs as identified by professionals using official data. The surveys carried out by Townsend, Beattie and others in the latter 1980s (see Chapter 3) used a set of standard criteria by which to assess deprivation. The Jarman index also measured levels of deprivation according to a set of criteria which, although different from those used by Townsend, measured deprivation against a 'norm'. Part of this process may include the establishment of relative needs by comparing the health needs of one locality with another. In any organisation where resources are limited priorities need to be established and an equitable way of achieving this is to measure the relative needs of each area or unit requiring resources. Every organisation makes these policy judgements about priorities and in recent years they have become more visible and public within health care.

A taxonomy of needs

Bradshaw (1972) drew attention to four types of need: normative, comparative, felt and expressed. Normative needs, as we have noted, are those defined by professional experts and reflect professional judgements and standards. Using the medical model, for example, doctors may define some people's health or behaviour as falling within a 'normal' range while others may be entitled to (or required to undergo) treatment on the basis of their identified health needs.

Normative definitions of need reflect professional views about the nature of health problems and there may be considerable discrepancies between these views and those of lay people. In research on the Corkerhill estate in Glasgow, for example, professionals' views about improving children's safety focused only on better child and parental education, whereas parents' views also included calls for traffic calming and safe play areas (Roberts et al., 1995). Health promoters' views will reflect their own judgements about priorities and will be underpinned by values about what constitutes 'good health' and what the goal of health promotion should be (see Part 1, Chapters 5 and 6). In addition, professionals 'will judge a need relative to what they are able to provide' (Naidoo and Wills, 1994: 205). The remit of health visitors on the Corkerhill estate was very much focused on education rather than making infrastructural changes in the environment.

Assessing comparative needs usually involves estimation by professionals of which groups are in greater need of available services or resources. One aspect of national health strategies that many welcomed was that they set out clearer priorities for health promotion by creating targets for disease reduction and for improving people's quality of life, although some critics have suggested that this unduly restricted the scope of health promotion (Adams, 1994). Whether working to targets or not, it is generally professionals who are assessing people's comparative needs and lay people have until recently had little involvement.

Comparative need raises important questions about rationing. Only so many human and financial resources are available and health promoters have to prioritise. There has been an extensive debate within public health about how this should be done (Smith and Jacobson, 1988). There are considerable advantages, for example, in prioritising high risk groups so that health promotion can be focused on those in most immediate danger. This runs the risk of stereotyping and stigmatising some groups but potentially can deliver more support and advice than general whole population campaigns. Within coronary health campaigns in the 1980s the high risk approach had some success in targeting and working to change eating and exercise habits in at-risk groups such as middle-aged overweight males (Rose, 1981). Whole population strategies, by contrast, may deliver greater overall benefits without stigmatising particular groups but at an individual level these benefits may be very small. This has been termed the 'prevention paradox' (Rose, 1981).

The benefits are likely to vary depending on the issues involved. In relation to seat belt legislation, for example, the benefits in terms of reduced morbidity and mortality were gained by most of the population but in relation to cardiovascular disease it might be argued that national campaigning would be less effective than more intensive individual focused interventions. Other whole population approaches, such as greater regulation of food production to reduce fat levels in foodstuffs, might be more effective in combating cardiovascular disease.

Felt needs, the third type of need discussed by Bradshaw (1972), are those which people themselves identify. These may be uncovered by questions addressed to individuals or perhaps by surveys of local residents but their characteristic feature is that they are perceived by users themselves and generated by their own life experiences. In many cases such needs may be described as hidden or 'latent' because, without knowledge of what services or support is available or how needs are being defined in the wider world, people may not believe themselves to be 'in need'. Latent need may be felt by the local population or by groups or families within a local area, but may not show up in a survey of need or be expressed to the health worker.

Expressed need is what people say they need; it is the turning of a felt need into a request, call or even demand for action. For example, people may grumble for years about the restricted opening hours of the local health centre without doing anything about it. However, if they are consulted about opening hours the grumbles turn into expressed demands for change. Local mothers may feel the need for a safe crossing place on a busy road and find out that on other roads traffic has been better controlled. This may turn their felt but latent need into an expressed need and they will begin to make demands for traffic controls. The level of complaints in the health service increased dramatically when the Patient's Charter was introduced in 1991 and people were given licence, as it were, to complain.

Expressed needs may reinforce normative needs because the process of channelling the felt need into an expressed need may itself be mediated by professionals and may reflect the realistic options open for action. Some surveys of people's needs may be fairly closed and focused on professional agendas (Bowling, 1997). On the other hand, people's expressed needs may conflict with health promoters' priorities. Attempts to encourage people to cut down their smoking may conflict with users' own expressed needs, such as the need to create pockets of 'time out' in a hectic day of unsupported child care by undertaking the pleasurable activity of smoking a cigarette (Graham, 1987). In addition, expressed needs from users may be in conflict with each other. A broad-based local needs assessment in Kirkstall, Leeds, found not only that health, social service professionals, police and probation officers were in open disagreement about the value they attached to aspects of physical and mental health and to factors underpinning health status but that community representatives disagreed with each other and with 'ordinary local people' in the survey area (Percy-Smith and Sanderson, 1992).

Two issues follow from this. If health promoters use consumer surveys to enable people to 'make their voices heard' in health promotion planning, then such surveys need to be sensitive and inclusive rather than quick, closed snapshots of local opinion. The Patient's Charter has spawned lots of questionnaire-based patient satisfaction surveys since 1993 although it is arguable that more sensitive studies of patients' views would have been more valuable. Second, it does not follow that expressed need necessarily translates easily into normative need and leads to new policy priorities but it may trigger more research to estimate the 'real' level of concern.

15.4 Developing needs assessment in health promotion

Assessing an individual's needs

You will remember from Chapters 8 and 9 that some of the most important skills in communicating and counselling individuals were concerned with *listening* rather than telling people what to do. Listening is important if individuals are to express their own health needs and priorities rather than having the health professionals priorities imposed upon them. Other skills explored in those chapters were the skills of clarifying and summarising health needs and helping individuals to form plans of action. The health check which, since 1990, GPs are required to offer to people over 75, provides such an opportunity. It is supposed to take place in the person's own home and be wide ranging. So instead of a cursory urine and blood pressure check it should be an occasion for the older person to express their own anxieties about their health and include an assessment of their social and economic circumstances. Expert and professional assessment of needs should be reviewed against the expressed (and, if possible, the felt) needs of the older person.

This view translated to the population as a whole was put forward by the National Health Service Management Executive in its discussion paper 'Listening to Local Voices' (Sykes *et al.*, 1993) in which it was argued that purchasers should listen to local people's views and take them into account when making decisions about priority services and rationing in health care.

Assessing the needs of the community

There are various ways in which this might be done, from radio phone-ins, postal questionnaires, focus groups, rapid appraisal techniques, user representation on PCG/PCT boards, high street surveys and even newspaper advertisements. In one health authority in Birmingham local consultation was put into effect through a full page advertisement in the local evening paper asking readers to vote for one of three packages. The alternatives were a 'high tech' package of hospital care, a 'mid tech' package of hospital and community-based care and a 'preventive' package of community care, preventive services and health promotion (*Birmingham Evening Mail*, 23 January 1995). Readers were given a number to phone before midnight to register a vote for their chosen package, and the winner was the high tech package.

Do you think this is a legitimate way of listening to local voices?

Two groups of health work students were asked the same question and they generally said 'no!' But a few thought it was better than not asking for views even though the questions were 'loaded' and the packages very muddled. They also agreed with the critics in the group who thought that the health authority would probably 'take little notice' of the results and that it was the health authority management's job to decide on priorities.

Listening to and interpreting local views correctly remains a very difficult process. The local media can whip up enthusiasm for particular policies or, more likely, project outrage against plans, but that does not necessarily reflect local views. The quality of surveys and types of respondents are important to check before deciding how much weight to attach to them. The local needs assessment survey in Kirkstall found that community representatives tended to align themselves with expert views about the importance to be attached to factors underpinning health status, such as a work environment free from hazards, economic security and appropriate health care, whereas ordinary local people had markedly different ideas (Percy Smith and Sanderson, 1992).

Assessing local needs and listening to local voices is not a simple matter. Local people do not speak necessarily with one voice. Although they may share common problems or interests they may have different agendas and express different needs. Some may speak louder than others, some may find it hard to express themselves, others may not be interested at all. Inviting people to comment or vote, as in the example from Birmingham, may fulfil the requirements of democracy but the result may not reflect the needs of the local people. Much depends on the size and scale of the locality. Dealing with one block of flats on a housing estate would allow for the interviewing of each flat dweller. A tenants meeting could accommodate all of the residents and, through discussion, the collective needs and priorities could possibly be arrived at. Achieving consensus will not always be possible but at least it should be possible to learn the views of most involved. If one was dealing with the whole estate or the borough or whole city then it becomes a much more difficult matter. As well as the familiar questionnaires phone-ins and high street surveys mentioned above, there are a number of ways that health promoters have adopted to try to overcome the difficulties and tap as comprehensive a local voice as possible. These include using key informants, focus groups and setting up health forums.

Working with key informants

This resembles the grapevine approach where key individuals are interviewed because they have particular access to local knowledge. They may be formal or informal leaders or the landlord of the local pub who has an 'ear to the ground'. Religious or cultural leaders might be in a similar position or the head teacher at the local school.

Can you think of the possible limitations of this approach?

It may provide a distorted or biased view because it may not be possible to disentangle the informant's own interests from the interests of the local population. It may provide only a superficial picture of the local community and not represent the views of minority groups or groups with special concerns.

Focus groups

Focus groups are thought to be a useful way of accessing a range of different interest groups within a community. They may represent the interests of older people, women or people from a minority ethnic group. Adiaha Antigha, the health promotion co-ordinator for the King's Cross Health Project in London, used focus groups when carrying out a health needs assessment in what is a very diverse and disparate community. They aimed to work with 25 groups.

Examples of the kinds of focus groups included:

- several groups of older people attending local day centres who were interested in forming focus groups around their health needs
- a Bengali Women's Health Group
- a Chinese Women's Health Group
- a Buddies Befriending Scheme set up with the help of the Terence Higgins Trust. This is a scheme for befriending people with HIV and AIDS
- a men's therapy group
- an African-Caribbean group.

Antigha felt that the groups should be very loosely structured because they were very different in their composition. Some of the groups were actually facilitated by the health promotion team, others worked independently and reported back. From the first set of meetings common themes and concerns were drawn together. These included drugs and drug taking, safe neighbourhoods and children's play areas. The purpose of the health needs assessment was to feed into and inform the purchase and planning of local services (Antigha, 1994).

Health forums

A health forum for a particular locality would comprise a mixture of professionals, members of voluntary organisations, community groups and local residents. It differs from a focus group in that the forum is a cross-section of the community rather than a special interest group. Once set up, a health forum would meet regularly, deal with health issues as they arise and have a finger on the pulse of the local community and its health needs.

What do you think might be the relative strengths and weaknesses of focus groups and health forums in assessing the needs of the community?

Focus groups have special access to the needs of specific groups in the community whose voice may not otherwise be heard but they, of necessity, have their own agenda which may well conflict with other group (Bowling, 1997). Reconciling those different agendas may be very difficult. A health forum can bring together different interest groups but they run the risk of becoming elitist and dominated by the professionals.

The Liverpool Healthy Cities Initiative used all of the methods described above to consult local people about their proposed draft health plan for the city. They trained facilitators to try to ensure that some of the possible pitfalls we have identified could be overcome. This was an example where national health priorities as set out in the Health of the Nation document were used as the basis for the city plan but which were then set in the context of the local people's health priorities. Mapping the priorities of local people against the Health of the Nation targets was an illuminating exercise as many of the local people's concerns could be identified as underlying causes of the diseases and conditions targeted by Health of the Nation.

The top ten concerns from the people of Liverpool about their health are shown below:

> The comments were categorised into 50 different themes. The rank order was derived from the percentage of responses where particular themes are mentioned at least once.
>
> | | | |
> |---|---|---|
> | 1 | Environment | 60 per cent |
> | 2 | Poverty | 45 per cent |
> | 3 | Mental health | 43 per cent |
> | 4 | Housing | 42 per cent |
> | 5 | Health services | 35 per cent |
> | 6 | Education/training | 35 per cent |
> | 7 | Young people | 34 per cent |
> | 8 | Diet/nutrition | 32 per cent |
> | 9 | Accidents | 31 per cent |
> | 10 | Transport | 30 per cent |

The draft health plan for Liverpool was based on preliminary work which had built up a health profile for Liverpool broken down into local areas. This would draw on morbidity and mortality statistics which were discussed in the previous chapters. Other information might be about the housing stock, the availability of health services, the provision of social services such as the availability of day centres for old people or for people with mental health problems. Thus a picture of the community can be built up.

Community profiling

This need not be on such a large scale as a city-wide profile. Indeed many GPs are being encouraged to adopt a community profiling approach to the services which they offer. Primary care groups are also involved in the developing health improvement programmes, which incorporate community profiling. This community-oriented primary care approach is very much about planning rather than responding to patients who present themselves at the surgery. The term 'community profile' is broader than an assessment of needs as it takes account of the resources available.

> A comprehensive description of the needs of a population that is defined, or defines itself, as a community, and the resources that exist within a community, carried out with the active involvement of the community itself, for the purpose of developing an action plan or other means of improving the quality of life in the community.
>
> (Hawton *et al.*, 1994)

The authors stress the need to engage the active involvement of the community. A community profile then is more than a health audit. Annett and Rifkin (1990) have designed an information profile which schematically builds up knowledge about a community (see Figure 15.3).

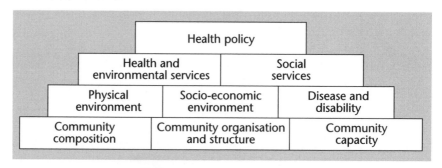

Figure 15.3 **Community information profile**

Rapid appraisal

A methodology which recently has become popular as a way of collecting information upon which priorities can be based is called rapid appraisal. Rapid appraisal does not rely solely on gathering new information but can collect secondary data (from demographers, epidemiologists and large-scale social surveys) as well as information from any source deemed appropriate. An example of such a study was that undertaken by Dale *et al.* (1996) who used rapid appraisal methods to create an interagency, community-oriented approach to service development. Their stated objective was to identify the views of users and providers about the strengths and weaknesses of out-of-hours medical care. The study took place in a socially deprived, multi-ethnic district in south-east London.

The Health for All 2000 philosophy underpinned the methods used in the study, emphasising the importance of the local community participating in decision-making about priority setting and resource allocation. The project team listed all local health and social service providers and community groups, and held agenda-setting meetings with key agencies and community representatives who in turn nominated someone as the link person. Local stakeholders then reviewed and commented on a draft outline of the project which was then refined.

The use of rapid appraisal methods was seen as effective in this study as it facilitated the delineation of issues, the understanding of service use, and the implications of potential service developments. This method provided a fast, reliable and collaborative method of accessing community perspectives without having to resort to large expensive surveys. This study was concerned to identify themes and issues, rather than produce results that might be generalisable. This was meant to ensure that needs were not overlooked in the very large and disparate population with whom the study group was concerned. The rapid appraisal, whilst not providing exact information about limited questions, provided a broad perspective on the issue at hand: out-of-hours medical services. More importantly, however, this type of methodology provides the basis upon which partnerships can be established across the professional/provider and consumer/stakeholder divide.

One of the problems that has been identified with rapid appraisal methods is that they mainly rely on key informants who may or may not represent the local population well. It is important that the wider community is involved. Setting priorities *with* rather than *for* people seems eminently sensible if people are to feel committed to a plan of action. But there may also be conflicting interests when setting priorities – there are those that are set by others, as well as the practical or real interests on the ground.

15.5 Programme planning

Setting priorities

As you will recall from Part 1, the Saving Lives: Our Healthier Nation strategy document identified four target areas. Consequently many health promoters are urged to work within these, as well as respond to what has been identified as a local priority or a health issue, for example diabetes, or groups such as young children or older people (Naidoo and Wills, 2000). In addition, in many people's work and in real-life situations a number of influences impact on the setting of health promotion priorities. These might include:

- the managers decided on this policy some time ago
- it's an established and long-standing initiative
- public pressure
- political pressure
- someone's hobbyhorse
- a response to a crisis
- it was necessary to demonstrate that the organisation was responding to the issue
- work done in this area had proven effective
- there is a national initiative (e.g. World AIDS day)
- a staff member had expertise in this area
- the unit had to economise and be more efficient.

(adapted from Ewles and Simnett, 1999: 109)

This indicates that setting priorities is dependent on the interests of both the people setting up the initiative and outside influences and pressures.

Setting up a planning group

It is possible that for small-scale interventions the planning and organisation will be taken on by the health promoter on his or her own. For example in setting up a series of group discussions with older people as discussed in Chapter 10, it was important to consult with the target group to find out their needs but the planning and organisation of the sessions could be done by the group facilitator.

Other programme plans may need the participation of a variety of people. Let us assume that you are planning to set up a food co-operative in order to provide access to fresh food at affordable prices to the residents of a council estate which only has a newsagent who sells milk and some frozen food. You will need to assemble a group of individuals willing to participate in the plan. You might call this group the advisory panel.

Appointing people to this panel is a sensitive endeavour and is usually directed by a key health professional keen to get the programme off the ground. However the composition of the panel may be determined by the funders or the agency under whose auspices the programme will run. The funder in this case might be a Cash and Carry which not only funds the project but provides a discount for the bulk buying. Wherever possible it is preferable to have members of the target group on the panel.

Can you think of other likely candidates for an advisory panel for the setting up of a food co-op?

As well as members of the target group there are a range of people with specialist knowledge who might be useful to the plan. Someone who has a knowledge of bookkeeping and dealing with VAT returns would be helpful. A dietition or nutritionist and an environmental health worker could give advice to ensure that the products were indeed likely to contribute to a healthy diet. Local situations will dictate different types of groups but it is always worth checking out any likely opposition and inviting them on to the advisory panel in order to get them on your side.

Once the group is assembled it will be necessary to discuss how the process of planning will work and familiarise the members with health promotion interventions. As the group becomes oriented, there will be some role negotiation of necessity so that each person understands what contribution they can usefully make. It is essential that each member of the group feels valued and useful otherwise tensions could set in which undermine the goals being pursued. Responsibility for different tasks will need to be delegated bearing in mind a fostering of a group responsibility for the whole undertaking. The next step is to work on the aims and objectives.

Setting aims and objectives

Aims or goals are broad statements that set out what the programme expects to achieve. Objectives are statements that map out the tasks needed to reach those goals including a time frame for the achievement of each task.

Table 15.1 identifies some major goals for health education and health promotion interventions.

The aim of a food co-operative – to improve the health and well-being of a given community by promoting a healthy diet, would involve the health education goals identified in Table 15.1, i.e. increasing levels of knowledge as well as attitudes and beliefs about what constitutes healthy eating. In terms of the health promotion goals, behaviour change would be aimed for such as a change in eating habits. But a food co-operative would also be concerned to increase participation and to change the local environment by making healthy foods affordable and accessible.

It is essential that the aims or goals, which provide the framework for the programme planning, reflect the expressed and felt needs of the target population, not only the normative needs of the health professionals on the planning group. Many food co-operatives have developed precisely because a local community has identified the lack of affordable and accessible food such as fresh fruit and vegetables.

Table 15.1   Some goals for health education and health promotion interventions

---

Health education goals
- related to increased levels of knowledge
- concerning attitudes and beliefs
- skills or pyscho-motor objectives concerning skills acquisition and competence.

Health promotion goals
- behaviour change including changes in lifestyles and increased take-up of services
- aiming for changes in policy
- concerning increases in participation and working together
- concerning changing the environment to make it more healthy.

(Ewles and Simnett 1999; Naidoo and Wills, 2000)

A prime objective for a food co-op might be organising a mobile van to sell fresh fruit and vegetables cheaply at various accessible locations. Objectives should be stated in terms of (a) the time-scale within which an intervention will take place and (b) the tasks needed to achieve the objective. A food co-op might set six months as the time-scale for having the mobile fruit and veg van operational. Before that it will be necessary to carry out the task of purchasing a van and organising drivers and suppliers of fruit and vegetables. In defining the objectives it is essential that they are appropriate and precise as well as realistic and manageable. This means being aware of the resources available and identifying likely constraints.

Resources exist in a variety of forms, and may include hard cash, availability of volunteers, political responsiveness or particularly useful skills possessed by colleagues, members of the advisory board or the target group (such as vehicle maintenance to keep the van in good order). For many interventions the primary constraint is lack of funds, with planning following the allocation of resources rather than determining resources (Naidoo and Wills, 2000). The constraints would basically include any feature that inhibits the implementation of a programme. In the case of a food co-op objections from local shopkeepers might act as a constraint.

Throughout the planning process it is helpful to keep a record of all decisions made and it is useful to prepare a coherent written planning document which will be multi-purpose, serving both as a funding document and a consultation document for discussions with the target and other audiences. This should include: an introduction setting out the background to the plan and the assessment of need on which it is based; the aims and objectives with a statement of the time-scale and the tasks to be achieved; a note of the resources and constraints. Along with programme planning you should be considering how to evaluate – if evaluation is not built in, it will be ignored and this may have implications for the funding of future interventions. Hawe *et al.* also believe that planning and evaluation are part of good health promotion practice. 'Planning, to take in the needs of the target group and the best of current knowledge as to how to meet these needs. Evaluation, to find out the effect of the programme, who has benefited and who has not' (1995: 5). This and other issues relating to evaluation are explored in Part 4.

15.6 Implementation

Putting the plan into action is the exciting and nerve-racking part. It is always worth making a final check to note that no significant changes have occurred during the planning process. For instance, if a supermarket chain has decided to locate a new venture on the estate then a plan to provide a mobile fruit and veg co-op may need to be rethought. At another level, changes in government or NHS policy may need to be taken into account and plans adjusted accordingly. If a lot of effort has been put into a plan then it can be difficult to jettison or redesign parts or all of it. But the need to adapt and be flexible is essential even after the plan has been put into action. Doggedly going on with a plan when circumstances have changed is a waste of time and resources. If evaluation is built into each step of the plan then changes can be integrated and plans revised.

15.7 Conclusions

The planning of any health promotion intervention needs to be thorough yet remain flexible. But above all planning should be based on sound information, and that information should include the knowledge and views of those involved whether individuals or communities. Planning should be done *with* rather than *for* people. We have somewhat artificially separated planning and evaluation. This is because evaluation is a complex and important process and needs detailed exploration. Part 4 is dedicated to this exploration.

Part 4
Evaluating health promotion

Introduction

Part 3 advocated taking a critical stance towards health information. This critical stance is equally important when we consider the value of the whole range of activities, programmes and projects that can promote health. Whether the focus is on building healthy alliances, engaging in health education in schools or running a group for people who want to stop smoking, it is essential to ask how things are working out and what might be improved. Such questions can be addressed at a number of levels and with varying degrees of formality and rigour. At the individual level, this kind of questioning is part of good reflective practice. Where it becomes more formal and consciously structured it can best be described as evaluation.

In Part 4 you will find that Chapters 16 and 18 are intended to equip you with the knowledge and background to plan and carry out evaluation on a fairly small scale. Chapters 17 and 19 focus on larger-scale debates about evaluation and health promotion and should help you critically review published evaluations and present trends.

Chapter 16
Evaluation in health promotion: why do it?

16.1 Introduction

Evaluation arises out of practice and is aimed specifically at reflecting on and influencing practice. This chapter will discuss, in a largely non-technical way, the nature and purpose of evaluation so that you may cast a critical eye over evaluations of the kinds of health promotion activities you are already involved in or might wish to consider. If you work in the health field it could be that much of the health promotion activity in which you are engaged is small-scale and semi-formal and the kinds of evaluation you are most likely to use may be equally small-scale and *ad hoc*. So this chapter seeks to stress the principles and the purpose of evaluation regardless of scale and style.

16.2 What is evaluation?

Evaluation is the process by which we judge the worth or value of something ...

(Suchman, E., *Evaluative Research*, cited in Hawe *et al.*, 1995: 6)

... (E)valuation is concerned with assessing an activity against values and goals in such a way that results can contribute to future decision making and/or policy ...

(Tones and Tilford, 1994: 49)

Although this basic definition is cast in straightforward terms, the language used in professional discussions of evaluation can at times be quite obscure and alienating. So it is important to begin by recognising that evaluation is something in which we are already actively involved, both professionally and in our daily lives. If evaluation is basically about judging the worth of an activity, then we are engaged in evaluation whenever we reflect critically upon our actions to decide whether to continue or modify what we are doing. Whenever you ask yourself questions such as: 'How did that session go?', 'Did I achieve what I set out to do?', 'Did that patient or client really understand what I was explaining to her or was she just being polite when she said she did?', you are engaged in evaluating your activities.

Think for a moment about how you travel to work (or somewhere else you regularly visit). If you are asked to consider whether your way of getting there is a good way, you are being asked to carry out an informal evaluation. It will involve deciding on and ranking your criteria, a choice that depends on what you most value (for instance, reliability, comfort, speed, economy, quiet, an opportunity to take exercise, an unwillingness to add to air pollution, or whatever) and then assessing the way you travel in the light of these criteria. Similarly, if you sit down with a colleague to review the way you have led or facilitated a group discussion you will do so in relation to particular criteria you either already share or have to begin by agreeing upon.

In all evaluation there are two fundamental elements: identifying and ranking the criteria (values and aims) and gathering the kind of information that will make it possible to assess the extent to which they are being met. Though these procedures and thought processes are familiar, working through them in the context of formal evaluation may not be. For instance, choosing the criteria which will guide the evaluation can be especially difficult and complex where there are no clearly stated aims or where there are diverse stakeholders with competing or conflicting perspectives. Decisions about the kinds of information that should be gathered and how best to gather it will need to take into account a large number of practical, ethical and methodological considerations; so they require careful thought and discussion.

A distinctive characteristic of formal (as distinct from informal) evaluation is its potentially public nature. It is 'not necessarily published or publishable, but open to inspection by an outsider and therefore capable of being made public' (Thorpe, 1988: 6). This openness is important and necessary because it means the process and findings can in principle be scrutinised and repeated, and this gives them a certain objectivity: it is possible for others to check and confirm or refute them. It is also possible for others to put into action what has been learned and thus to benefit from it.

Despite the potential benefits of evaluation, its ability to disturb preconceptions and vested interests means that not everyone feels enthusiastic about it, as the following 'tongue-in-cheek' story illustrates.

The Origin of Evaluation

In the beginning God created the heaven and the earth ...

And God saw everything He made. 'Behold,' God said, 'it is very good.'

And the evening and the morning were the sixth day

And on the seventh day God rested from all his work.

His archangel came then unto Him asking:

'God, how do you know what you have created is "very good"?

What are your criteria? On what data do you base your judgement? Aren't you a little close to the situation to make a fair and unbiased evaluation?'

God thought about these questions all that day and His rest was greatly disturbed.

On the eighth day God said, 'Lucifer, go to hell.'

Thus was evaluation born in a blaze of glory.

(Halcolm's The Real Story of Paradise Lost, quoted in Patton, 1981)

How else might the story have ended?

In this particular story the project manager and the evaluator are different actors who become separated by an enormous gulf. Evaluation, according to this model, is entirely external to the project and offers a final and fixed judgement when the only way of improving things would be to start again. But evaluation can also be integral to the development of a particular project and part of an ongoing process of review and reform. In this contrasting model, evaluation is seen as part of a cyclical process (Figure 16.1). In reality these two contrasting models represent two ends of a continuum with many, but by no means all, evaluations containing aspects of both.

What is the relation between evaluation and monitoring? Monitoring involves the systematic and continuous surveillance of particular aspects of a project or service. Often such monitoring is required in relation to externally set targets and as such may not be part of an evaluation process, though it may alert people to problems calling for further investigation. Sometimes, however, monitoring is an integral part of a formative evaluation. Evaluation is always wider than monitoring: it not only gathers information but also involves judgements about values. One way of summing up the difference is to say that evaluation responds to the question 'Are we doing the right things?', whilst monitoring is more narrowly concerned with answering the question 'Are we doing things right?'

If monitoring refers to a smaller-scale activity than evaluation, quality assurance is broader, referring to both the undertaking of evaluation and the implementation of findings. In the context of health services it has been defined as: 'The measurement of the actual level of the quality of the services rendered plus the efforts to modify when necessary the provision of these services in the light of the results of the measurement,' (Vuori, 1982). In one sense this statement begs the questions of what quality means and whose values and criteria are being used to define quality. Frequently quality is said to mean effectiveness, efficiency, equity, appropriateness and acceptability, though whether these provide a commonly agreed and feasible set of criteria is open to debate. How these criteria may be used in evaluation is a question we return to later but first let's consider some of the reasons people give for carrying out evaluation.

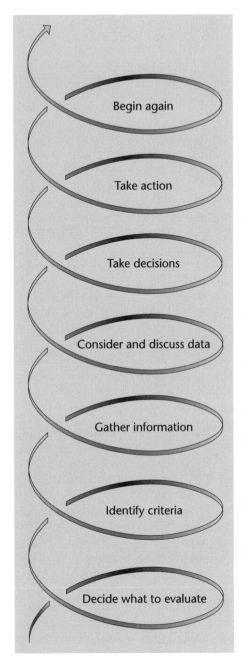

Figure 16.1 **Evaluation cycle**
(adapted from Edwards, 1991: 12)

16.3 Why evaluate?

If you ask a number of people why they evaluate their work they will give different answers. Figure 16.2 sets out some of the answers people have given to this question.

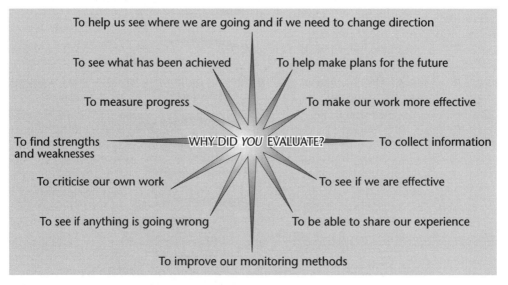

To help us see where we are going and if we need to change direction

To see what has been achieved   To help make plans for the future

To measure progress   To make our work more effective

To find strengths   WHY DID YOU EVALUATE?   To collect information
and weaknesses

To criticise our own work   To see if we are effective

To see if anything is going wrong   To be able to share our experience

To improve our monitoring methods

Figure 16.2 **Why we evaluate** (adapted from Feuerstein, 1986: 2)

There are many possible reasons for wanting to evaluate activities aimed at promoting health. These include questions about effectiveness, the desire to improve practice and a willingness to be self-critical and do as good a job as possible by consciously learning from experience. There is often a link between evaluation and planning. Indeed in an ideal world evaluation and planning are inextricably linked as parts of an ongoing cycle.

In addition to the desire of individuals to learn lessons that will improve practice, there may also be financial and political pressures that encourage or demand evaluation. Increasingly projects are required to have an evaluation component in order to be eligible for funding. In Scotland, for instance, the Primary Care Development Fund, which offered £4 million pump-priming finance, stipulated that an evaluation plan must form part of any funding proposal (Shiroyama *et al.*, 1995).

The increasing pressure for evaluation is linked with reforms initiated by NHS and community care legislation in the early 1990s. The creation of an internal market in which purchasers were given the responsibility of 'buying' services that were effective, efficient and appropriate placed considerable pressure on people to demonstrate the value of what they were doing. In such a competitive climate it was said that the future of health promotion depended on evaluation:

> With the development of an internal market in the NHS 'the purchasers'
> new role... offers the opportunity for preventative strategies to make
> their case for additional resources on an equal basis with curative
> interventions. However, in order to effectively compete for resources it is
> necessary to obtain hard irrefutable evidence of the health gains arising
> from preventative strategies. All health interventions must undergo
> rigorous evaluation to assess their value in an environment in which
> resources have become increasingly constrained.
>
> (Haycox, 1994: 5–6)

From this perspective, evaluation has become an essential and central tool
in a system aimed at providing a rational, evidence-based way of meeting
needs. The World Health Assembly in its meeting of May 1998 urged all
member states to 'adopt an evidence-based approach to health promotion
policy and practice, using the full range of quantitative and qualitative
methodologies'. In current UK health service provision, clinical governance is a key feature, with the emphasis on demonstrating 'best practice'
in health interventions based on evaluation of the available evidence. But
in a number of important respects, the evaluation of health promotion
tends to be more complex and difficult than the evaluation of health
services and therapeutic interventions. Although often judged by the same
criteria, health promotion has rather different tasks and goals, which are
for a number of reasons harder to measure. The effects of the medical
treatment of sick individuals are more obvious and immediate than the
effects of health promotion interventions upon medically well groups and
populations.

Some commentators argue that the growing culture of evaluation has a
directly political and ideological function, legitimating unpopular actions
by governments:

> As economies falter and governments lose legitimacy, evaluation has
> been a tool for informing and legitimising the actions that governments
> must take, particularly budget cutting.
>
> (House, 1993: xi)

Before moving on let's summarise the main reasons for evaluation
discussed so far.

Box 16.1: Some reasons for evaluating health promotion activities

1 to secure funding

2 to check that a programme is having the desired effect

3 to improve methods, procedures and materials

4 to assess whether the resources invested are being used efficiently

5 to demonstrate that an activity is worth continuing

6 to inform future plans

7 to assess whether an intervention is ethically justifiable

> 8 to increase knowledge and understanding of the value and limitations of health promotion
>
> 9 to develop theory
>
> 10 to ration resources or legitimate budget cuts.
>
> (based on Downie *et al.*, 1990: 73–74)

16.4 Who should evaluate?

Evaluation may be carried out either by independent, external researchers or by practitioners. Much evaluation of health promotion activities is done by the very people who carry out the health promotion. There are advantages and disadvantages with either pattern. An external evaluator may be fairer and more objective perhaps, but also may take longer to understand the issues and establish contacts. It can also be argued that when people evaluate their own practice they learn more easily what they can improve and how, but perhaps only when they are committed to improvement rather than self-justification. Capitalising on the strengths of both kinds of evaluator, there are those who argue that it is desirable for evaluation to be carried out on both an external and an internal basis; 'this is the best guarantee of validity and authority in the evaluation and can be a stimulus to the dialogue that is essential in reflecting systematically on questions of worth' (Beattie, 1990: 231). In planning an evaluation of a drop-in centre in Milton Keynes a combined approach was taken both because there was insufficient money to pay for an entirely external evaluation and because training the centre workers to carry out interviews themselves was felt to be valuable career development for them.

A further and important consideration is the role of users and clients. To what extent are the people for whom the intervention or service is designed going to play an active part in evaluating it? Will they act as evaluators themselves; as consultants to the evaluation, helping to shape and guide it; as one source of information amongst others; or will they be completely passive recipients? Where they are being used as informants, how might they respond differently to external and internal evaluators? There are several possibilities here that require exploration. Sometimes people feel able to talk more freely to external evaluators, perhaps because they are seen as more neutral. Sometimes external people are mistrusted; sometimes their unfamiliarity means communication proves too difficult. These and other possibilities have to be considered in relation to particular groups and contexts.

16.5 When and what to evaluate?

The question of when to evaluate is closely bound up with the kind of role an evaluation is to play. Is it to be a final judgement or a contribution to what is happening? There are technical terms to be aware of here. Considering the worth of an intervention when it has reached its final form is known as summative or an *outcome* evaluation, whereas an evaluation that involves feed-back during the course of a project, when things are still taking shape, is termed formative or an evaluation of *process*. A formative evaluation will usually involve stage-by-stage comparison between stated objectives or criteria and what is actually happening, which has the advantage of creating opportunities for things to be changed for the better before the form is entirely fixed. Many evaluations incorporate both kinds by having two aspects or phases, the formative stage focusing on the process (the way things are done) and the summative on the outcome (the consequences).

Some evaluations are entirely concerned with process. In the field of health education, for instance, an evaluation might focus entirely on the quality and nature of the communication between professionals and their clients by questions such as: is the communication culturally appropriate? is the information perceived as credible and relevant? is there a good match between the aims of the professional and the needs of the client?

When an evaluation is primarily concerned with outcomes, decisions about timing will need to take into account questions about the short- or long-term nature of the outcomes. For example, evaluation of an intervention aiming to assist weight loss might decide to evaluate immediately after the intervention and then again one year later, so that it could speak with some confidence about both short- and longer-term influences. In some of the literature about evaluation the immediate effects of an intervention are described as the impact or outputs and longer-term effects as the outcomes. For instance, with a programme designed to teach parents of young children about household safety and accident prevention, increased recognition of dangerous conditions in the home might form the impact whilst the longer-term intended outcome would be taking action to make changes in the home to prevent accidents.

Decisions about the focus of the evaluation and, in particular, whether to concentrate on process, impact or outcome will depend on the resources and funding available, the underlying questions and, most importantly perhaps, the criteria guiding the evaluation.

16.6 Evaluation criteria

It has already been noted that evaluation necessarily involves identifying criteria against which to measure or assess the worth of the activities being evaluated. Frequently, the aims or goals of the activity, project or programme provide the criteria, though it is also possible to assess worth in relation to external standards and values such as public acceptability, cost-effectiveness or efficiency.

Consider the following influential attempt to identify a general set of criteria for evaluating quality. Originally designed for health care, rather than for health promotion, it provides a checklist which for the moment we present in an uncritical way simply to suggest some possible general criteria. Some have argued that the list may be used in a different way, as a common set of criteria that should be used in health promotion to assess performance and quality right across the board (Catford, 1993) but here it is introduced to illustrate the kinds of evaluative question that might be asked.

Box 16.2: Evaluation criteria

effectiveness – the extent to which aims and objectives are met

appropriateness – relevance to need

acceptability – to the people concerned and society at large

equity – equal provision for equal needs

efficiency – the ratio of costs to benefits

(adapted from Maxwell 1984, summarised in Philips *et al.*, 1994: 19)

Let's consider what is meant by each of these criteria, beginning with the first, effectiveness. This lies at the heart of evaluation and quite rightly tends to be what most people have in mind when they hear or use the word evaluation.

Effectiveness

Effectiveness is concerned with whether an activity has achieved what it set out to do. This is sometimes described as the evaluation of outcomes in relation to aims and objectives. Aims are the planned, or hoped for, effects of an activity and outcomes are the actual effects, both intended and unintended. So, for example, if a teacher says that the main aim of providing sex education at school is to reduce the risk of unwanted pregnancy then an evaluation of its effectiveness will involve trying to find out whether this aim has actually been achieved. It will also need to take note of other outcomes that were not part of that aim. Some may be welcome, for instance increased understanding of how HIV is transmitted, but others may not be, for example, a group of parents withdrawing their children from the school.

In everyday conversation we often use the terms aims and objectives interchangeably. In principle there is an important difference, though in practice it is sometimes difficult to draw a clear distinction. Aims tend to be *general*, and they may be broken down into *specific* objectives which contribute to the aim. They may refer to the long- and/or short-term consequences of a programme or project (Downie *et al.*, 1990: 67). Often they include intentions and hopes about the way a project will operate (the process) as well as about its outcomes, and sometimes the focus is almost entirely on style and ethos when this is the desired immediate outcome or impact. An example of the latter can be seen in the following extract from an evaluation of an open meeting designed for Asian women with, or with an interest in, diabetes (Kaur and Bedford, n.d.: 7):

Aim

The central aim of the event was to bring together Asian women with diabetes and those with an interest in diabetes, e.g. carers, to share experiences, to identify concerns and to gauge interest in a self-help/ support group.

Objectives

- to create a comfortable and positive atmosphere for women to actively participate in the event
- to ensure participation from representative groups of Asian women with diabetes and those who care for someone with diabetes
- to ensure the diverse language and cultural needs of each participant are appropriately and sensitively met
- to explore the possibility of setting up a self-help/support group for informal, personal and emotional support
- to raise awareness about the incidence of diabetes amongst the Asian community in the Borough.

Notice that the first three objectives specify the manner in which the event should be conducted so that it is inclusive and enables active participation, whilst the last two are more obviously about outcomes.

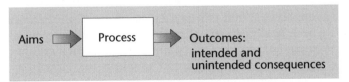

Figure 16.3 **The relationship between aims and outcomes**

Identifying aims and objectives is not always straightforward. Certain kinds of aims and objectives are by their nature easier to describe than others, and not all programmes and projects have an explicit and agreed set of aims, though if there is to be an evaluation of effectiveness it is important that the various parties involved should try to be explicit and specific about what they are aiming to achieve.

> **Do you think the aims and objectives of the Asian women and diabetes meeting are specific and clear enough? What further information or detail would be helpful?**

One possible difficulty is that whilst the second objective refers to representative groups these are not identified, which means it may be difficult to agree how far it has been achieved. Does it refer to age groups, religious groups, language groups or groups defined by the kind of diabetes they are concerned with? Also the main aim makes no mention of the number of women they hope will attend, which leaves open the question of how many will be regarded as a satisfactory number. If five women turn up and feel they have a useful meeting, will this be seen as a great success? Then there is the question of whether the objectives are all of equal importance.

A project that intends to be open to evaluation would be wise to try to formulate its aims and objectives with at least some of the following considerations in mind:

Box 16.3: How to formulate aims and objectives in order to assess effectiveness

Wherever possible they should be –

- **explicit**: discussed and written down

- **specific**: not general and vague

- **scheduled**: operating within a definite period

- **prioritised**: placed in order of importance

- **related** to one another rather than in conflict

(adapted from Philips *et al.*, 1994: 71–73)

The aims and objectives of the Asian group do seem to conform to the guidelines in many respects, though they aren't listed in order of importance (but maybe they are all equally important) and it might have been helpful to be more specific about the number of women they might reasonably hope would participate and which groups they hoped would be represented. For evaluation to take place, aims have to be made testable (operationalised), which involves not only identifying smaller-scale objectives that contribute to an aim but also finding a way of assessing or measuring the extent to which these objectives have been achieved. The evaluation of the Asian women's meeting was based on a debriefing of participants at the end of the event and a more detailed debriefing of the group that planned the event. One conclusion arrived at in the evaluation was:

> ... more time should have been spent in the early stages of planning, regarding expectations. Within that clear aims and objectives of the event should have been discussed ... disparities in expectations ranged from members expecting 'possibly 100 women for education and information' to women with diabetes expecting 'even if just another woman talked about it ... it is worth it.
>
> (Kaur and Bedford, n.d.: 16)

Of course individuals will always differ in their expectations and needs but for this very reason it is helpful for those planning an event such as this to try to agree on a measure of what precisely would be regarded as adequate participation.

Acceptability

An important but sometimes overlooked evaluation criterion is acceptability. There are a number of reasons why, and levels at which, questions about acceptability may be relevant and important in an evaluation. For instance, an intervention that has been acceptable to a particular population may encounter difficulties elsewhere if in a different geographical, economic, cultural or ethnic context the language and imagery prove highly problematic. Much of the original UK health education material on HIV/AIDS, which depicted the origin of HIV as being firmly African and Third World, reinforced racist stereotypes and caused great offence to many black and minority ethnic groups. 'The portrayal of "where AIDS comes from", which to many health educators was unnecessary and incorrect, left many groups angry and not prepared to participate in HIV/AIDS education programmes' (Elliott, 1994: 207) .

Methods can be generally effective without being generally acceptable in relation to aesthetic, religious, or moral values. Health education that involves the use of fear or sexually explicit material, for instance, may well run into problems that an evaluation can and should identify. Health promotion that unintentionally reinforces unhealthy stereotypes needs to become more aware of its potential impact so that more acceptable alternatives may be sought.

Box 16.4

One example of the unacceptable use of fear was an advertising campaign in the south of England by SANE (Schizophrenia – a National Emergency). This campaign was intended to influence health policy and thus may be seen as an aspect of health promotion. Aiming to stop closures of psychiatric hospitals, it depicted psychiatric patients as frenziedly dangerous and thus carried very negative images not only of people diagnosed as schizophrenic but also of mental illness in general.

> The campaign had powerful backers, enjoyed the patronage of Prince Charles and was heavily financed by, amongst others, P&O Ferries and Rupert Murdoch. Conscious of the potential effects of such a campaign on public perceptions of people experiencing mental illness, it fell to mental health users groups to lobby the Advertising Standards Authority.
>
> (Rogers *et al.*, 1993: 5)

A formative evaluation which asked questions about the acceptability of the campaign to the general public, including those diagnosed as mentally ill, might well have identified the possible difficulties before the campaign got fully under way. (The benefits of formative evaluation before the production of advertising material are widely acknowledged in the literature about health promotion: see, for instance, McCron and Budd, 1981; Flay, 1987; Leathar, 1987.)

Appropriateness

The criterion of appropriateness differs from that of acceptability. Is an activity appropriate to the particular health needs of the people being targeted rather than culturally and ethically acceptable to their world view? For instance, funding an expensive campaign encouraging cyclists to wear safety helmets may well be generally very acceptable, but highly inappropriate in a retirement area with very few cyclists but a great need for a lunch club and meals-on-wheels. You will recall that appropriate targeting is central for the social marketing approach to health education discussed in Chapter 11 and also that needs assessment, described in Chapter 15, provides the foundation for making informed decisions about appropriateness. It is important to remember that external and internal perceptions of need may differ greatly, so evaluations may have to distinguish between people's own perceptions of their needs and those held by others such as doctors or health workers who are drawing on a different understanding or model of health. If, for example, regular visits to the local pub are part of what it means to me to be healthy I may well judge TV adverts about the dangers of alcohol to be inappropriate and irrelevant to my health and well-being, even though a medical model of health need would make the opposite judgement.

Equity

At the minimum, concern for equity involves asking how accessible to all a particular health intervention is. An evaluation concerned with equity will not be content to learn simply about the numbers of people who have been involved in a project but will also wish to identify the social composition of the population reached. Health information that is only available in English is a fairly obvious example of an inequitable approach. Similarly, written information, whatever the language, may exclude people who are visually impaired or who have low literacy skills.

You will recall from Chapter 4 that the reduction of health inequalities has been a major theme in WHO policy statements. *Health 21 Strategy* (WHO, 1998), for instance, has as its first two targets improvement in the health of disadvantaged nations and groups and reduction of health inequalities by at least 25 per cent within countries and one third between member states. During recent years statements on healthy public policy, such as the Adelaide and Ottawa charters, have made explicit reference to developing health, income and social policies that foster greater equity and this is reflected in present UK government policy. In an editorial discussing the signs of quality in health promotion, John Catford draws an important distinction between equity and equality, placing equity at the top of the list: 'Striving for equity, not always equality, is the guiding principle and needs to be explicitly demonstrated.' (1993: 67). As Catford's statement indicates, pursuing equity may not always mean aiming for equal access but rather the deliberate targeting of groups who are particularly disadvantaged.

Efficiency

During recent years questions about the relation between costs and effectiveness in the field of health promotion have become important. In a world of limited resources costs clearly have to be taken into account. If, for instance, a health education programme is entirely effective in changing the health behaviour of a small group of people but achieves this success by drawing on an enormous amount of human and financial resources, this fact is relevant in evaluation. Once cost is made explicit a number of comparisons become possible, in principle at least. For example, a comparison may be made between a project and equally effective but cheaper projects; between this project and projects that are slightly less effective but considerably cheaper; between this and projects that reach larger numbers with similar success and similar cost, and so on.

In this context there are two main forms of analysis of which you need to be aware. *Cost-effectiveness* analysis (CEA) compares the costs of similar interventions that achieve a given goal (for instance, smoking cessation clinics compared with family doctors providing routine advice on giving up smoking). If different interventions meet with similar success then it becomes important to know which is cheaper. But the comparison becomes more complex if there are differences in degrees of success *and* differences in cost, and in such a case a calculation needs to be made in terms of 'cost per unit of effect' or 'effects per unit of cost'. Here *Cost-benefit* analysis (CBA) provides a way to compare the cost of the intervention with the financial benefits resulting from achieving the goal (for instance the cost of various kinds of anti-smoking advice with the financial benefits of giving up smoking.) The two are summarised in Box 16.5.

Box 16.5: Cost-effectiveness and cost-benefit analysis

1 Cost-effectiveness analysis compares the efficiency of similar interventions to achieve a given goal by stating the different financial costs involved.

2 Cost-benefit analysis not only states the costs but also seeks to place a monetary value on the benefits accruing from a programme. A calculation of the cost per given benefit is then possible.

(adapted from Tones and Tilford, 1994:113)

It could be argued that at one level an informal use of the ideas is already part of our everyday decision-making. Whenever we make a decision about how much of our time to spend on a particular activity or person we are implicitly applying a cost-benefit analysis (perhaps based more on guesswork than on evaluation). For example, a community worker may find herself having to choose between a range of requests made on her limited time, for instance between spending six hours a week counselling a small number of adults who want support in losing weight and using the same amount of time setting up a playgroup for children living in a very overcrowded area with no play facilities. Deciding which of these is going to be a better use of her time and therefore of her employer's budget involves trying to calculate the long-term health benefits of the two projects.

One important limitation of purely economic cost-effectiveness and cost-benefit analyses is the assumption that economic costs and benefits matter to the exclusion of other dimensions. But when we look at individual decision-making about health this is clearly not what we find. This means that the calculations purchasers, managers and practitioners make when deciding how best to use scarce economic resources may well need to include non-economic considerations, such as pleasure and anxiety, as well as the more obvious ones relating to money. For instance, one invisible cost of a screening programme could be the raising of anxiety levels to a degree that impairs not only people's sense of well-being but also their health as medically defined. An evaluation that failed to take into account such apparently non-economic effects would provide an unsatisfactory basis for planning.

The formal application of economic analysis to health promotion is a quite recent phenomenon. For example, in 1979 a review of 250 health education studies contained no instances of cost-benefit or cost-effectiveness analysis (Gatherer *et al.*, 1979). Only in the 1990s has the language of health economics begun to enter the discourse of health promotion. The extent to which we can in practice carry out the very rigorous calculations required here is explored further in Chapter 19.

16.7 Conclusion

This chapter has outlined the basic principles and tasks of evaluation, namely the identification of values and criteria and the gathering of appropriate information. It has been argued that in both *ad hoc* activities and large-scale, formal projects and programmes, evaluation is an important tool for improving practice and planning (though it has to be acknowledged that, at times, an over-emphasis on evaluation may be unhelpfully burdensome). So far we have discussed five different criteria that may be used in evaluation and in the next chapter we move on to consider ways of assessing or measuring the extent to which such criteria are being met.

Chapter 17
Evaluation design

17.1 Introduction

This chapter considers how to plan evaluations of various kinds of health promotion, what sorts of information are needed and how such information can be organised and used to assess how far a health promoting activity is measuring up to the criteria that have been chosen. The first part focuses on evaluation design and the second on the role and choice of indicators which permit the kind of measurement that best fits the evaluation in question. Although this chapter is primarily about formal evaluation, it also has implications for small-scale and semi-formal evaluations. Regardless of the scale and level of an evaluation, there are certain fundamental questions that need to be considered before beginning to plan an evaluation.

> **If you have ever planned an evaluation or envisage doing so in the future, what initial questions need to be considered?**

Here are some that would seem to be essential (with a few examples of answers):

- What are the **purposes** of the evaluation? (Check effectiveness; plan the next stage; justify continued funding; understand what is happening.)
- What **criteria** will be used? (Achieving aims and objectives; cost-effectiveness; acceptability to clients; open access.)
- What **information** is required? (Views of clients; annual accounts; referral rates.)
- What **methods** can be used to gather the information? (Postal surveys; group discussions; interviews; consulting records.)
- How should the information be **reported** and used to achieve the original purpose? (Verbally at a meeting with your line manager; by written report; at a staff workshop.)

It is important to consider these questions from the outset so that you can plan a coherent and feasible evaluation. If you are already experienced in evaluation perhaps you thought of other more detailed questions, some of which may be contained in the following checklist:

Table 17.1 **Checklist for planning an evaluation**

1   Who are the principal groups and individuals involved?
2   What is the purpose of the evaluation?
3   What approach, model or framework will be used to provide direction?
4   What are the main evaluation questions or issues?
5   What political and ethical considerations need to be taken into account?
6   By what standards or criteria will the evaluation be judged?
7   What resources are available for the evaluation?
8   Who should carry it out?
9   What sort of data (information) is needed?
10 What will be the methods of enquiry?
11 How is the data to be analysed?
12 How will the data be checked for its validity and reliability?
13 How will the findings be presented?
14 To whom are the findings to be made available?

(adapted from Philips *et al.*, 1994: 67, based on Patton, 1981)

A number of these questions were considered in the previous chapter, where attention was paid in particular to the identification of criteria (item 6 above) and who should conduct evaluations (item 8). In this chapter the focus is on evaluation design (item 3) and the sort of information needed (item 9). Chapter 18 considers methods of enquiry (item 10) and the presentation of findings (items 13 and 14).

17.2 Evaluation design

There are very different views as to the best way of carrying out evaluation. Some of the differences can be highlighted by contrasting two different approaches to knowledge and understanding. On the one hand there is the perspective that tries to apply the rules and procedures of the physical and medical sciences to the area of evaluation; on the other is a more holistic, qualitative approach which challenges the appropriateness of applying physical science methods to complex human phenomena.

You will recall from Chapters 4 and 5 that the nature of health promotion is highly contested. Ewles and Simnet, for instance, distinguish five main approaches (see Table 5.1). If you turn back to this table and pay particular attention to the values and aims accompanying each of the five approaches, you will notice that whilst the first two (the medical and behaviour change models) sit most comfortably with a physical/medical science approach to evaluation, the educational and client-centred models of health promotion are likely to favour a more qualitative style of evaluation. This means that people involved in funding, managing and carrying out particular kinds of health promotion will have certain expectations and assumptions about what evaluation means and what kind of evaluation is needed in relation to their areas of work. So, for example, where there is an emphasis on medical approaches to health promotion, evaluation will tend to be regarded as a way of demonstrating reductions in mortality and morbidity that can be attributed to health promotion interventions. In contrast, client-centred approaches might expect evaluation to describe and illuminate health-promoting interactions so that practitioners can reflect on the way they work and understand more about the processes involved.

Designing a formal evaluation means choosing a research plan that is appropriate to the purposes of the evaluation, and, as we have just noted, this choice will be influenced by the kind of health promotion being pursued and the values and assumptions underlying it. Hawe *et al.* (1995) state: 'Evaluation is not an absolute science. There is no right or wrong way to evaluate a programme, because people have different ideas about what sort of information about a programme is important. If the main emphasis of the evaluation is on participant satisfaction, for example, the evaluation method will differ from that when the main emphasis of the evaluation is an assessment of costs and benefits' (pp. 7–8). There are three broad (and in practice often overlapping) categories from which to choose: (quasi) experimental designs concerned to establish cause and effect; survey designs which aim to identify significant patterns; and qualitative designs which focus on description and interpretation. Quasi-experimental designs and survey designs are quantitative methods which are attempting to measure change (e.g. health status, health behaviour, health knowledge). Qualitative methods, on the other hand, attempt to examine the experience and meaning of the intervention for the people involved. It is important to be aware of the choices that are available and the possibilities and problems inherent in each. In planning any particular evaluation it might well be appropriate and useful to adopt a mixture of styles by, for example, using qualitative methods to fill out the detail of a general pattern revealed by a large-scale survey.

1 (Quasi) experimental designs: establishing cause and effect

Given the complexity of factors that influence human activity, it is often very difficult to ascertain the extent to which a particular intervention has brought about a particular consequence. So, for instance, if the introduction of health warnings on cigarette packets is followed by a reduction in smoking, it can't be assumed that the reduction is a consequence of health warnings, because smoking might have decreased anyway for other reasons. Acknowledging this difficulty, the evaluation of the Health Show (the television health education programme described in Chapter 11) contains the following caveat:

> Assessing the effectiveness of an intervention such as a television show and supportive literature upon an individual's behaviour is difficult. This is particularly problematic when lifestyle issues such as healthy eating,

exercise and smoking have a complex interplay of continuous, uncontrolled, unmeasured and sometimes unmeasurable variables.

(Wallace, 1993: 222)

What would be the essential features of an evaluation design capable of demonstrating that the Health Show had led directly to changes in lifestyle?

Where an evaluation is trying to demonstrate the effectiveness of a particular health education intervention in achieving specific outcomes, then in theory at least, an experimental design is the strongest that can be used. (As we shall see later, this was not the design used in the evaluation of the Health Show.) An evaluation using an experimental design would subject the programme and its viewers to scientific assessment in much the same way as new drugs are tested by means of randomised control trials. This would involve comparing the experience of a group randomly allocated to participate in the initiative with that of a similarly randomised group not participating (Cochrane, 1972). Individuals would be randomly assigned so as to distribute evenly other factors that might affect the outcome. There are, however, many problems in doing this, and it is often argued that the experimental approach assumes a greater degree of control over extraneous factors than is usually possible or desirable in social research (Smith and Cantley, 1984). (You may have noticed the reference to unmeasurable variables in the Health Show evaluation extract above.)

Here is one useful summary of what is meant by an experimental design written by an experienced evaluator who sees it as the ideal that is rarely realised in practice:

> The basic elements of experimental design are pretest studies to establish baseline measurements; the use of a representative sample of the target population; random assignment of subjects to intervention and control groups; the use of a clearly defined intervention; and post-test studies to identify change from the baseline measurements.
>
> (Nutbeam *et al.*, 1990: 85)

An example of an evaluation using a simple experimental design is a study by Basler *et al.* (1991) of nicotine gum therapy with smokers. Smokers identified as having an increased risk of coronary disease were randomly allocated between two groups and pretest measures were made (as a basis for comparison with outcome measures). One group then received the therapy, which used nicotine gum together with nutritional information, training in self-management techniques and the prescription of a date to stop smoking. The other group (the control) received no intervention but were offered it after the experimental groups completed their treatment. A follow-up three months after the treatment of the experimental group found 64 per cent were not smoking compared with 3 per cent of the control group (Tones and Tilford, 1994: 57).

Experimental design has been largely restricted to single-factor interventions, especially smoking cessation, and interventions in closed
systems such as schools (Flay *et al.*, 1983), workplaces (Sutton and Hallet,
1988; Glasgow *et al.*, 1984) and health clinics (Sanders *et al.*, 1989),
because these are contexts in which it is possible to exercise more control
and to have more knowledge about the various factors that may influence
outcomes.

What are likely to be the main problems with trying to use an experimental design in evaluating health promotion?

There are several. The random assignment of individuals in a community
to intervention and control groups is problematic in a number of ways.
For instance, there are ethical difficulties relating to consent. There are
also practical difficulties relating to the fact that people are social and
cultural beings whose lives cannot become artificially sealed off from one
another. When members of one group share parts of their lives with
members of the other, through neighbourhood, work, and so on, there is
inevitably considerable interaction, exchange of information and sharing
of new experiences. In evaluating mass media, for example, it is almost
impossible to arrange things so that it is only the members of a randomly
selected population group who see a particular programme, though this
has been achieved in a community with two completely separate cable
television networks (Robertson *et al.*, 1974). Also, many interventions are
meant to influence whole communities and in these situations the
problem of trying to create experimental conditions is even greater.
Nutbeam comments that 'contamination' of communities by interaction
and external factors is more likely than with individuals and that 'the
causal chain in a community system is longer and harder to trace than in a
clinical research study on volunteers' (Nutbeam *et al.*, 1990: 85).

One response to some of these difficulties has been the use of a
modified or quasi-experimental design. For instance, instead of using a
control group formed by random assignment, an evaluator may choose a
highly comparable, but not randomly selected, comparison group. This
has been the path taken in American and European community-based
heart disease prevention programmes where the population forming the
experimental group has been matched for health and demographic
variables with a geographically separate population (see, for instance,
Nutbeam *et al.*, 1987; Farquhar *et al.*, 1983). Whilst geographical
separation has the advantage of minimising the impact of social
interaction and shared cultural influences, such as that of mass media,
at the same time it reduces the ability of these programmes to attribute
change to the intervention (rather than to other variables).

Given all these practical difficulties, are experimental and quasi-
experimental designs the ideal methods some have suggested them to
be (e.g. Nutbeam *et al.*, 1990; Green and Lewis, 1986)? Perhaps the clue to

this question lies in the two meanings of the word 'ideal' as used in everyday language (both 'best' and 'unrealisable'). Here is one view relating to health education that reflects on the gap between experimental design and the demands of normal practice settings:

> In practical terms it can be difficult to plan and implement fully controlled experimental studies of health education activities. The use of laboratory type conditions can be both artificial and inappropriate and where interventions have been tested in such artificial situations we have to ask questions about the generalizability of findings to the real world. Even when experimental studies in health education have taken place in normal practice settings the outcomes which result from the extra efforts which typically go into an evaluation study may be an unrealistic guide to what can be achieved in routine practice. Finally, while experiments can establish statistical significance it may be more important to focus on practical significance.
>
> (Tones and Tilford, 1994: 59)

In short, even where it is *possible* to create situations approximating to the rigorous requirements of an experimental design, the effort may not be worthwhile if these situations are far removed from the realities of everyday practice.

Choosing an appropriate research design is not usually an 'off-the-peg' activity and each study is, in a sense, unique, though much can be learned from the experience of others. Perhaps one lesson to be learned from major experimental studies is that evaluation of human activities will usually tend to indicate areas, directions and degrees of influence rather than provide water-tight evidence of causal relationships. But experimental studies also act as a useful reminder that whatever the design and methods selected it is important to aim at being as careful and systematic as possible.

2   Survey designs: identifying significant patterns

A survey involves making systematic 'measurements' (of attitudes, actions, knowledge, blood pressure, or whatever) over a series of cases (individuals, communities, publications etc.) in such a way that the information can be analysed to discover significant patterns. Survey designs come in many shapes and sizes, may be concerned with process and/or outcome and may employ any of a range of methods, including face-to-face interviews, telephone interviews, postal questionnaires, detailed analyses of written material and observations of individuals and groups. Although the purpose is to identify patterns and to understand more about the way things are related, in contrast with experiments, surveys can't be expected to establish definitively cause and effect relation. They are, however, often a good way of gathering quantitive and (to a lesser extent) qualitative data. Practically everyone has been asked at some time to participate in a survey of some kind, whether about shopping habits, train services or political preferences. It can be helpful to reflect on those experiences as you consider the possible uses and limitations of survey designs in evaluation.

The Health Show evaluation, conducted by a market research agency, used a survey described below. (On the night of screening the show achieved an average audience of eight million and generated altogether 1.6 million telephone responses):

Box 17.1: The Health Show evaluation

The quantitive phase consisted of a two-stage telephone survey among a sample of people who had requested a copy of the Health Show Guide (or on whose behalf a copy was requested). 500,000 copies of the guide were sent out in response to telephone requests.

Stage 1: 750 telephone interviews were conducted. The main objectives were to collect profile information, brief details of the recall of the programme and the guide and some basic information about the extent to which The Health Show and The Health Show Guide had stimulated claimed behavioural changes among recipients of the guide.

Stage 2: 250 interviews with Stage 1 respondents who fulfilled certain criteria were conducted. The criteria included:

1 willing to be re-interviewed

2 having received the Health Show Guide

3 having requested the booklet for themselves (or themselves and other people)

4 having read at least some of the booklet

5 claimed to have changed their behaviour in the areas of healthy eating, physical activity or smoking since The Health Show was screened.

The main objectives were to expand on the information gained in Stage 1. This involved exploring in more detail the claimed behavioural changes and influences on change and collecting more comprehensive information about attitudes towards the Health Show Guide including suggestions for improvement. All respondents were sent a second copy of the guide so that detailed questions could be asked of it.

(adapted from Wallace, 1993: 22)

You will probably have noticed that the sample was self-selected (people opted in by being sufficiently interested to phone and request the guide), which means they are unlikely to be representative of the audience.

What might be the advantages and disadvantages of sampling from amongst those who requested the guide rather than from the audience or from the general public?

Under the heading 'caveats to the research', the evaluation makes clear the untypical nature of the sample and acknowledges that selecting a random sample of the audience would have been a better strategy:

Box 17.2: The Health Show evaluation continued

Requesters of the guide should not be confused either with the audience of The Health Show or the population in general. They differ both demographically and attitudinally and are characterised by an above average awareness and interest in health issues ... Compared with the population as a whole, the television audience ... was skewed towards women and the over 45s. This sex bias was even more accentuated among respondents from Stages 1 and 2 of the quantitative survey: over four in five of those interviewed were women. In terms of age, 45–64s were strongly over-represented, as were those from ABC1 households. These same respondents also appeared to be more health conscious than the general population, tending to have a more positive attitude to health and lifestyle issues, particularly diet and physical activity... In terms of the evaluation of any future enterprise, such research should obviously aim to obtain the views of the audience as a whole, rather than an elite minority.

(adapted from Wallace, 1993: 222–3, 226)

There are a number of ways to select a sample, ranging from random selection from a total population to an entirely opportunistic selection that makes no attempt to cover a range of potentially influential factors such as age, gender, race and social class. When the evaluation of The Health Show moved into its qualitative phase, which consisted of group discussions focusing on health and healthy living and reasons for watching the programme, four of the twelve groups were recruited not from the people who had requested a copy of the guide but from the general population and specifically from social classes under-represented in the self-selected sample. In other words, this was a non-random sample that aimed to redress some of the imbalance created by the main method of sampling.

Where it is possible (and considerations of time and money will be very relevant in this decision), random sampling of the target population (whether geographical or not) is advantageous, especially if it is important to be able to make generalisations from an evaluation. So, for example, if the target population is one town or area, the electoral register might be used as a basis for the sample. An evaluation of a one-year health education campaign in Corby followed this procedure. The aim of the programme (Healthy Choices) was to stimulate discussion on a variety of health-related issues and the venture was seen as an undertaking that might be replicated in other locations if the outcomes were promising. This meant it was important to feel confident about the nature and range of the conclusions. A major element in the evaluation was a general population study, carried out over ten days, using a structured interview administered by 15 students and two staff members from a local college. From a total population of 33,466 Corby electors a sampling fraction of 1 in 50 gave a potential sample of 400 individuals. In fact, 301 interviews were successfully completed (a response rate of 75 per cent) (Spratley, 1982). The evaluation report stresses the time demands of the evaluation process.

Gaining access to names and addresses, other than through an electoral register, presents practical and ethical difficulties. One alternative to the electoral register is the telephone directory, though response rates and gaining access to particular sub-groups are both problematic. One example of the use of a telephone survey focusing on a specific social category ('opinion leaders') can be seen in the following formative evaluation of a campaign aiming to promote moderate alcohol use in New Zealand.

This campaign sought to focus the policy debate on the negative consequences and costs associated with alcohol consumption and was directed at people regarded as influential 'opinion leaders'. After the first phase of the campaign an evaluation took place in which a series of advertisements were placed in selected magazines. This formative evaluation was comprised of telephone interviews and had three strands: a large-scale survey to obtain quantitive data and two small-scale semi-qualitative studies aimed at identifying the nature of the response to the advertisements. The first survey involved over 1,000 interviews with people 15 years and over, randomly selected from telephone directories. The response rate was only 35 per cent, and where contact was successfully made it was 49 per cent. From this general population sample, sub-groups of 188 high socio-economic level men and 172 high socio-economic level women were identified. (The top socio-economic grouping was considered to be the most likely to contain opinion leaders and those who move in circles where they may have some influence on policy makers (Wyllie and Casswell, 1992: 157).)

Just over a third of calls made were answered and, of these, almost a half agreed to be interviewed. Do you think the low response rate matters?

Arriving at the qualitative samples was a very time-consuming and costly procedure, yet even in such a large-scale and technically sophisticated design the results may be no more reliable than in a less ambitious study. The studies referred to so far in this section have been large-scale but survey design may also be appropriate in smaller-scale evaluation. If, for instance, you want to evaluate a particular relaxation class or counselling service with, say, 30 clients and haven't the resources to interview all of them you might choose to distribute a questionnaire to everyone and conduct individual interviews with a sample of five. In this situation it may be especially important to try to get representation of the different kinds of people involved. Random sampling alone (e.g. interviewing every sixth person on an alphabetical list of clients) might not achieve this without first dividing the total population into sub-groups or strata in terms of, say, age, gender, race and occupation and then random sampling each sub-group. This approach to sample selection, known as stratified random sampling, may also be neccessary in larger populations from whom it is important to ensure that particular kinds of people are represented in the final sample; and a simple random sample may not yield this. An obvious example would be a survey of cultural responses to health information leaflets in which it would be important first to identify the different ethnic and cultural groupings involved to ensure that the final sample contained sufficient numbers from each. The summary box below gives an overview of the various sampling options.

Box 17.3: Sampling options

A sample may be

random:	all begin with an equal chance of being chosen
stratifed random:	the sample is chosen from different layers or strata of a population
multi-stage random:	the samples are selected randomly but at different times or stages
purposive:	the selection is made according to the purpose
quota:	an interviewer goes to a location and selects interviewees up to a set number

(adopted from Feuerstein, 1986)

---

3   Qualitative designs: describing and interpreting what has happened

Qualitative design is most obviously relevant when the underlying questions are as much or more about 'what happened?' than about 'does it work?' A design that uses qualitative data and brings to the forefront people's experiences and perceptions may be variously described as illuminative, qualitative or ethnographic. The emphasis here is on understanding with a degree of depth and detail that is not possible in most other evaluation design. For the evaluator it involves more direct contact with participants: methods most often used within this design include participant observation, focus groups, interviews, documentary analysis and case-studies (the meaning of each of these terms will be explained later). The analysis of qualitative data is complex but the general aim is to draw out themes from the data and in doing this researchers try to be open and clear about their procedures so that others are able to assess their accounts.

A qualitative design is likely to be relevant to an evaluation that is interested in processes (the detail of what happens) either for its own sake or as a way of understanding the nature of the outcomes. A design focusing on (rather than simply including) qualitative data tends to cast the evaluator in the role of one who provides interpretative summaries:

> The evaluator assumes the position of being an orchestrator of opinions, an arranger of data, a summarizer of what is commonly held, a collector of suggestions for changes, a sharpener of policy alternatives. Illuminative evaluators do not act as judges and juries but, in general, confine themselves to summing up arguments for and against different interpretations, policies and possible decisions.
>
> (Parlett, 1981, quoted in Tones and Tilford, 1994: 64)

It has been argued that qualitative design 'allows values to re-enter evaluation openly' (Weiss and Rein, 1983) in contrast to experimental design, in which, it is said, the evaluation criteria are embedded in the programme from its inception and there is no incentive to use alternative criteria.

In health promotion, a predominantly or entirely qualitative design is most often found either in very small-scale studies or in evaluations of community development initiatives (an area of evaluation discussed in detail in Jones and Sidell, 1997, Chapter 6). A review of evaluation reports in the field of community development over the ten-year period 1979 to 1989 identified several distinct qualitative styles of evaluation including the following:

- A historical approach, assembling a chronological narrative.
- Participatory evaluation, giving priority to the views of lay people in the process of evaluation.
- Action research, allowing the evaluator to contribute formatively to processes of project management and steering.
- Goal-free evaluation, focusing on the processes of the project (not the outcomes).
- Negotiated evaluation, checking accounts with key informants.

(adapted from Beattie, 1990: 226)

As this list indicates, qualitative design may be chosen as part of a commitment to redistribute power and find ways of enabling ordinary people's voices, values and priorities to be heard. But it may also be used simply because of the descriptive detail and depth needed in a particular evaluation.

A clear and fairly typical illustration of this fact, can be seen in the following extract from the evaluation report of a programme of workshops for primary health care teams, designed to help those working in primary health care enhance their activities in prevention and health promotion by developing plans and strategies relevant to their circumstances.

> The challenge to the evaluation programme has been to map the development, implementation and management of the ... workshop

strategy through an illustrative, descriptive process ... In developing the
evaluation programme, a number of research methods have been
involved including participant observation, interviews, documentary
analysis and interactive approaches including the provision of interim
feedback, reflections, and observations to planning groups in order that
they might avail themselves of the information and experience that has
been accumulating throughout the development of the ... workshop
programme as a whole, as well as having the opportunity to reflect on
their own experience of organising such events.

(Spratley, 1989: 12)

The strengths and limitations of qualitative design are closely connected.
Very intensive methods that can deal with detail and complexity are costly
and time-consuming. They may also be open to the charge that they give
evaluators too much scope to impose their own values and perceptions
and are too concerned with process at the expense of outcome. The
richness of the data provided by qualitative methods can be very difficult
to make sense of, especially if there is a lot of it. Increasingly researchers
are using a combination of qualitative and quantitative methods to
evaluate health promotion outcomes.

Evaluation design and pragmatic pluralism

This chapter has looked at three main designs, experimental, survey and
qualitative, which may be drawn on when planning an evaluation. The
choice of design has very practical consequences because it influences the
kind and range of information or data that the evaluation will consider
relevant. It will be partly linked with the extent to which an evaluation is
intended to be either goal-oriented (mostly concerned with measurable
outcomes) or process-oriented (using a more open-ended documentation
of relationships and values). It may also be affected by the extent to which
the terms of reference are internal or external in origin. But in the end
each design has to be decided according to its appropriateness to each new
undertaking. An evaluator needs to be aware of the choices available so
that the advantages associated with each feature of the design may be
balanced against any sacrifices that each choice entails.

The design, therefore, becomes a matter of planning for allocation of
resources (time and money) based upon a selection of questions that are
considered to be most apt and guided by practical and political
considerations.

(Shrinkfield, 1983: 357)

It is worth noting here that many evaluations in the field of health
promotion use a mixture of designs and methods and may be described as
pluralist (in varying degrees), though it should also be noted that pluralist
methodology is not without its critics. Some researchers have argued that
the logic, values and rules underlying experimental and quantitive design
on the one hand and qualitative, illuminative design on the other are so
different that the two cannot, with integrity, be added together (e.g. Smith

and Heshusius, 1986), though others, whilst remaining sensitive to the differences, have argued that methodological pluralism is possible, but 'requires its practitioners not to violate the strengths of each approach...' (Rennie and Toukmanian, 1992: 247). The European Guidelines on Evaluation (WHO, 1999) stress the importance of using a range of methodologies and not focusing purely on randomised controlled trials.

17.3 Information and indicators

The checklist in Table 17.1 includes crucial questions about the standards or criteria providing the basis of an evaluation (item 6) and the kind of information that will make it possible to assess the extent to which they are being met (item 9). In all three of the evaluation designs discussed in the first part of this chapter these questions have to be considered: what sort of evidence counts and what kind of measurements are possible? Considering them leads us to look at the role and importance of *indicators*. It may help to think of an indicator as a marker. It can be compared to a road sign, which shows whether you are on the right road, how far you have travelled and how far you still have to go (Feuerstein, 1986). Sometimes indicators provide ways of measuring outcomes, sometimes they provide evidence of steps believed to be essential stages in reaching the desired aim or goal and sometimes they indicate whether prodecures and processes are going as planned. They may be either quantitive or qualitative, and decisions about the kinds of indicator to use will be influenced by the values and assumptions underlying the various approaches to health promotion and evaluation already outlined.

Let's think about the choice of indicators in the context of health education. Suppose you want to assess whether a piece of health education has been effective. What kind of information will you need? Probably the first questions to ask yourself are: what was the education aiming to do? What would indicate it had been successful? If, for instance, you had been teaching children about the need to eat fruit and vegetables each day then ideally you would want to find out whether their behaviour had changed, whether they were actually eating them more than before. To measure this kind of change you would need to decide on some sort of *outcome indicators*. The best and most reliable evidence of behaviour change is likely to be found in real-life situations, but these are, of course, very difficult, time-consuming and expensive to observe systematically; and so, instead of trying to observe the eating patterns of the children directly, you might settle for an indirect indicator using the children's own accounts of whether their eating patterns had changed.

Self-reported change (i.e. change people perceive they have made and are willing to report) is a very popular measure in this kind of evaluation and sometimes a project's aims and objectives are framed in terms of self-reported changes in knowledge, attitudes and behaviour. For instance, an

AIDS educational programme for young adults (Streetwise UK) aimed to 'increase knowledge, generate positive attitudes towards condom use and increase *self reported* safer sexual practices involving condom use' (Bellingham and Gillies, 1993). Of course, it is difficult to see how information about sexual behaviour can be reported other than by those actually involved. But even in more public spheres self-reported behaviour is frequently an important source of information. You may have noticed that self-reported change was the main measure in the evaluation of the television programme The Health Show, described earlier .

Another kind of information that might be gathered is change in knowledge and attitudes. Improvements in these areas do not necessarily mean that people will go on to behave differently. But at least it means that people are better informed and have the kinds of attitudes that predispose them towards a particular line of action, even though other factors might inhibit change. So, returning to the first example of teaching children the value of eating fruit and vegetables each day, you might choose to regard change in the children's knowledge as an indicator of success rather than reports of changes in eating patterns.

If changing knowledge does not necessarily lead to changes in behaviour, how is it possible to use it as an intermediate indicator?

There is no necessary connection between knowledge, attitude change and behaviour though the three are not unrelated. Keith Tones describes the relationship this way: once people become aware of a message (such as that it is good to eat fruit and vegetables each day) there are a number of stages which may or may not be passed through before they adopt new patterns of behaviour. First they need to understand the message, secondly they need to believe it and see it as relevant to them, and thirdly they need to assess the costs and benefits of acting upon it. If and when these three steps are successfully negotiated, a positive attitude to the change will emerge. But for attitudes to be translated into practice other things are needed, such as access to a healthier diet, and factors such as family income will then come into play. In the case of children who don't themselves do the weekly shopping the issue is complex. Figure 17.1 shows how Tones summarises this process:

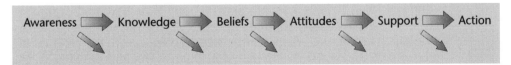

Figure 17.1   (adapted from Tones, 1995: 65)

The term support includes economic and structural factors as well as the psychological support provided by peer groups and so on. On the basis of Tones's model it could be argued that knowledge change is a better indicator of the effectiveness of an educational programme than behavioural change, which depends on many factors in addition to knowledge. To improve its effectiveness the educational programme would have to be supplemented by a number of other interventions, including an appropriate healthy public policy that allowed for the easy and cheap purchase of, say, fresh fruit and vegetables.

Health education according to the 'modern' or 'empowerment' models discussed in Chapter 5 will tend to focus on what Tones describes as the support stage in assessing effectiveness. From this perspective, how effective health promotion improved nutrition levels would ultimately be judged by such measures as decrease in poverty, successful campaigns against food manufacturers who operate unhealthy marketing practices, the provision of healthy foods at prices people could afford and good labelling of food.

Deciding what will be an appropriate and feasible measure of effectiveness or change is a crucial step in planning and carrying out an evaluation. Where it is difficult to gather information directly about the outcome of an activity and where it is not possible to demonstrate a direct link between health promotion activities and the desired outcome, *intermediate and indirect indicators* are often used. For example, HIV/AIDS health promotion's ultimate aim is to reduce the incidence of infection, but trying to measure change along the way and, in particular, identifying changes that are directly linked with the activity being evaluated involve choosing intermediate and indirect indicators as well as lower-level outcome indicators. The choice of indicators will depend on the objectives of the activity as well as on an understanding of the relation between health and factors influencing behaviour.

An example of this is an evaluation of the Cambridge AIDS Programme (Armstrong and Hutton, 1992). The programme itself had four elements: an AIDS helpline, a needle exchange, an HIV testing and counselling service and an AIDS education unit. The long-term aim of a programme such as this is to reduce the transmission of HIV by changing the behaviour of individuals. But in selecting indicators the evaluators decided that within the period of the evaluation evidence of identifiable changes in individual behaviour was unlikely to be available and would also be difficult to interpret. They chose, instead, to focus on one stated aim of the programme, 'to facilitate positive change in social consciousness about HIV infection and AIDS among agencies and communities in Cambridge'. The task then became one of choosing indicators that would measure changes in knowledge, attitudes, agency policies and practices amongst the various groups and agencies who were in contact with the programme, the underlying premise being that such changes would eventually lead to the kinds of changes in individual behaviour that would reduce transmission.

To give you an overview of the possibilities, Table 17.2 summarises the range of indicators that have been used to evaluate HIV/AIDS health promotion activities.

Table 17.2 **Indicators that can be used to evaluate HIV/AIDS health promotion**

Type of indicator	*Example*
Outcome indicators	
Health status indicators	Incidence of HIV infection
Behavioural measures	Reported safer sex practice
	Reported injecting behaviour
	Reduction in risk taking
Attitude/knowledge measures	Knowledge of HIV transmission
	Knowledge about risky behaviour
	Attitude towards people with HIV
Self-concept measures	Empowerment to negotiate safer sex
	Confidence in talking about safer sex
	Values and beliefs about sexuality
	Measures of self-esteem
Intermediate indicators	
Output indicators	Number of materials produced
	Number of training sessions run
	Number of staff trained
Input indicators	Amount of human and financial resources devoted to the activity
Health/social policy indicators	Extent of workplace policies
	Extent of legislation in relation to non-discrimination
Process indicators	Extent of involvement of group members
	Relationship between participants

(adapted from Aggleton *et al.*, 1992)

In the area of large-scale plans and healthy public policy, indicators are often explicitly related to and closely linked with targets and goals. An example of this can be seen in Australian policy initiatives aiming to improve health through the creation of healthier environments (as advocated in the WHO Health for All strategy). In 1993, *Goals and Targets for Australia's Health in the Year 2000 and Beyond,* presented a framework for expressing goals and targets relating to transport, housing and so on in ways that could be measured. This was done by identifying *intermediate indicators.* So a very large-scale goal such as 'to increase the proportion of people living in adequate housing' was focused on the most disadvantaged communities (Aboriginal and Torres Straits Islanders living in rural communities and settlements), and in the indicators specific minimum requirements for adequate housing were spelt out. These included the provision of adequate water, electricity and sewage disposal. Box 17.4 summarises the indicators chosen in two main areas: housing and work.

Box 17.4: Examples of goals and targets and intermediate indicators for healthy environments

Housing, home and community infrastructure

Goal:

To increase the proportion of people living in adequate housing.

Priority populations:

Aboriginal and Torres Strait Islanders in rural communities and settlements.

Target:

To reduce exposure to risks to health associated with poor living conditions.

Intermediate indicator:

To increase the proportion of Aboriginal and Torres Straits Islanders living in remote and rural communities who live in dwellings which have:

• potable water for drinking/cooking

• adequate water supply

• electricity

• bathing and laundry facilities

• waste and sewage disposal.

Work and the workplace

Goal:

To reduce the impact of unemployment on health.

Priority populations:

Young people aged 14–25.

People who have been unemployed for 12 months.

Target:

To increase the proportion with opportunities for paid employment and/ or training programmes.

Intermediate indicator:

The proportion of target populations in paid employment or training programmes.

(Nutbeam and Harris,1995)

In Britain, Friends of the Earth have spelt out targets and indicators in a similar manner for reducing vehicle emissions and saving energy. Identifying indicators for community development projects as distinct from public policy programmes presents equally interesting but not insurmountable challenges. Measureable objectives and intermediate indicators can be selected even where an activity's or project's main aim is something as general and seemingly abstract as empowerment, though in such situations it may be important for the manner of selection to reflect the aim. A reviewer of community intervention evaluation suggests this can be done by

> an interactive dialogue between evaluator and program workers which shows how a common but indistinct objective ... 'to empower residents' can be broken down and translated into more practical and recognisable terms ... (which) represent specific things happening to specific people. There may, for example, be attitudinal changes across the community as a whole, skills changes within the immediate group involved, changes in the makeup of advisory boards or groups.
>
> (Hawe, 1994: 205)

Identifying and using indicators is possible not only in areas that do not appear to lend themselves to quantification; it may enhance the whole activity by stimulating discussion and debate about the direction being followed. Sometimes this will involve making explicit some quite divergent views that have been lurking beneath the surface.

17.4 Conclusion

This chapter has focused on questions of evaluation design, setting out the main choices and suggesting that, for the most part, evaluation in the area of promoting health is not a matter of creating designs that establish cause and effect, and that qualitative designs are at least as important as the more experimental designs used in drug trials and so on. The second half of the chapter has stressed the value of searching for appropriate ways to measure progress. Whatever the criteria guiding an evaluation, information has to be gathered and in some way measured against these criteria. This usually involves selecting indicators which allow you to assess the extent to which criteria or standards are being met and these may relate to outcome, progress or process. There is a growing literature on health promotion research and evaluation, and the examination of qualitative and quantitative approaches to evaluating the effectiveness of health promotion interventions (Scott and Weston, 1998; Thorogood and Coombes, 2000). The use of qualitative data through methods such as focus groups, interviews and case studies is acknowledged to be as important as randomised control trials. Questions of how to go about gathering this information in contexts where randomised control trials are inappropriate are the subject of the next chapter.

Chapter 18
Enquiring and reporting

18.1 Introduction

This chapter is about the practicalities of evaluation and focuses on three issues. It begins by discussing some methods you might consider using in an evaluation: observation, interviews, focus groups and questionnaires. It then looks at several ways of reporting evaluation findings and at the importance of shaping reports to the needs of particular groups. Finally it considers some ways to influence the implementation of results. Placing reporting and implementation *after* methods reflects the order in which things actually occur, though not their order of importance. Almost by definition, the usefulness of an evaluation depends much more on the degree to which people become aware of its findings, consider them to be plausible and act upon them, than on the academic respectability of the methods and procedures followed. A technically admirable evaluation that fails to be noticed and implemented might be good research but isn't good evaluation.

18.2 Methods of enquiry

Let's begin with methods most likely to be used in evaluation with a qualitative dimension or design. Qualitative methods enable close attention to detail so, for example, a qualitative interview will go into greater depth and is often much more open ended than the tightly structured interviews or questionnaires normally used in a large-scale survey.

> Imagine you are invited to advise on the methods that might be used in a small-scale, unfunded evaluation of nurse-patient consultations in your local GP practice. What are some of the important questions that should be asked? (Remind yourself of the questions listed at the beginning of Chapter 17.) What are the possibilities and constraints?

Probably the first questions you would need to ask are: who wants this evaluation and why? Are the nurses themselves seeking to improve their practice? Is there a desire to identify training needs? Has there been a complaint? Has the GP recently developed a passion for quality control? In short, what is the evaluation's *purpose* and what are those involved going to feel about the activity?

Once you have a clear view of these issues (and if you agree an evaluation would be helpful, appropriate and feasible) you can begin to discuss criteria, potential indicators, the kind of information that is needed and who will do the work. The final choice of methods will depend on the answers to all these questions as well as on constraints of time and so on.

Methods you are likely to consider are observation, interviews, group discussions perhaps, and case studies, so let's think about what each of these may involve.

Observation

Observation can be a very useful way of teasing out the detail of conversations and consultations and, perhaps, of discovering what people actually do compared with what they recall doing, what they believe they do or what they would ideally hope to do. In addition, it provides insights and information about non-verbal communication and about ways in which understandings are shaped and maintained through particular kinds of interaction. An evaluation concerned with the quality and pattern of the communication between a practice nurse and her patients might well consider using observational methods. The evaluator would probably sit in on or video consultations, subject to the agreement of the individuals concerned.

When you are acting as an observer there are decisions to be made about the kind of role to adopt. Logically there are four options (Junker, 1960). At one end of the spectrum is the intensely involved role of the complete participant who acts as a full and ordinary member of the group being studied, whilst at the opposite end is the complete observer who has no contact at all with those being studied (such as one watching a group through a one-way mirror). Between the two lie 'participant as observer' and 'observer as participant' (depending on the degree of involvement with the people being studied). As a general rule observation with a high degree of involvement tends to be especially useful when there are important differences between the views of outsiders and insiders (as with a minority ethnic group) and when the phenomenon is hidden from public view (for instance illegal drug use). In situations that are less culturally removed from the everyday world of the observer a less intense degree of participation is often sufficient.

One possible difficulty with observation is that it may change or influence what is being observed. So, for instance, a patient may feel inhibited and unusually silent if an observer is present; a nurse who is aware of the focus of an evaluation may respond much more positively to patients' questions than normally. These problems of interference and distortion are not unique to observational methods and may be just as great when questionnaires and interviews are used. It is sometimes assumed that observation and participation are necessarily in competition and conflict with one another and that accuracy and reliability are best achieved by minimising participation and involvement (Junker, 1960: 36). But lack of participation may well bring difficulties in interpretation: 'the potential for misunderstanding and inaccurate observation increases when the researcher remains aloof and distanced physically and socially from the subject' (Jorgensen, 1989: 56). It is important to try to strike a balance and ask what level and style of observation will be appropriate, useful and acceptable in a particular situation (Peberdy, 1993).

How observations are recorded depends to a great extent on the criteria being used and the issues being addressed. If, for instance, the focus of an evaluation is to find out how well nurses encourage and respond to patients' questions, the observer may well need to tape-record the conversations (for subsequent analysis) and make notes on non-verbal cues and responses, perhaps under headings reflecting various aspects of facial expression, gaze, body position and so on. If more than one observer is used it will be especially important to agree precisely on the way the observation will be recorded by perhaps using a very detailed observation sheet specifying the full range of facial expressions that are to be recorded and when this should happen (for example when the patient enters the room, then every 60 seconds and/or whenever a question is asked and answered).

Interviews

Interviewing is a good way to find out in some depth about people's perceptions, views and priorities. As with observation, this method may be highly or loosely structured. In structured interviews the intention is that each person will be asked the same questions, in the same way and in the same order, whilst unstructured interviews simply identify the main areas and issues to be pursued. An unstructured interview is most appropriate when there is a need to explore various facets of an interviewee's concerns and when the interviewee's perceptions are regarded as more important than the interviewer's expectations and preconceptions (Mahoney *et al.*, 1995: 4).

Unstructured, in-depth interviews require a great deal of planning, sensitivity and concentration if they are to be productive and reliable. In addition to planning the questions it is important to explain and set up the interview in a manner that helps the interviewee to understand its purpose and feel valued. The interview itself calls for skill in attentive listening, framing questions, drawing out relevant responses and recording answers. After the interview there comes the central and time-consuming task of analysing what has been said to identify the key themes and patterns.

Giving sufficient time and thought to analysis is important. A study using unstructured interviews exploring the health beliefs and practices of a group of middle-class Americans was able to uncover several important themes underpinning their accounts. For example, it was shown that in their common-sense view of the world health was grounded in an understanding of the body and self as twin aspects of one entity rather than as two entities. The researcher illustrated each of the themes with a range of extracts from respondents' accounts, and the differences between accounts were explored in terms of gender and so on (Saltonstall, 1993, cited in Secker *et al.*, 1995: 84).

Questionnaires

A method most commonly associated in people's minds with evaluation is the questionnaire. For instance, the circulation of a short evaluation questionnaire at the end of a workshop has become normal practice and, as you are aware from your own experience, questionnaires come in a variety of shapes and sizes. To avoid some pitfalls it is important to be familiar with some basic principles and guidelines underlying the design of questionnaires. Clarity and brevity are important words to keep in mind, though perceived relevance or saliency has the greatest impact on response. Developing a questionnaire is often a demanding and laborious process involving several drafts. It is important to test out (pilot) a questionnaire on a few people to find out how well it works in practice before using it more widely. It is also always necessary to check that a questionnaire has been designed in such a way that it is possible to analyse and make use of the kind of information that is gathered.

Questions may be either open (any answer can be given) or closed (the answer has to be chosen from a fixed number of options). Examples of the second occurred in the Nottingham Health Profile, referred to in Chapter 2, which attempted to allow respondents some scope to make subjective assessments of their health by recording scores in a range of categories selected by the researchers. The information gained through closed questions is quicker to record and easier to analyse, but unless it includes the gist of the answer that would have been given to an open question the data will be less significant and reliable. The boxes contain questions taken from the survey that formed part of the evaluation of the Corby Healthy Choices Programme mentioned in Chapter 17. The first offers a straight yes/no choice and tells the interviewer what to say if the person is unsure.

---

4   Do you remember seeing the Health Choices caravan parked in the Market Square and other parts of Corby for short periods over the past year? Yes / No

(Prompt – *the caravan was giving out information on various health topics.*)

The next example has to list more categories but again there can be only one answer for each respondent. Notice the way the categories don't overlap.

> 1   How long have you lived in Corby?
>
>   11 months or less
>
>   1 year – 5 years 11 months
>
>   6 years – 9 years 11 months
>
>   10 years – 14 years 11 months
>
>   15 years – 19 years 11 months
>
>   over 20 years

In some questions the respondent may agree with more than one of the options, as in the next question. Notice also the open nature of the list at the end.

> 19e. Who did you talk to about the information?
>
>   husband/wife/partner
>
>   friend(s)
>
>   neighbour(s)
>
>   child/children
>
>   parent(s)
>
>   other(s) (write in) ....

Some of the questions in the questionnaire were entirely open.

> 11b. What did you think was the purpose of the caravan? (write in)
>
> ....

Here is a useful summary of the pros and cons of open and closed questions:

Open questions leave the field wide open. There is little risk of directing or channelling interviewees to think in particular ways. There is little chance of you missing out something important. With gentle inquisitive prompting you can invite your interviewee to keep adding to the opinion.

Closed questions are particularly useful if you are seeking factual information (who, where, when, how many) or if you don't have much

Table 18.1 **Types of interview**

Type of interview	Characteristics	Strengths	Weaknesses
Informal, conversational interview	Questions emerge from the immediate context and are asked in the natural course of conversation. There is no predetermination of topics or wording.	The salience and relevance of questions is increased. Interviews are built on and emerge from observations. Interviews can be matched to individuals and circumstances.	It is less systematic and comprehensive if certain questions don't arise naturally. The organisation and analysis of data can be quite difficult.
Interview guide approach	Topics to be covered are specified in advance, in outline form. The interviewer decides the sequence and working of questions in the course of the interview.	The outline increases the comprehensiveness of the data and makes its collection somewhat systematic for each respondent. Logical gaps in the data can be anticipated and closed. Interviews remain fairly conversational and situational.	Important and salient topics may be inadvertently omitted. The interviewer's flexibility to sequence and word questions can result in substantially different responses, thus reducing the usefulness of their comparison.
Standardised, open-ended interview	The exact wording and sequence of questions are determined in advance. All interviewees are asked the same basic questions in the same order.	Respondents answer the same questions, thus facilitating the comparison of their responses. For each person the data is complete on the topics addressed in the interview. It reduces the interviewers' influence and bias when several interviewers are used. It permits decision-makers to see and review the instrumentation used in the evaluation. It facilitates the organisation and analysis of the data.	It allows little flexibility to relate the interview to particular individuals and circumstances. The standardised wording of questions may limit the naturalness and relevance of questions and answers.
Closed, quantitive interviews	Questions and response categories are determined in advance. Responses are fixed, and respondents choose from among them.	Data analysis is simple: responses can be directly compared and easily aggregated. Many questions can be asked in a short time.	Respondents must fit their experiences and feelings into the researcher's categories. The interview may be perceived as impersonal, irrelevant and mechanistic. It can distort what respondents mean or have experienced by so completely limiting their response choices.

time to let the interviewee think about her/his answers (e.g. in the street). They direct attention to particular key points rapidly. Their main limitation is obvious – people might have come up with very different answers, but, because you have not asked, they can only answer what you have asked. The other limitation of Yes/No, or even Yes/No/Don't know, is that it is just too rigid a way to answer lots of questions.

(Edwards, 1991: 121–2, adapted)

Analysing open questions can be very time-consuming. It is important to begin by getting an overview of the kinds of answers that have been given by rapidly reading through the responses (perhaps from only a sample). Look for patterns that will allow you to think up some general headings under which you can note the replies. It will be important to find a way of recording how frequently a particular kind of response has been made. Remember also to identify quotations which may be useful in your report.

The summary table, which compares different types of interview, may help you weigh up the strengths and weaknesses of some of the methods.

Case studies

Case studies provide very detailed information about and insights from the experiences of particular individuals and may be especially helpful in revealing the dynamics and processes at work. There are a number of different ways to carry out case studies. Probably the most relevant here is the narrative case study, which is concerned to make sense of the stories people tell of their experiences.

One way to use a case study method in the evaluation of nurse-patient interactions would be to interview a few patients several times, over a period, to learn more about the development of the relationships and how they connect with and are influenced by other aspects of the patients' lives and health. The emphasis here might be on the building up of a narrative, based as much on patients' perspectives and categories as on the evaluator's framework. A less ambitious and time-consuming use of the case study is to complement the findings of interviews by describing in some detail the experiences of one or two individuals selected from all those who have been interviewed (purposive selection). Box 18.1 contains some thoughts on what makes for a good case study.

The criteria identified by Yin are derived from case-study research in management, education and sociology. Case studies have long been an important tool in the fields of counselling and psychotherapy, but the new interest in the case study approach in other areas is accompanied by an awareness that there are systematic ways of using this method. Its central features are: the use of multiple sources of the data; a variety of perspectives on the data and consideration of competing perspectives; procedures that are clear and explicit; backing up conclusions by evidence (McLeod, 1994: 119). The case study method need not only be used with individuals, but can be used in an organisation such as a school or a GP practice.

Box 18.1: Criteria for a good case study

Significance: A study will have more meaning and impact if it focuses on fairly common experiences or if it is unusual and reveals largely hidden factors and processes.

Completeness: It should give the reader a sense of the whole by providing sufficient contextual information.

Evidence: The reader must be given sufficient evidence to make his or her own judgement.

Effective representation: It is important that the style should be lively and engaging.

(adapted from Yin, 1989)

Focus groups

Focus groups can be quicker than individual interviews at gathering the views and perceptions of a small number of people, and the stimulus of hearing other views can encourage people to express their own perspectives. This may be especially true in situations where power is imbalanced as, for example, in relationships between children and adults, when group discussion with peers may be less inhibiting than individual interviews with an adult (see, for instance, Davis and Jones, 1996).

In most studies that use focus groups several groups are organised, each with six to twelve people who share some characteristics or experiences. The discussion needs to be facilitated or moderated either by the evaluator or by someone with special skills in group work, so that the group is encouraged to explore and express views on the topics under scrutiny and every individual is able to contribute. Often members do not know each other and it is the job of the facilitator to make introductions, orient the group to its task and ensure it is carried out. Usually the discussion is taped and then analysed by themes. The analysis may use software packages such as Ethnograph, NUD.IST or Atlas.

The evaluation of the Cambridge AIDS Programme referred to in the previous chapter made extensive use of focus groups. The evaluators felt that the group setting was both realistic and illuminative, highlighting differences of perspective and drawing attention to common patterns of response. The focus of that particular evaluation was the impact the programme was making on the community and on local agencies and groups within it. So what happened within the group (the ways people worked and contributed to the group) was regarded as 'a demonstration as

well as a description of the impact the programme was making'
(Armstrong and Hutton, 1992: 51).

How appropriate would a focus group be for the evaluation of nurse-
patient relationships in a local GP practice? It will certainly be much
cheaper and quicker than individual interviews. But it won't gather the
same kind of information, although if patients are experiencing some
obvious and widespread difficulties with the practice nurses, these will
tend to emerge quite quickly. It will probably be much better at
identifying general views and perceptions than at gathering material
about particular experiences. Whilst it may be especially useful in allowing
the evaluator access to the patients' culture and priorities, it risks not
revealing difficult, sensitive issues that make people feel vulnerable and
becoming dominated by the views of more talkative or confident
members. One useful role of focus groups may be to help set the agenda
for subsequent individual interviews although, if there isn't the time or
money for such interviews, then the focus group might be a good second
best. Sometimes a mixture of group discussion and individual interviews
can be a fruitful strategy, providing both depth and breadth.

**Pause and consider the advice you would give about appropriate ways to evaluate
nurse-patient consultations.**

Having discussed some of the main ways to gather information for
evaluation, we now move on to consider how to report the findings of an
evaluation.

The importance of participatory evaluation

Participatory evaluation and participatory action research are approaches
that have been used to evaluate community development programmes.
These approaches seek to actively involve participants in the process of
evaluation (Springett, 2000). They are discussed further in K301 Book 2.

18.3 Reporting and implementing

Small-scale studies

In small-scale, informal evaluation the question of what to report and to
whom is usually straightforward because you are familiar with the people
concerned and with the ways they best communicate and make decisions.
The important task will be to make sure that time and attention is given to
the reporting and implementing aspects of the evaluation. In a semi-

formal, internally conducted evaluation, it may be necessary to adopt a more formal style deliberately when it comes to finding ways to implement changes that need, say, management support, additional funding or a different relationship with the public. This doesn't mean you will have to produce a hefty, technical written report, but you will need to consider how best to communicate effectively and persuasively with, perhaps, a variety of groups and individuals. Because you are seeking to influence people who are in a position to make things different, how much time and effort to spend and which people and groups to spend it on are largely political decisions. If you have received some financial backing for the evaluation then for reasons of accountability you will need to report back to funders in some way.

There will be other reasons too for wishing to share your experience and findings. Below is the opening paragraph of the report of an evaluation of the Asian Women and Diabetes event described in Chapter 16.

> Our main reason for having a report is to make sure that all the hard work which has gone into this project gets some recognition. Quite often in community based work, there is no time to write things up and the good ideas don't get passed around. So this report is for the women involved in the work and for others who may be interested in this particular model of community development.
>
> (Kaur and Bedford, n.d.: 4)

Larger-scale studies

Sometimes with commissioned evaluations, there may never have been any intention to act on their findings. Perhaps arranging for an evaluation is simply a public relations exercise ('it's good practice to conduct evaluations'); perhaps it is a piece of window-dressing (publicising existing achievements); or maybe it is just satisfying a contractual requirement without any desire to improve practice. In these situations, failure to implement recommendations clearly says nothing about the quality of the evaluations or the political astuteness of the evaluators.

But in a more open situation, the way in which an evaluator works and communicates may make a huge difference to whether or not its findings are implemented. Where evaluation is for other than private use, the question of how best to communicate its findings so that it may lead to action is vital. To begin answering it, the evaluator has to be clear about who needs to be communicated with. Knowing who makes what decisions is crucial. Several different groups who should be considered are:

- users and potential users (those on the receiving end and who are meant to benefit)
- those whose job it is to provide the activity being evaluated (health or welfare workers, educators and so on)
- managers and policy-makers

- funders (whether of the activity, the evaluation or both).

From the beginning, involving and relating well to all these groups is important if the evaluation and its findings are to stand a good chance of not being ignored:

> At the outset of an evaluation therefore, it is important to consider and develop mechanisms by which the findings of the evaluation can be discussed, not only with those involved in the activity but also with stakeholders and funders. It is also important that the level of institutional support ... is scrutinised before and during the evaluation. It may be necessary to include those 'higher' in the institutional hierarchy in the evaluation, so that the findings and recommendations are not, and cannot, be ignored.
>
> (Aggleton *et al.*, 1992: 69)

Yet, however politically astute an evaluation, success cannot be guaranteed. In some situations implemetation will remain blocked by entrenched vested interests with strong reasons for not making changes that have been recommended.

Selective reporting

Many issues compete for people's attention and an evaluation report rarely gets a thorough reading. This means that the reporting task of the evaluator is different from the task of the professional researcher. Whereas the researcher reports to a select audience with a common language and style of thought, the evaluator may need to address numerous and scattered audiences. The question of who needs to learn from the experience of a particular evaluation and what it is that different groups and individuals need to know will influence the choice of ways in which this is done. It is important, therefore, to keep in mind the many different uses to which evaluation results can be put as this will clarify the range and nature of the audiences. These uses include:

- improving programme organisation and management
- improving planning
- assisting in decision-making and policy-making
- indicating where further action and research are needed
- indicating approaches for training
- providing information for publicity.

Reporting, whether of anecdotal information or formal measurement and statistics, is necessarily highly selective and, therefore, it makes sense to select consciously on the basis of the needs and interests of particular audiences. Alan Beattie makes the same point in a different way, 'in seeking to stake a claim on the attention of a variety of audiences ... the authors of evaluation reports need to engage seriously with the politics of presentational styles' (1990: 230).

When thinking about who needs to know what, you need to consider the providers, the potential providers, the recipients and the potential recipients. It may also be helpful to distinguish between specialist and general areas of interest within each of these categories. Issues of time and areas of responsibility will also be relevant. Bear in mind the proportion of an individual's time and work-load allocated to the kind of activity being evaluated when you decide whether to provide a full report or a summary.

Sometimes it helps to design a flow of information matrix. The one in Table 18.2 was drawn up for an evaluation of a community development project in Latin America. The project was partly funded by overseas agencies. Local village people were directly involved in planning and carrying out the evaluation together with the programme staff.

Table 18.2 **Flow of information matrix**

Who?	*Role in evaluation*	*What results?*	*How?*
Neighbouring villages	Answer questions	Summary to create interest and support	Meetings Newsletters Pictures
Village directly involved	Central in planning and carrying out evaluation	Full results and recommendations so that the village can act on them	Meetings Newsletters Pictures
Community workers	Co-ordinate and facilitate evaluation	Full results and recommendations as above	Meetings Study of report
National-level departments, agencies and organisations	Can disseminate lessons learned and support future action	Full results or summary	Study report Discussion with evaluation co-ordinators

(adapted from Feuerstein, 1986: 154)

Creative presentation of findings

It is helpful to see the evaluator as to some extent like the journalist who judges what will receive public attention and packages it in a form that will attract that attention (Cronbach, 1982). This may involve conveying a feeling for the health promotion intervention and the experience of the participants, and awareness of this will influence the manner in which the evaluation is carried out, gathering material that will add colour and realism. Depending on the context, press releases, speeches and even the use of drama may prove to be appropriate ways to communicate evaluation findings and evaluation reports.

Sometimes it may be appropriate to present findings in the form of a dialogue between advocate and adversary, in which the issues presented are culled from interviews and other material. The dialogue form invites participation, to some extent leaves the conclusion open and allows for different views, unresolved conflicts and discrepancy but might provoke antagonistic responses.

Alternative forms of presentation include:

- summarising findings in a tape-slide format
- combining a statistical analysis with a diary written by a participant
- a collage of quotes
- photographic records.

What other forms of presentation might be useful?

Presentations that do not rely primarily on the written word will be especially useful and appropriate when communicating with people with certain disabilities, with young children and in places where literacy is low or writing is a fairly alien medium. In Peru, village women acted out a drama to communicate results about coastal merchants selling over-priced food to highland women who could not speak Spanish. The idea was to expose how the merchants were taking advantage of the women. Sometimes a comic-strip format combining pictures and words communicates more powerfully than a more formally written document.

Evaluation reports

Written reports

In most cases there is some kind of evaluation report, usually, but not invariably in written form. A report of a completed evaluation answers the evaluation questions, describes how the answers were obtained and then translates the findings into conclusions and recommendations.

If a report is being submitted to a funding agency the composition and format may be set. Otherwise evaluators are free to choose the appropriate length and structure for their particular projects. Sometimes a very valuable but simple evaluation exercise can be completed in a short time with few resources. Then the process and results may well be adequately covered in a very short report. On the other hand, really major and expensive evaluations may require a long document, but do beware of using a report to tell the world how much hard work has gone into the evaluation and how many difficulties you faced. The purpose is to *communicate the findings* in a way that demands attention and credibility, not to switch readers off or drown them in a weight of words.

Box 18.2: The structure of a written report

A report will usually need the following sections in some form:

1   Summary

2   Introduction

This will describe the project being evaluated and its purpose. It will identify those aspects of the project that have been chosen for evaluation and the particular questions the evaluation has been concerned to answer. It also needs to be clear about the economic, political and strategic context of this particular evaluation, the funding of both the project and evaluation, the position of the evaluator in relation to the project and the people and interests who have instigated the evaluation.

3   Methods or process

This describes how the evaluation was carried out. It gives details of the methods used and the reasons for selecting them. Where the evaluation has used very specialised or quantitive techniques you will need to define the terms used and describe its design, sample, measures and analysis.

4   Results

As far as possible present quantitive and qualitative results, both in detail and in summary, so that they speak for themselves. Where appropriate, use tables, graphs and diagrams to summarise results. As a general rule do not interpret data in this section. Statements such as 'These results contradict the findings of previous evaluations' belong in the discussion.

5   Conclusions or discussion

Here you interpret the results by answering questions such as:

- Taking the broadest perspective, what can you conclude from the evaluation?

- Is the project any good? For whom? In what circumstances?

- Which aspects of the project were most and least effective (or whatever the criterion chosen)?

- How do the results compare with the findings of other studies?

- What can be learned about health promotion projects and evaluation from this evaluation?

- What gaps in knowledge and understanding have been revealed?

- What are the limitations of the evaluation and how do these affect the conclusion?

> ### 6 Recommendations
>
> These will obviously depend greatly on what has gone before but might involve answering questions such as:
>
> - If the project were to be improved whilst retaining its main goals and objectives, what are the five main changes or additions that should be considered?
>
> - If the project were applied to another group or setting who would be likely to benefit most?
>
> - What objectives might be changed or added to the project to expand its scope or effectiveness?
>
> (summarised from Fink, 1993)

Oral reports

An oral report will usually consist of an account of some or all of the objectives of the evaluation, the methods used and the main findings. To accompany an oral presentation it often helps to prepare visual aids such as overhead transparencies or slides. The visual aids are there to help listeners focus on the main points of your talk and not to distract their attention from what is being said; so they must be clear and succinct.

Each visual should have a title and should be clearly visible to all members of the audience. It is important to check visibility and the layout of your room well in advance. It is also a good idea to allow time to rehearse your presentation before creating the final copies of the visual aids, and then to rehearse again after you have them. The length of the presentation will depend on the nature of your audience and the amount of information they really need.

Implementation

This chapter has considered a number of ways of reporting an evaluation's findings and recommendations clearly and engagingly. But if you want decision-makers to act upon your recommendations you will need to think how best to gain their involvement and interest. Zweig and Mann (1981: 11–22) argue that evaluators need to take into account the culture and practices of the people they wish to influence. The task becomes one of finding how to present a case for implementing the recommendations that respects their point of view. They also suggest that evaluators should recognise the secondary place of evaluative information in day-to-day decision-making. This means finding ways to spell out the uses of the evaluation and its recommendations to the decision-makers in terms of their main interests. Sichel (1982: 82–84) goes further and advises evaluators to give key individuals previews of their reports to increase the chances that the material will be accepted by those in a position to influence what happens. When this is done care has to be taken not to give the impression that they are being invited to influence a report.

What should happen when an evaluation produces inconclusive or negative findings? If findings have implications for future initiatives or research then it will be important to disseminate rather than 'bury' the findings. One example is given by the Family Heart Study Group, which conducted a study measuring the change in cardiovascular risk factors achievable in families by cardiovascular screening and intensive lifestyle intervention (Family Heart Study Group, 1994). It found that the implementation of the government's cardiovascular screening programme for primary care was not justified. Such negative results are as useful in informing policy as positive results.

18.4 Conclusion

This chapter has looked at some very practical questions that have to be addressed when carrying out and reporting on an evaluation. Whilst the information about methods of enquiry is far from exhaustive, it indicates the main options and provides a basis on which decisions may be made and further questions asked. The importance of appropriate and effective reporting of results has been emphasised. The main challenge is to be clear about who needs to know what, why and how. When these aspects are properly addressed the chances of implementing the findings are significantly increased.

The next and final chapter returns to broader questions about the significance and place of evaluation in health promotion and the kinds of interests and values underlying different approaches.

Chapter 19
Evaluation and the future of health promotion

19.1 Introduction

Evaluation provides a formal means of relating knowledge and practice so this final chapter begins by asking how far evaluation is contributing to decision making in relation to health promotion. It looks first at the evaluation of effectiveness and then at cost-effectiveness. To what extent are these kinds of evaluations providing a rational and adequate basis for decisions that have to be made by commissioners? To what extent is it feasible and desirable that they should do so in the future? The chapter then goes on to ask what values in addition to those implicit in the economic rationality approach come into play in decisions relating to evaluation of health promotion; we explore what might be termed an emancipatory or social justice perspective on evaluation. Then, finally, we consider how values, such as partnership and critical awareness, can be brought more fully into the process of evaluation.

Each health promotion agency has placed emphasis on evaluation of health promotion interventions. This approach is reflected in each national strategy for health promotion. Since the introduction of targets in The Health of the Nation in England, the Saving Lives: Our Healthier Nation strategy has reduced the number of targets and made them broader. Evaluating effectiveness of interventions still forms a central part of health promotion work, and the future of health promotion is dependent upon being able to demonstrate the effectiveness of health promotion interventions. 'The professional development of health promotion depends on evaluation. Evaluating activities helps inform future plans and contributes to the building up of a knowledge base for health promotion' (Naidoo and Wills, 2000: 371).

19.2 Evaluation of effectiveness: the present state of knowledge

It was noted in Chapter 16 that evaluation has come to be regarded as an essential and central tool in the provision of a rational, evidence-based way of meeting health needs. Such a view rests on the belief that the findings of evaluations somehow 'add up' in a way that can improve our understanding of how health promotion works and, in particular, our knowledge about the effectiveness of particular kinds of intervention. So it is important to ask whether, by reviewing a range of evaluations, it is possible to find generalisable results which can be used to guide health promotion in the future (Speller *et al.*, 1998).

We try to answer this question in relation to two very different areas which have been the subject of published reviews and in England formed part of the Health of the Nation targets. The first is the quite sharply defined area of smoking and pregnancy. The second is the much broader field of childhood accidents which includes the whole range of domestic, leisure and road accidents that may be experienced during the first 14 years of life.

Smoking and pregnancy

It is well established that smoking during pregnancy can damage the health of a foetus. One of the Health of the Nation targets, for example, related specifically to smoking and pregnancy. The target was '... at least 33 per cent of women smokers to stop smoking at the start of their pregnancy by the year 2000' (DoH, 1992). In order to see how to move towards this it was important to identify the kinds of intervention and support which help women stop smoking.

With this aim in mind, the Health Education Authority published a review of interventions that have attempted to reduce smoking amongst pregnant women (HEA, 1994). The focus of this review was on evaluation of effectiveness using studies which conformed to a rigorous experimental design. 'In order to draw firm conclusions about the effectiveness of an intervention it must be subjected to a randomised controlled trial with a sample size sufficient to detect a clinically significant effect, and an outcome measure that is an unbiased indicator of the smoking status.' (HEA, 1994: 10). Many studies which used a randomised control trial design were regarded by the reviewer as insufficiently rigorous because, for instance, they relied on self-reported change without seeking biochemical confirmation, or they had insufficient numbers of subjects to demonstrate a clinically significant effect. Such studies were discarded as methodologically unsound.

It was decided that of the eighteen evaluation studies examined only seven had reliable, interpretable results. On the basis of these remaining studies it was concluded that an intervention using self-help material and/ or individual (not group) counselling can increase the number of women who stop smoking during pregnancy. (As there is concern that nicotine might entail some of the risks to the foetus associated with tobacco smoking, none of these interventions used nicotine replacement.) It is worth noting that all of the selected studies were conducted in either North America or Scandinavia. Recognising the difficulties of generalising from these to British contexts, the report called for methodologically sound trials to be undertaken in Britain.

The report also recommended that future studies would benefit from a systematic analysis of the attitudes and beliefs of smokers at the time of the intervention so that styles of intervention (whether using coercion, persuasion or assistance) can be matched to types of smoker. Although British surveys have consistently shown a social class gradient with regards to smoking in pregnancy (and the opening chapter of the review takes note of this), no mention of social class was made either in the analysis of the intervention evaluations or in the recommendations relating to British trials.

Interestingly the final chapter of the report was not based on the evaluation review which had provided little by way of generalisable findings. It focused instead on monitoring and surveillance procedures without making any attempt to demonstrate their value or explain why and how they might be linked with effectiveness. It is important for us to pause and consider why these procedures are presented as self-evidently valuable. Whilst monitoring might well be used as an indicator of *commitment* to the reduction of smoking during pregnancy, in the absence of an accepted knowledge-base about what helps women stop smoking during pregnancy they can't be used as process indicators of effective preventive services. Some reasons for the official popularity of monitoring and performance indicators are suggested later in this chapter (see Section 19.4).

Reducing childhood accidents

Domestic and road accidents are the leading cause of death and a major cause of ill-health amongst children. Targets for reducing childhood accidents were not set in every national health strategy but in England, in the Health of the Nation strategy, there were specific targets relating to childhood accidents where the aim was to reduce the death rate by one-third from 6.7 per 100,000 population in 1990 to no more than 4.5 per 100,000 population by the year 2005. To provide information about the most effective forms of health promotion interventions in this area, a review of over a hundred relevant studies encompassing health education, environmental modification and legislation was published in 1993 (Towner *et al.*, 1993).

Towards the end of the review key points were identified to provide a basis for future action. These covered the characteristics of effective preventions, the relationship between education, environmental modifications and legislation, and the role of healthy alliances. To provide a picture of the kinds of conclusions reached, the findings relating to road accidents are summarised in Box 19.1. You may recall from reading Chapter 5 that people's perceptions of the causes of road accidents, and therefore of the kinds of preventive action to take, are influenced by their particular position. Teachers and road safety officers tended to focus on the role of education, whilst children and parents gave priority to structural changes such as safer crossing places (Roberts *et al.*, 1995) The review attempts to cover the whole range of factors from policy-making to education and individual protection.

The authors note that very few of the studies reviewed pay attention to the measurement of process and they suggest this is a major omission: 'Very often the intervention is seen as a "black box" ... Process measures such as network analysis (tracing the process through the community) or programme exposure may help in answering the more difficult questions of why a programme works in specific circumstances or localities ... successful interventions reported from the USA or Sweden may not necessarily be applicable in Britain' (p. 43).

Box 19.1: Summary of key points arising out of a review of studies aiming to reduce childhood road accidents

Policy makers need to recognise the impact that broad land use and transport policies have and act accordingly.

In England, area-wide engineering schemes have resulted in reduction in accidental injuries for child pedestrians and cyclists.

Drivers are unprepared for the unpredictable behaviour of child pedestrians and need to be more responsible in law for their actions. There are no evaluated studies.

Vehicle speed has a strong relationship to the severity of pedestrian injuries.

There is a need for operational road safety programmes to have an empirical base.

Children's traffic clubs have shown mixed results but injury reductions demonstrated elsewhere have not been replicated in the UK.

Lack of co-ordination between agencies has led to a very fragmented road safety education in the past.

There is fairly strong evidence that it is possible to increase cycle helmet wearing rates by concerted campaigns.

There is some evidence that increased wearing of cycle helmets leads to a reduction in casualty reductions and should be extended.

Infant and child car restraints should be available to all and their widespread use promoted.

(Towner *et al.*, 1993: 49)

Compare the range and presentation of these findings with the approach taken in the review of the smoking and pregnancy studies.

As in the pregnancy and smoking review the authors draw attention to a lack of methodological rigour in many of the published studies, commenting 'In this review it has not always been possible to assess the strength of the evidence of interventions because too few details are provided or because trials have been insufficiently controlled' (p. 42). At the same time there is an acceptance that experimental designs are by their very nature usually limited to single measure interventions such as cycle helmets and 'closed systems' such as schools and health centres. They note that the relative speed and ease of demonstrating positive results in single measure interventions can distract attention from the importance of community-wide measures. Such measures, which may involve the formation of alliances between individuals, policy makers and communities require a much longer period before effects become visible. In general conclusion to the review, the authors call for more evaluation. 'The whole area of injury prevention is still at an early stage of development – there is an urgent need for well-designed and evaluated studies to underpin the priority attached to this in *The Health of the Nation*.' (Towner *et al.*, 1993: 46)

So both reviews paint a picture in which the results of evaluation studies do not at the moment provide a solid basis for decision-making in health promotion and both call for more work in this area. But their advice about what precisely is most needed differs. Whereas the smoking and pregnancy report recommends UK-based, rigorously conducted, randomised control trials, Towner *et al.* take the view that for many interventions such trials are inappropriate and may draw attention away from initiatives which do not lend themselves to this kind of evaluation but which might in the long term have far greater potential to reduce childhood accidents.

In a similar vein, speaking about the long-term nature of much of his work (and interestingly using the language of economics to do so) one health promotion specialist quoted in a study by Nettleton and Burrows summed up the situation in relation to evaluation thus:

> The difficulty is that the way in which clinical effectiveness is being measured or looked at is being linked back into research and development and people running controlled trials and everything being scientifically based, and all the rest of it, which is fine for an intervention that has a short term outcome. But I'm trying to argue that health promotion is not so much intervention as an investment and it should be looked at almost in parallel to the money market where you put something in and you don't see very much coming back for some considerable time but you can see where you've put it and you can begin to see things beginning to happen, but you're not actually going to get your return for some period of time, which is longer than a 'Financial Year'.
>
> (a health promotion specialist in Nettleton and Burrows, 1997)

Speller *et al.* (1997) argue that the selection of studies for inclusion in many health promotion effectiveness reviews is based on the quality of the research and not the quality of the health promotion intervention, and that this can produce anomalous results. They further argue that process evaluation using qualitative research should complement outcome evaluation. Whereas initially systematic reviews of effectiveness were based on randomised control trials, there has been growth in research evidence on the effectiveness of health promotion using a wide range of research methodologies in addition to randomised control trials.

19.3 Is health promotion and prevention cost-effective?

The problem with the 'longer-term investment' approach expressed above is that it very clearly does not meet the immediate needs of commissioning authorities and others who are expected to ground or make legitimate their decisions in evidence of effectiveness and value for money. But as we have just noted in relation to both smoking during pregnancy and childhood accidents, to a large extent the evidence requirements of commissioning authorities are not adequately provided for even in relation to the kinds of situations that appear to lend themselves to experimental evaluation designs. Moreover, if effectiveness is proving difficult to demonstrate then it is hardly surprising that proof of cost-effectiveness is an even rarer commodity. Without this evidence some health promotion advocates fear that health promotion and prevention will not be able to argue their corner vis a vis curative medicine.

> Is prevention better than cure? Which prevention strategies are cost effective? Purchasers require some answers to these questions if prevention is to be given a higher priority than in the past. Information is however very limited.
>
> (Godfrey, 1993: 183)

In principle at least, a number of different kinds or techniques of economic evaluation can be undertaken in this field. Common to them all is the task of identifying and measuring – in economic terms – inputs, processes and outcomes. In order to consider how far this is possible and what kinds of calculations and decisions might be involved, it may help to focus on one particular area: mass media HIV/AIDS health education programmes.

HIV/AIDS education

The calculation of costs and benefits is complicated partly because they can be very wide ranging and difficult to quantify. Even the valuing and measuring of inputs, which might at first glance seem to be a relatively straightforward task, is in practice often very difficult. There are different kinds of costs to consider and calculate, direct, indirect and intangible, each of which may have hidden dimensions (Godfrey and Tolley, 1992). In calculating direct costs for instance, in addition to those that clearly appear on the balance sheet, there may well be *hidden* direct costs that need to be included, such as existing staff time which could have been used in alternative ways. If capital and labour costs are shared between a number of programmes or voluntary services are involved, or where health education occurs within a current affairs programme or a television soap opera, the calculation of direct costs is far from simple. Then there is the question of the indirect costs of health education which may include the cost of demands generated by the programme, such as increased demands for screening or counselling. Where a society-wide perspective is adopted, the costs to all individuals receiving the intervention should be included. These will involve intangible costs such as the anxiety individuals experience in undertaking a blood test or the social and economic costs of being identified as HIV-positive, such as being unable to get employment or insurance (Rovira, 1990). In short, '(t)his process of costing is, in practice, extremely difficult if not impossible to carry out.' (Burrows *et al.*, 1995: 246.)

With regard to the calculation of outcomes and economic benefits it is equally important to consider direct, indirect and intangible dimensions and similar problems arise. In the case of HIV/AIDS education a society-wide perspective is normally taken because HIV/AIDS has a wide range of effects on individuals, non-health agencies and the economy. Questions of where to draw the line and how to predict the future are highly problematic. For instance, an important potential economic benefit of health education is savings in health care costs, a calculation requiring some anticipation of the future costs of treatment which are in fact very uncertain. Even with the major hoped for benefit of saving lives there are debates about quantification – whether by numbers of deaths or by life years lost (since the age at death tends to be quite low). Improving the quality of the lives of those diagnosed with AIDS is a further important, but difficult to quantify, potential outcome. What to count and how to do so is clearly a matter of choice and value judgement. 'Value judgements, affected by social attitudes, are involved in costing studies, and therefore it is especially important to state clearly what assumptions are being made.' (Godfrey and Tolley, 1992: 124.)

Table 19.1   **Costs and benefits in HIV/AIDS health education programmes**

Inputs		*Outcomes*
Costs	*Health effects*	*Economic benefits*
direct costs	morbidity	direct
indirect costs	mortality	indirect
intangible costs		intangible

(based on Godfrey and Tolley, 1992)

Pause for a moment to consider where and how values enter into the calculation of costs and benefits in HIV/AIDS health education programmes.

Although economic evaluation might seem to be an entirely rational, technical exercise it is rarely so. However sophisticated the techniques it is the case that most questions of effectiveness and therefore of cost-effectiveness remain largely unanswered. Is this inconclusiveness because not enough work has been done or because the enterprise is in some way misconceived? In a trenchant and closely argued critique of the relevance of economics to the evaluation of health promotion, Burrows *et al.* conclude '... although conceptually coherent ... it is, and we argue will remain, empirically unoperationalizable because of the nature of the phenomena to which it is being directed... In short the problem is not one of methodological refinement ... ' (1995: 247). The point they are concerned to make is that the object of study in the evaluation of health promotion (human interaction and behaviour) is an 'open system' subject to very complex patterns of determination at a number of levels.

At the individual level, values, intentions and perceptions of risk all play a major part alongside the determinants most frequently focused upon in health education campaigns and evaluations. For instance, much HIV/AIDS education rests on the assumption that information about the risks of infection together with the removal of any barriers, such as price, will lead those at risk to adopt a safer lifestyle. But this is to assume that unhealthy lifestyles are valueless to those who pursue them, which may well not be the case (Birch and Stoddardt, 1990). Understanding more about people's perception of risk and the meaning and value they attach to medically defined risky behaviour requires attention to lay perspectives and an ethnographic approach to research and evaluation. Questions also need to be raised about the adequacy of a simple rational choice model of human action. As a Norwegian academic studying unsafe sex among young gay men commented: 'the world is not that simple ... a wider understanding of rationality is needed: including longing and love as motives for action.' (Prieur *et al.*, 1990: 12 quoted in Aggleton *et al.*, 1991: 19.)

At the level of structures and systems, not only is there enormous diversity in the meanings and values attached to health and health promotion (as we saw in the opening chapters of this book), there is also a wide variety of values and interests associated with particular perspectives on evaluation. The next section places the rational, technical approach in a wider perspective.

19.4 Values and evaluation

The values of the market-place

As we noted in Chapter 16, the creation of an internal market in the health service led to a competitive environment which increasingly required people to demonstrate the economic value of what they provided. This trend, visible in all public service areas and agencies, was part of what has been described as the development of the 'Evaluative State': the installation of a culture of management based on economic concepts of rationality (Cave and Kogan, 1990). Movement towards this more market-based framework with its system of competitive contracting placed great emphasis upon monitoring and performance indicators which were said to 'play a vital role in this type of system, not only as a way of making institutions accountable and allocations transparent but also as a mechanism for defining the nature of the ... "product" for which contracts are made.' (Cave and Hanney, 1990: 81.) In this view formal evaluation became a new form of cultural authority (House, 1993: viii).

Within this culture the explicit purpose of evaluation was to provide a rational basis for decision-making so that money and effort were chanelled towards the most effective and economical initiatives. But as we have seen in relation to smoking and pregnancy and childhood accidents, for the most part this is not actually what is happening at present. Moreover it may be that too great an insistence on scientifically rigorous studies of effectiveness may distract attention and resource from possibly more promising interventions which do not lend themselves to this kind of evaluation. One of the questions that has to be raised is whether the application of economic concepts of rationality to the fields of health promotion is the objective way forward that advocates claim it to be. We have seen that attempts to apply economic analysis involve very complicated decisions about what to include in the calculations. The basis for such decisions rests on values and assumptions that arise 'outside' of the rational-economic model so the question of which values to use remains. In short, evaluation is not and cannot be a purely rational-technical exercise. But if this is the case then why does it tend to be regarded as so necessary and sufficient?

Managerial evaluation

One line of argument is that the rational-technical ideal works in the interests of managers and government and this is the main reason for its official popularity. Monitoring, audit, effectiveness and detailed account-ability all work to enhance managerial control. Parton makes the point thus:

> The increased emphasis on management, evaluation, monitoring and
> constraining professionals to write things down, is itself a form of
> government of them ...
>
> (Parton, 1994: 26)

Some commentators argue that managerial evaluation with its pressure to
measure and record performance against set criteria and to establish cause
and effect relationships has the consequence of discouraging people from
asking the kinds of questions about worth and purpose which might
threaten the status quo (Everitt, 1995). Thus managerial evaluation might
be said to preclude moral debate and to support or intensify the existing
distribution of power, driving values 'into the critical unconscious, where
they continue to exercise force but without being available for analytical
scrutiny' (Connor 1993: 34). What alternatives exist?

Critical evaluation

In contrast to managerial evaluation, critical evaluation attempts to foster
moral debate by recognising the impact of power differentials and using
dialogue as a method of consciousness raising and empowerment. In this
view, emancipatory dialogue is the way of arriving at truth. Going one step
further, critical post-modernist thinkers would argue that as truth is
inextricably linked with power, evaluation far from being a way of
revealing the truth in fact contributes to its construction by means of
deconstructing ways of knowing that consistently render some people less
powerful than others. But post-modernism has been criticised for lapsing
into total relativism. If there is no truth, just many 'truth claims'
constructed through discourses, then is there any way of knowing
whether an activity intended to promote health is worthwhile? In
response to this dilemma Everitt simultaneously argues for the centrality
of values and warns against the dangers of absolutism,

> ... values must be treated with care, ... we must strive for making
> judgements in the direction of the 'good', just as we must strive for
> 'truth' but we must be tentative about the status of 'a value' and 'the
> truth'.
>
> (Everitt, 1995: 15)

Others are prepared to be less tentative. House, for instance, writing in a
North American context, is willing to claim social justice as a fundamental
value:

> Here is a test for evaluation. If this were 1920 and female suffrage were
> being debated, should evaluators remain neutral ... Or should evaluators
> represent the interest of those ignored, in this case women, in their
> evaluations? I believe the latter is morally correct.
>
> (House, 1993: 126)

In his view a central value in evaluation is that of helping to give a voice to
those who are least heard. This has a number of implications for the

conduct of evaluation. The evaluator, far from being a neutral middle-person, actively seeks out the experience and perspectives of the least powerful parties or 'stakeholders'. The task is not simply to ensure that less influential people are given a chance to answer questions but also to find ways of enabling them to shape decisions about the nature and purpose of the evaluation. It is important to be aware that this perspective differs not only from managerial evaluation but also from the liberal evaluation model based on a pluralist-equilibrium theory of democracy. In this latter model the role of an evaluator is simply to identify and present the views of various, possibly competing, groups or 'stakeholders' in an entirely neutral way. But as House comments of this model of evaluation: 'Although the reality of multiple stakeholders who have legitimate and sometimes conflicting interests is recognised, how these interests should be adjudicated remains unresolved. The practice of decribing various interests in a neutral fashion seems inadequate ... The critical political question remains: Whose interests does the evaluation serve?' (House, 1993: 10) And, we might add another question: who defines the interests and health needs of particular groups in the first place? You may recall that Chapter 15 considered some issues of practice and principle in relation to this question.

19.5 Conclusion

Views about what counts as good evaluation are likely to be closely influenced by the meaning and value we attach to health and health promotion as well as the professional culture in which we work. This brings us round full circle to the issues which were raised in the first part of this book. For instance, people who draw on a predominantly medical model of health will usually be concerned with disease reduction, risk factor analysis and regard establishing relationships of cause and effect through randomised control trials as the ideal approach to evaluation. Quantification and objectivity will be emphasised and the role of social structures minimised or completely overlooked. The reviewer of the smoking and pregnancy studies discussed earlier provides an example of this approach. You may recall the recommendation that future studies might usefully include reference to 'types' of smoker, by which is meant psychological type, but that no mention is made of social and economic circumstances, social class or family structure.

But as the opening chapters of this book sought to emphasise and explore, the medical model of health is only part of the picture. The salutogenic approach, for instance, described in Chapter 2, focuses on the dynamic relationship between people and their environment. It maintains that fostering an atmosphere of autonomy and participation is a major way of enhancing health. Being healthy depends not just on personal resources but on relationships, social support and supportive environments.

The question of how health promoting values such as participation and critical awareness can be built into the process of evaluation could usefully be placed higher on the agenda, especially by those who regard the medical model of health as insufficient. This chapter has argued that the 'high status' and apparently most rational approaches to evaluation are in many contexts not productive. It may well be that instead of devoting more time and money to such projects the way forward is to adopt a more creative approach which acknowledges the centrality of values and makes no claim to be neutral.

There is a continuing debate about 'evidence' in health promotion, particularly as the achievement of targets for Saving Lives: Our Healthier Nation and other national strategies for health promotion depend to some extent on the commissioning and implementation of effective health promotion programmes. However, 'whilst few would argue about the principle that all health promotion practice should have its basis in sound evidence, there is lively discussion about exactly what this means and what are the best ways of achieving it' (Perkins et al., 1999: 1).

People who work in the area of community development approaches to health place great emphasis on the importance of participation and working in ways which value process as much as outcome. It is in the context of community work that the importance of questions about who conducts evaluation and whose interests evaluation serves have been most directly acknowledged and addressed. (Issues relating to the community health movement and participative evaluation are explored in detail in Jones et al., 1997) Participatory methods of evaluation are regarded as valuable because they offer relatively powerless groups and individuals an opportunity to articulate and reflect on their experience, influence what happens and develop new skills, knowledge and confidence. They are, in short, actively health promoting.

McQueen (2000) argues:

> Gathering evidence for the value of health promotion remains a challenging task. However, we need to have a broad vision of evidence that embraces the inherent complexity of health promotion as a field. Also we need to understand that the knowledge of what works and is successful is embedded in a complex neural network. Rather than retreating to limited rules for what constitutes evidence, there is a need to look toward analytical frameworks that recognise the complexity of the field. It is a challenge for health promotion to convince its enthusiasts and detractors that there are no easy answers to complex human phenomena.

References

Aakster, C.W. (1993) 'Concepts in alternative medicine', in Beattie, A. *et al.* (eds) *Health and Wellbeing: A Reader*, Macmillan.

Abramson, J.H. (1990) *Survey Methods in Community Medicine*, Churchill Livingstone.

Adams, L. (1994) 'Health promotion in crisis', *Health Education Journal*, 53: 354–60

Aggleton, P., Hart, G. and Davies, P. (eds) (1991) *AIDS: Responses, Interventions and Care*, Falmer Press.

Aggleton, P., Moody, D. and Young, A. (1992) *Evaluating AIDS/HIV Health Promotion*, Health Education Authority.

Ahmad, W.I.U. (ed) (1993) *'Race' and Health in Contemporary Britain*, Open University Press.

Ajzen, I. and Fishbein, M. (1980) *Understanding Attitudes and Predicting Social Behaviour*, Prentice Hall, New Jersey.

Allen, P. (1996) 'Health promotion, enviornmental health and the local authority' in Scriven, A. and Orme, J. (eds) (1996) *Promoting Health: Professional Perspectives*, pp. 89–94, Macmillan.

Allsop, J. (1984) *Health Policy and the National Health Service*, Longman.

Amos, A. (1993) 'In her own best interests? Women and health education: a review of the last fifty years', *Health Education Journal*, 53, 3, Autumn.

Anderson, D. (1986) *A Diet of Reason*, Social Affairs Unit.

Anionwu, E. (1993) 'Genetics - A philosophy of perfection?', in Beattie, A. *et al.* (eds) *Health and Wellbeing: A Reader*, Macmillan.

Annett, H. and Rifkin, S. (1990) *Improving Urban Health*, World Health Organisation.

Antigha, A. (1994) 'Communities for better health': Proceedings of a seminar 'Building Healthy Alliances', Health Promotion Wales.

Antonovsky, A. (1987) *Unravelling the Mystery of Health: How People Manage Others and Stay Well*, Wiley, New York.

Antonovsky, A. (1993) 'The sense of coherence as a determinant of health' in Beattie, A. *et al.* (eds) *Health and Wellbeing: A Reader*, Macmillan.

Argyle, M. (1994) *The Psychology of Interpersonal Behaviour*, Penguin.

Armstrong, D. (1993) 'From clinical gaze to regime of total health', in Beattie, A. *et al.* (eds) *Health and Wellbeing: A Reader*, Macmillan.

Armstrong, D. (1995) 'The rise of surveillance medicine', *Sociology of Health and Illness*, 17, 3: 393–404.

Armstrong, D. and Hutton, P. (1992) 'A systematic model for evaluating local HIV/AIDS health promotion programmes' in Aggleton, P., Young, A., Moody, D., Kapila, M. and Pye, M. (eds) *Perspectives on the Evaluation of HIV/ AIDS Health Promotion*, Health Education Authority.

Ashton, J. and Seymour, H. (1988) *The New Public Health*, Open University Press.

Ayres, J. (1994) 'Asthma and the atmosphere', *British Medical Journal*, 309: 619–20.

Backett, K., Davison, C., Mullen, K. (1994) 'Lay evaluation of health and healthy lifestyles: evidence from three studies', *British Journal of General Practice*, 44, 277–80.

Basler, H.D., Brinkmeier, U., Buser, K. and Gluth, G. (1991) 'Nicotine gum assisted group therapy in smokers with an increased risk of coronary heart disease - evaluation in a primary care setting', *Health Education Research*, 7 (1): 87–96.

Beattie, A. (1984) 'Health education and the science teacher: invitation to a debate' *Education and Health*, January, pp. 9–15.

Beattie, A. (1990a) 'Community development for health: the British experience' in Smithies, J. and Adams, L., *Community Participation in Health Promotion*, pp. 46–60, Health Education Authority.

Beattie, A. (1990b) *A Picture of Health (For All?) – A Review of the First Cohort of Reports on Public Health*, Faculty for Public Health Medicine, London.

Beattie, A. (1990c) *Roots and Branches*, Papers from the Open University/Health Education Authority, 1990, Winter School in Community Development and Health Education. The Health Education Unit, Department of Community Education, The Open University.

Beattie, A. (1991) 'Knowledge and control in health promotion: a test case for social policy and social theory' in Gabe, J., Calnan, M. and Bury, M. (eds) *The Sociology of the Health Service*, Routledge.

Beattie, A., Gott, M., Jones, L.J. and Sidell, M. (eds) (1993) *Health and Wellbeing: A Reader*, Macmillan.

Beauchamp, T.L. and Childress, J.F. (1995) *Principles of Biomedical Ethics*, Oxford University Press.

Beck, U. (1992) *Risk Society: Towards a New Modernity*, Sage.

Becker, H. (1963) *Outsiders: Studies in the Sociology of Deviance*, The Free Press, New York.

Becker, M.H. (ed.) (1974) *The Health Belief Model and Personal Health Behaviour*, Charles B. Slack, New Jersey.

Bedell, G. (1991) 'The only right way to grieve', *Independent*, 27 October.

Bellingham, K. and Gillies, P. (1993) 'Evaluation of an AIDS education programme for young adults', *Journal of Epidemiology and Community Health*:134–8.

Bennett, N. *et al.*, quoted in Health Education Authority (1995) *Health Update 5 Physical Activity:* 10, Figure 2.2.

Bennett, P. and Hodgson, R. (1992) 'Psychology and health promotion', in Bunton, R. and Macdonald, G. (eds) *Health Promotion: disciplines and diversity*, Routledge.

Benzeval, M., Judge, K. and Whitehead, M. (1995) *Tackling Inequalities in Health: An Agenda for Action*, Kings Fund.

Berkman, L.F. and Syme, S.L. (1979) 'Social networks, host resistance and mortality: a nine year follow-up of Alameda County residents', *American Journal of Epidemiology*, 104.

Birch, S. and Stoddardt, G. (1989) 'Promoting health behaviour: the importance of economic analysis in policy formulation for AIDS prevention' in Drummond, M. and Davies, L. (eds) *AIDS: The Challenge for Economic Analysis*, pp. 53–58, The Health Services Management Centre, Birmingham.

Blackburn, C. (1994) *Poverty and Health, Working with Families*, Open University Press.

Blackburn, C. (1999) 'Poor health, poor care' in Purdy, M. and Banks, D. (eds) *Health and Exclusion : Policy and Practice in Health Provision*, Routledge.

Blaxter, M. (1983) 'The causes of disease: women talking', *Social Science and Medicine*, 17, 2: 59–69.

Blaxter, M. (1984) 'Equity and consultation rates in general practice', *British Medical Journal*, 288: 1963–7.

Blaxter, M. (1990) *Health and Lifestyles*, Tavistock.

Blaxter, M. and Paterson S. (1982) *Mothers and Daughters: A Three Generational Study of Health Attitudes and Behaviour*, Heinneman.

Blythe, M. (1986) 'A century of health education', *Health and Hygiene*, 7, 3: 105–15.

Bopp, M. (1989) 'Spiritual barriers in health promotion in family nursing assessment: meeting the challenge of health promotion' Hartrick *et al.* (1994) *Journal of Advanced Nursing* 20: 85–91.

Boseley, S. (1995) 'Nutrition specialist warns against BSE beef products' *Guardian*, G2: 16.

Bowes, A.M. and Meehan Danokos, T. (1996) 'Pakistani women and maternity care: raising muted voices', *Sociology of Health and Illness*, 18, 1: 45–65.

Bowling, A. (1991) *Measuring Health : A Review of Quality of Life Measurement Scales*, Open University Press.

Bowling, A. (1997) *Research Methods in Health: Investigating Health and Health Services*, Open University Press.

Bradford, M. and Winn, S. (1993) 'A survey of nurses' views of health promotion' *Health Education Journal*, 52, 2: 91–5.

Bradshaw, J. (1972) 'The concept of social need', *New Society*, 19; 640–3.

British Association of Counselling (1989) *Invitation to Membership*, BAC.

British Medical Journal (1996) 312: 67–68.

Brown, C. (1984) *Black and White Britain: The Third PSI Survey*, Heinemann.

Bryan, B. *et al.* (1985) *The Heart of the Race: Black Women's Lives in Britain*, Virago.

Buckman R. with Kason Y. (1992) *How to Break Bad News: A Guide for Health Care Professionals*, Macmillan.

Bunton, R. and Macdonald, G. (eds) (1992) *Health Promotion: Disciplines and Diversity*, Routledge.

Bunton, R., Baldwin, S. and Flynn, D. (1999) *The Stages of Change Model and its Use in Health Promotion: A Critical Review*, Health Education Board for Scotland.

Burrows, R., Bunton, R., Mercer, S. and Gillen, K. (1995) 'The efficacy of health promotion, health economics and late modernism', *Health Education Research*, 10 (2): 241–9.

Byrne, P.S. and Long, B.E.L. (1976) *Doctors Talking to Patients*, HMSO.

Calnan, M. (1987) *Health and Illness: The Lay Perspective*, Tavistock.

Calnan, M. (1990) 'Food and health: a comparison of beliefs and practices in middle-class and working-class households', in Cunningham-Burley, S. and McKeganey, N. (eds) *Readings in Medical Sociology*, Tavistock/Routledge.

Calnan, M. and Gabe, J. (1991) 'Recent developments in general practice: a sociological analysis' in Gabe, J. *et al.* (eds) *The Sociology of the Health Service*, Routledge.

Calnan, M. *et al.* (1994) 'Involvement of the primary health care team in coronary heart disease prevention', *British Journal of General Practice* 44: 224–8.

Campbell, D. (1997) 'World's first national health promotion web site from Scotland', *British Journal of Healthcare Computing and Information Management*, 14.

Caplan, R. (1993) 'The importance of social theory for health promotion: from description to reflexity' *Health Promotion International*, 8, 2: 147–57.

Castle, P. and Jacobson, B. (1988) 'The health of our regions: an analysis of strategies and policies of regional health authorities for promoting health and preventing disease' *A Report for the Health Education Council*, Birmingham, NHS Regions Health Promotion Group.

Catford, J.C. (1995) 'The mass media is dead, long live the multi-media', *Health Promotion International*, 10, 4: 247–51.

Catford, J.C. (1993) Editorial, *Health Promotion International* 8: 2: 67–8.

Cave, M. and Hanney, H. (1990) 'Performance indicators for higher education and research' in Cave, M., Kogan, M. and Smith, R. *Output and Performance Measurement in Government. The state of the art*, Jessica Kingsley.

Cave, M. and Kogan, M. (1990) 'Some concluding observations' in Cave, M., Kogan, M. and Smith, R.,*Output and Performance Measurement in Government. The state of the art*, pp. 179–87.

Centre for Health Promotion Studies (1999) *The National Health and Lifestyle Surveys* (SLAN/HBSC), Galway, National University of Ireland.

Chadwick, E. (1842) *Report on the Sanatory Conditions of the Labouring Population of England*, Vol. 26, HMSO.

Chapman, S. and Egger, G. (1993) 'Myth in cigarette advertising and health promotion' in Beattie, A. *et al.* (eds) (1993) *Health and Wellbeing: A Reader*, pp. 218–27, Macmillan.

Chapman, S. and Lupton, D. (1994) *The Fight for Public Health: Principles and Practice of Media Advocacy*, BMJ Publishing Group.

Chapman, S. and Lupton, D. (1995) *The Politics of Public Health*, British Medical Journal.

Cochrane, A.L. (1971) *Effectiveness and Efficiency: Random Reflections on Health Services*, Nuffield Provincial Hospitals Trust.

Coid, J. (1991) 'Interviewing the agressive patient', in Corney, R. (ed.) *Developing Communication and Counselling Skills in Medicine*, Routledge.

Coleman, A. (1992) 'Pre-retirement education and the role of the GP', in George, J. and Ebrahim, S. (eds) *Health Care for Older Women*, Oxford University Press.

Collins, T. (1993) 'Models of health: pervasive, persuasive and politically charged', *Health Promotion International*, 10, 4: 317–24.

COMA (Committee on Medical Aspects of Food Policy) (1984) *Diet and Cardiovascular Disease*, Report on Health and Social Subjects No. 28, HMSO.

Connor, S. (1993) 'The necessity of value' in Squires, J. (ed.) *Principled Positions: Postmodernism and the Rediscovery of Value*, Lawrence and Wishart.

Cooper, C. and Payne, R. (1988) *Causes, Coping and Consequences of Stress at Work*, Wiley.

Cooper, D.B. (1994) *Alcohol Home Detoxification and Assessment*, Radcliffe Medical Press.

Copenhagen, City of (1994) *Healthy City Plan 1994–97*, Copenhagen, Denmark.

Cornwell, J. (1984) *Hard Earned Lives,* Tavistock.

Coronary Prevention Group (1986) 'Coronary heart disease and Asians in Britain', Coronary Prevention Group and Confederation of Indian Organisations.

Coward, R. (1984) *Female Desire: Women's Sexuality Today,* Paladin.

Cox, B.D. *et al.* (1987) *The Health and Lifestyle Survey: preliminary report,* The Health Promotion Research Trust.

Cox, B.D. *et al.* (1993) *The Health and Lifestyle Survey: Seven Years On,* The Health Promotion Research Trust.

Crawford, R. (1977) 'You are dangerous to your health; The politics and ideology of victim blaming', *International Journal of Health Services,* 7, 4: 663–80.

Cronbach, L.J. (1982) *Designing Evaluations of Educational and Social Programs,* Jossey-Bass, San Francisco.

Currer, C. and Stacey, M. (eds) (1986) *Concepts of Health, Illness and Disease: A Comparitive Perspective,* Berg.

Dahlgren, G. and Whitehead, M. (1991) *Policies and Strategies to Promote Social Equity in Health,* Institute for Future Studies, Stockholm.

Dale, J., Shipman, C., Lacock, L., Davies, M. (1996) 'Creating a shared vision of out of hours care: using rapid appraisal methods to create an interagency, community oriented approach to service development, *British Medical Journal,* 312: 1206–10.

Dalley, G. (1988) *Ideologies of Caring: Rethinking Community and Collectivism,* Macmillan.

Davey Smith, G. (1994) 'Increasing the accessibility of data', *British Medical Journal,* 308, 1: 1519–20.

Davies, C. (1988) 'The health visitor as mother's friend: a woman's place in public health, 1900–14', *The Journal of the Society for the Social History of Medicine.*

Davis, A. and Jones, L.J. (1996) 'Health and environmental constraints: listening to children's views', *Health Education Journal,* September 1996.

Davis, H. and Fallowfield, L. (eds) (1991) *Counselling and Communication in Health Care,* Wiley.

Davison, C., Frankel, S. and Davey Smith, G. (1992) 'The limits of lifestyle: Reassessing "fatalism" in the popular culture of illness prevention', *Social Science and Medicine,* 34, 6: 675–85.

Delamothe, A. (1991) 'Social inequalities in health', *British Medical Journal,* 303: 1–9.

Department of Health (DoH) (1991) *The Patient's Charter,* HMSO.

Department of Health (DoH) (1992) *The Health of the Nation,* HMSO.

Department of Health (DoH) (1993a) *Working Together for Better Health,* HMSO.

Department of Health (DoH) (1993b) *Targeting Practice: Contribtuion of Nurses, Midwives and Health Visitors,* HMSO.

Department of Health (DoH) (1994) *Nutritional Aspects of Cardiovascular Disease: Report of the Cardiovascular Review Group Committee on Medical Aspects of Food Policy,* (Report on Health and Social Subjects 46).

Department of Health (DoH) (1995) *Variations in Health, What Can the Department of Health and the NHS do?*, Report of the Variations Sub-Group of the Chief Medical Officer's Health of the Nation Working Group, HMSO.

Department of Health (DoH) (1999) *Saving Lives: Our Healthier Nation*, London, HMSO.

Department of Health (DoH), Northern Ireland (1993) *A Health Strategy for Northern Ireland*, HMSO.

Department of Health (Republic of Ireland) (1986) *Health – the Wider Dimension: a Consultative Statement on Health Policy*, Dublin, Stationery Office.

Department of Health (Republic of Ireland) (1995) *A Health Promotion Strategy: Making the Healthier Choice the Easier Choice*, Dublin, Stationery Office.

Department of Health and Social Security (DHSS) (1976) *Prevention and Health: Everybody's Busines*, HMSO.

Department of Health and Social Security (DHSS) (1980) *The Black Report on Inequalities in Health*, HMSO.

Department of Health and Social Security (DHSS) (1986) *Primary Health Care*, HMSO.

Department of Health and Social Security (DHSS) (1987) *Promoting Better Health*, HMSO.

Dignan, M.B. and Carr, P.A. (1994) *Programme Planning for Health Education and Promotion*, Lea and Febiger, Philadelphia.

DiMatteo, M.R. and DiNicola, D.D. (1982) *Achieving Patient Compliance: The Psychology of the Medical Practitioner's Role*, Pergamon Press.

Dines, A. and Cribb, A. (1993) *Health Promotion, Concepts and Practice*, Blackwell.

Dix, (1995) 'Promotional tactics', *Health Service Journal*, 23 Nov., p. 37.

Dix, A., Finlay, J., Abowd, G. and Beale, R. (1998) *Human-Computer Interaction* (2nd edn), Prentice Hall.

Doll, R. and Hill, A.B. (1950) 'Smoking and carcinoma of the lung', prelimary report, *British Medical Journal*, ii: 739–48.

Doll, R. and Hill, A.B. (1964) 'Mortality in relation to smoking: 20 years' observations on male British doctors', *British Medical Journal*; ii: 1525–36.

Doll, R. and Peto, R. (1981) *The Causes of Cancer*, Oxford University Press.

Doll, R., Peto, R., Wheatley, K., Gray, R., Sutherland, I. (1994) 'Mortality in relation to smoking: 40 years' observations on male British doctors', *British Medical Journal*, 309: 901–11.

Dorn, N. and South, N. (1989) 'Drugs and leisure, prohibition and pleasure: from sub-culture to the drugalogue' in Rojeck, C. (ed) *Leisure for Leisure: Critical Essays*, Macmillan.

Douglas, J. (1992) 'Black women's health matters', in Roberts, H. (ed.) *Women's Health Matters*, Routledge, pp. 33–46.

Downie, R.S., Fyfe, C. and Tannahill, A. (1990) *Health Promotion: Models and Values*, Oxford Medical Publications.

Doyal, L. and Gough, I. (1991) *Towards a Theory of Human Needs*, Macmillan.

Doyal, L. with Pennell, I. (1979) *The Political Economy of Health*, Pluto Press.

Draper, P. (1983) 'Tackling the disease of ignorance', *Self-health*, 1: 23–5.

Draper, P. (ed.) *Health Through Public Policy*, Merlin Press.

Draper, P., Griffiths, J. and Popay, J. (1980) 'Three types of health education', *British Medical Journal*, 281: 493–5.

Dubos, R. (1959) *Mirage of Health*, Harper, New York.

Dudgill, L. and Springett, J. (1994) 'Evaluation of workplace health promotion: a review', *Health Education Journal*, 53, 3: 337–47.

Durant, J.R., Evans, G.A. and Thomas, G.P. (1989) 'The public understanding of science', *Nature*, 340: 11–14 .

Edwards, J. (1991) *Evaluation in Adult and Further Education*, The Workers' Educational Association.

Egan, G. (1982) *The Skilled Helper*, Brooks/Cole.

Elliot, K. (1994) 'Working with black and minority ethnic groups' in Webb, P. (ed) *Health Promotion and Patient Education*, Chapman and Hall.

Engel, G.L. (1977) 'The need for a new medical model: a challenge for biomedicine', *Science*, 196: 129–36.

Entwistle, V. (1995) 'Reporting research in medical journals and newspapers', *British Medical Journal*, 310: 920–3.

Esland, G. (1973) 'Language and social reality', E262 *Language and Learning* Block 2, The Open University.

Everitt, A. (1995) *Developing Critical Evaluation* Social Welfare Research Unit, University of Northumbria at Newcastle, unpublished paper.

Ewles, L. and Simnett, I. (1999) *Promoting Health*, 4th edn, Balliere Tindall/RCN.

Family Heart Study Group (1994) 'Randomised control trial evaluating cardiovascular screening and intervention in general practice: principal results of British family heart study', *British Medical Journal*, 308: 313–20.

Farquhar, J.W., Fortmann, S.P., Wood, P. D. and Haskell, W.L. (1983) 'Community studies of cardiovascular disease prevention', in Kapler, N.M. and Stanmer, J.(eds) *Prevention of Coronary Heart Disease: Practical management of risk factors*, W.B. Saunders & Co.

Faulkner, A. (1992) *Effective Interaction with Patients*, Churchill Livingston.

Faulkner, A. (1993) *Teaching Interactive Skills in Health Care*, Chapman Hall.

Faulkner, A. and Macleod Clark J. (1987) 'Communication skills teaching in nurse education' in Davis, B. (ed) *Nurse Education: Research and Development*, Croom Helm.

Fennell, G. and Sidell, M. (1989) 'Social factors in problem drinking', Research Report, University of East Anglia.

Feuerstein, M. (1986) *Partners in Evaluation: Evaluating Development and Community Development Programmes with Participants*, Macmillan.

Fink, A. (1993) *Evaluation Fundamentals*, Sage.

Fitzgerald, T. (1985) 'The New Right and the family', in Loney, M., Boswell, D. and Clarke, J. (eds) *Social Policy and Social Welfare*, Open University Press.

Flay, B.R. (1987) 'Evaluation of the development, dissemination and effectiveness of mass media programming', *Health Education Research*, 2: 1213–29.

Flay, B.R. *et al.* (1983) 'Cigarette smoking: why young people do it and ways of preventing it' in McGrath, P. and Firestone, P. (eds) *Pediatric and Adolescent Behavioural Medicine*, New York.

Foucault, M. (1973) The *Birth of the Clinic: An Archaelogy of Medical Perception*, Tavistock.

Frazer, W.M. (1950) *A History of English Public Health 1834–1939*, Balliere Tindall and Cox.

Freidson, E. (1975) *Profession of Medicine*, Dodd, Mead and Co., New York.

French J. and Adams, L. (1986) 'From analysis to synthesis: theories of health education', *Health Education Journal*, 45, 2: 71–4.

French, J. (1990) 'Boundaries and horizons, the role of health education within health promotion', *Health Education Journal*, 49, 1: 7–10.

French, J. and Milner, S. (1993) 'Should we accept the status quo?', *Health Education Journal*, 52: 98–101.

Fries, J.F. (1980) 'Aging, natural death and the compression of morbidity', *New England Journal of Medicine*, 303, 3: 130ff.

Gatherer, A., Parfitt, J., Porter, E. and Vessy, M. (1979) *Is Health Education Effective?* Health Education Council.

Geuss, R. (1981) *The Idea of Critical Theory: Habermas and the Frankfurt School*, Cambridge University Press.

Gilman, E.A., Cheng, K.K., Winter, H.R., Scragg, R. (1995) 'Trends in rates and seasonal distribution of sudden infant deaths in England and Wales 1988–1992', *British Medical Journal*, 310: 631–2.

Glanz, K., Lewis, F.M. and Rimer, B.K. (eds) (1990) *Health Behaviour and Health Education: Theory, Research and Practice*, Jossey-Bass, San Francisco.

Glasgow, R.E. *et al.* (1984) 'Evaluation of a worksite controlled smoking program', *Journal Clinical Psychology* 52: 137–8.

Godfrey, C. (1993) 'Is prevention better than cure?' in Drummond, D. and Maynard, A. (eds) *Purchasing and Providing Cost-Effective Health Care*, Churchill Livingstone.

Godfrey, C. and Tolley, K. (1992) 'An economic approach to the evaluation of HIV/AIDS health education programmes' in Aggleton, P., Young, A., Moody, D., Kapila, M. and Pye, M. (eds) *Does it Work? Perspectives on the Evaluation of HIV/AIDS Health Promotion*, pp. 115–39, HEA.

Gott, M. and O'Brien, M. (1990) *The Role of the Nurse in Health Promotion: Policies, Perspectives and Practice.* Report of a two year research project funded by the Department of Health, The Open University.

Graham, A. (1994) *Teach Yourself Statistics*, Hodder.

Graham, H. (1984) *Women, Health and the Family*, Health Education Council/ Wheatsheaf.

Graham, H. (1986) *Caring for the Family*, Research Report No. 1, Health Education Council.

Graham, H. (1988) 'Women and smoking in the United Kingdom: implications for health promotion', *Health Promotion*, 3, 4: 371–82.

Graham, H. (1993) *Hardship and Health in Women's Lives*, Wheatsheaf.

Graham, H. and Blackburn, C. (1993) *Poverty and Health: Tools for Change*, Public Health Alliance.

Green, C. (1992) 'Liverpool' in Ashton, J. (ed.) *Healthy Cities*, Open University Press.

Green, L.W. and Lewis, F.M. (1986) *Measurement and Evaluation in Health Education and Health Promotion*, Mayfield Publishing Co., Palo Alto, California.

Gudex, C. (1986) *'QALYS' and their Use by the Health Service: A Discussion Paper*, University of York Centre for Health Economics: 14.

Habemas, J. (1984) *The Theory of Communicative Action*, Vol. 1 'Reason and the rationalization of society', Heinemann.

Hancock, T. (1998) 'Caveat partner: reflections on partnership with the private sector', *Health Promotion International*, 13, 3: 193–5.

Hannay, D.R. (1979) *The Sypmtom Iceberg: A Study of Community Health,* Routledge and Kegan Paul.

Haralambos, M. and Holborn, M. (1995) *Sociology Themes and Perspectives,* Harper Collins.

Hardey, M. (1998) 'Doctor in the home: the Internet as a source of lay health knowledge and the challenge to expertise', *Sociology of Health and Illness.*

Harrison, S. and Ashcroft, M. (1994) 'Health Promoting Hospitals' in *Health Service Journal.*

Hastings, G. and Haywood, A. (1991) 'Social marketing and communication in health promotion', *Health Promotion International,* 6, 2: 135–45.

Hawe, P. (1994) 'Capturing the meaning of 'community' in community intervention evaluation', *Health Promotion International,* 9, 3: 199–209.

Hawe, P., Degeling, D. and Hall, J. (1995) *Evaluating Health Promotion: a Health Worker's Guide,* Sydney, MacLennan and Petty.

Hawe, P. and Shiell, A. (2000) *Social Capital and Health Promotion: A Review,* Social Science and Medicine accessed at URL: http://www.msocmrc.gla.a-c.uk/SocialScienceMedicine/WorkshopF/SOCCAPHP.pdf [24 August 2000]

Hawton, M., Percy-Smith, J. and Hughes, G. (1994) *Community Profiling: Auditing Social Needs,* Open University Press.

Haycox, A. (1994) 'A methodology for estimating the costs and benefits of health promotion, *Health Promotion International,* 9, 1: 5–11.

Health Education Authority (HEA) (1989a) *Health for Life: The Health Education Authority Primary School Project,* Nelson.

Health Education Authority (HEA) (1989b) *Exploring Health Education,* HEA.

Health Education Authority (HEA) (1991, revised 1995) *Health Update 2: Smoking,* Figure 12, HEA.

Health Education Authority (HEA) (1992) *Tomorrow's Young Adults,* HEA.

Health Education Authority (HEA) (1993a) Certificate in Health Education Open Learning Resources: *Contemporary Issues in Health Promotion,* p. 29, HEA.

Health Education Authority (HEA) (1993b) *Peers in Partnership: HIV/AIDS Education with Young People in the Community,* Health Education Authority.

Health Education Authority (HEA) (1994a) Evidence from the national cot death campaign; personal communication.

Health Education Authority (HEA) (1994b) *Health Update 1: Coronary Heart Disease,* p. 7, HEA.

Health Education Authority (HEA) (1994c) *Health Update 4: Sexual Health,* p. 8, HEA.

Health Education Authority (HEA) (1994d) *Smoking and Pregnancy,* HEA.

Health Education Authority (HEA) (1995a) *A Survey of the UK Population Part 1: Health and Lifestyles,* HEA.

Health Education Authority (HEA) (1995b) *Health and Lifestyles in the UK,* HEA.

Health Education Authority (HEA) (1995c) *Health and Lifestyles: A Survey of the UK Population,* HEA.

Health Education Authority (HEA) (1995d) Pertussis notifications and immunisation (personal communication).

Health Education Board for Scotland (HEBS) (1992) Strategic Plan: a consultation document, HEBS.

Health Education Board for Scotland (HEBS) (1999) Review of research literature on ICT in health promotion, HEBS.

Health Education Council (HEC) (1968) *Annual Report*, HEC.

Health Education Council (HEC) (1971) Annual Report 1970/71, Health Education Council.

Health Education Council (HEC) (1978) *Look After Yourself* Campaign, HEC.

Health Education Council (HEC) (1983) *My Body*, Heinnemann Education.

Health Promotion Agency for Northern Ireland (HPANI) (1992) *A Health Promotion Strategy for Northern Ireland*, HPANI.

Health Promotion Wales (HPW) (1990) *A Health Promotion Strategy for Wales*, HPW.

Health Promotion Wales (1994) *The Health Promoting School in Wales*, Curriculum Council for Wales.

Heath C. (1986) 'Participation in the medical consultation', *Sociology of Health and Illness*, 6, 3: 311–38.

Heather, N. (1991) 'Foreword' in Robinson, R., Rollnick, S. and MacEwan, I. (eds) *Counselling Problem Drinkers*, Tavistock/Routledge.

Helman, C. (1986) 'Feed a cold, starve a fever: folk models of infection in an English suburban community, and their relation to medical treatment', in Currer, C. and Stacey, M. (eds) *Concepts of Health, Illness and Disease*, Berg.

Helman, C. (1990) *Culture, Health and Illness*, Wright.

Hensey, B. (1998) *The Health Services of Ireland*, Dublin.

Herbst, A.L. and Scully, R.E. (1980) 'Adenocarcinoma of the vagina in adolescence: a report of seven cases including six clear-cell carcinomas (so-called mesonephromas)', *Cancer* 25: 754–7.

Herbst, A.L., Ulfelder, H. and Poskanzer, D.C. (1971) 'Adenosarcoma of the vagina associated with maternal stilboestrol therapy with tumor appearance in young women', *New England Journal of Medicine*, 284: 878–81.

Herzlich, C. (1973) *Health and Illness*, Academic Press.

Hiley, C.M.H. and Morley, C.J. (1994) 'Evaluation of government's campaing to reduce risk of cot death', *British Medical Journal*, 309: 703–4.

Hill, F. (1993) 'HIV/AIDS education in six colleges. Report to the Health Education Authority, *HIV/AIDS and Sexual Health Programme Paper 14*, Health Education Authority.

Hirayama, T., Waterhouse, J.H. and Fraumeni, J.F. (1980) *Cancer Risk by Site, UICC Technical Report Series*, Geneva No. 41.

Hirst, M. (1995) 'Variations in practice nursing: implications for family health services', *Health and Social Care*, 3: 83–97.

Hochschild, A.R. (1983) *The Managed Heart: Commercialisation of Human Feeling*, University of California Press, Berkeley.

Hopson, B. and Scally, M. (1980) *Lifeskills Teaching Programme No. 1*, Lifeskills Associates, Leeds.

House, E.R. (1993) *Professional Evaluation: Social Impact and Political Consequences*, Sage.

Howlett, B., Ahmad, W.I.U. and Murray, R. (1991) 'An examination of Asian and Afro-Caribbean people's concepts of health and illness causation', paper presented at the *Annual Conference of the British Sociological Association*, Manchester, 25–28 March.

Hubley, J. (1993) *Communicating Health: An action guide to health education and health promotion*, Macmillan.

Hunt, S.M., McEwen, J. and McKenna, S.P. (1986) *Measuring Health Status*, Croom Helm.

Illich, I. (1976) *Limits to Medicine: The Expropriation of Health*, Marion Boyars (Penguin edition 1977).

Illsley, R. (1986) 'Occupational class, selection and the production of inequalities in health', *Quarterly Journal of Social Affairs*, 2, 2: 151–65.

Independent (1995) 'Food giant may sue BBC in beef scare', *Independent*, 7th December 1995.

Independent (1995) 'To beef or not to beef', *Independent*, 6th December 1995.

Independent (1995) 'Why we should all give up beef', *Independent*, 7th December 1995.

Inman, C.E. (1996) 'Analysed interaction', in Smith J.P. (ed) *Nursing Care of Children*, Blackwell Science.

Jacobson, B., Smith, A. and Whitehead, M. (eds) (1988) *The Nation's Health*, King Edward's Hospital Fund for London.

Jones, L.J. (1994) *The Social Context of Health and Health Care*, Macmillan.

Jones, L.J. (1995) 'Business interests and public policy making' in Jones, H. and Lansley, J. (eds) *Social Policy and the City*, Avebury.

Jones, L.J. and Bloomfield, J. (1996) 'Promoting health through social services' in Scriven, A. and Orme, J. (eds) (1996) *Health Promotion: Professional Perspectives*, pp. 95–105, Macmillan.

Jones, L.J. and Davies, A. (1996) 'Transport and the Health of Urban Children', unpublished research report.

Jones, L.J. and Rose, W. (2001) 'Promoting health through social services' in Scriven, A. and Orme, J. (eds) *Health Promotion: Professional Perspectives* (2nd edn), Macmillan.

Jones, L.J. and Sidell, M. (1997) *The Challenge of Promoting Health: Exploration and Action*, Macmillan.

Jones, R. (1997) 'A flavour of health computing in Scotland', *British Journal of Healthcare Computing and Information Management*, 14.

Joos, S.K. and Hickam, D.H. (1990) *How Health Professionals Influence Health Behavior: Patient-Provider Interaction and Health Care Outcomes*, in Glanz, K. et al. (1990) *Health Behaviour and Health Education: Theory, Research and Practice*, Jossey-Bass, San Francisco: 216–41.

Jorgensen, D. (1989) *Participant Observation: A methodology for human studies*, Sage.

Junker, B. (1960) *Fieldwork*, University of Chicage Press.

Kalpan, A. (ed) (1992) *Health Promotion and Chronic Illness*, WHO.

Kaur, J. and Bedford, J. (n.d.) *Asian Women and Diabetes: an evaluation report of a community based initiative*, Wolverhampton Asian Women and Diabetes Forum.

Kelly, M. and Charlton, B. (1995) 'The modern and the post modern in health promotion' in Bunton, R., Nettleton, S. and Burrows, R. (eds) *The Sociology of Health Promotion*, pp. 78–90, Routledge.

Kolasa, K.M. and Miller, M.G. (1996) 'New developments in nutrition education using computer technology', *Journal of Nutritional Education*, 28, 1: 7–14.

Kotler, P. (1975) *Marketing for Non-Profit Organisations*, Prentice Hall.

Lalonde, M. (1974) *A New Perspective on the Health of Canadians*, Ministry of Supply and Services, Ottawa.

Lambert, H. and McPherson, K. (1993) 'Disease prevention and health promotion', in *Dilemmas in Health Care*, Book 8, U205 Health and Disease series, The Open University.

Leathar, D.S. (1987) 'The development and assessment of mass media campaigns: the work of the advertising research unit: Part 1-Perspectives', *The Journal of the Institute of Health Education*, 25: 125–31.

Lefebvre, C. (1992) 'Social marketing and health promotion' in Bunton, R. and Macdonald, G., *Health Promotion, Disciplines and Diversity*, Routledge.

Leonard, J. (1995) *Interacting: Multi-media and Health*, Health Education Authority.

Lewis, J. (1980) *The Politics of Motherhood*, Croom Helm.

Ley, P. (1983) 'Patients' understanding and recall in clinical communication failure' in Pendeton, D. and Hasler, J. (eds) *Doctor-Patient Communication*, Academic Press.

Ley, P. (1986) 'Cognitive cariables and noncompliance', *Journal of Compliance in Health Care*, 1986, 1: 171–88.

Liverpool, City of (1988) *Liverpool Healthy Cities Conference Declaration*, City of Liverpool.

Lupton, D. and Chapman, S. (1991) 'A healthy lifestyle might be the death of you; discourse on diet, cholesterol control and heart disease in the press and among the lay public' *Sociology of Health and Illness*, 17, 4: 477–94.

Mackenbach, J.P. (1995) 'Tackling inequalities in health', *British Medical Journal*; 310: 1152–3.

Macleod Clark, J. (1981) 'Communication in nursing' *Nursing Times*, 1 Jan: 12–18.

Macleod Clark, J. (1993) 'From sick nursing to health nursing: evolution or revolution?' in Wilson-Barnett, J. and Macleod-Clark, J. (eds) *Research in Health Promotion and Nursing*, pp. 256–70, Macmillan.

Macleod Clark, J., Kendall, S. and Haverty, S. (1992) 'Effective use of health education skills' in Horne, E. and Cowen, T. (eds) *Effective Communication – Some Nursing Perspectives*, Wolfe.

McCluskey, D (1989) *Health: People's Beliefs and Practices*, Dublin: Stationery Office.

McQueen, D. (2000) 'Perspectives on health promotion: theory, evidence, practice and the emergence of complexity', *Health Promotion International*, 15, 2: 95–7.

Madaus, G., Scriven, M. and Stufflebeam, D. (eds) (1983) *Evaluation Models*, Kluwer-Nijhof Publishing.

Maguire, P. (1993) Audio Cassette 3, K260 *Death and Dying*, The Open University.

Mahoney, C.A., Thombs, D.L. and Howe, C.Z. (1995) 'The art and science of scale development in health education research' in *Health Education Research*, 10, 1: 1–10.

Majeed, F.A., Cook, D.J., Poloniecki, J., Griffiths, J. and Stones, C. (1995) 'Sociodemographic variables for general practices: use of census data', *British Medical Journal*, 310: 1373–4.

Marks, L. (1988) *Promoting Better Health? An Analysis of the Government's Programme for Improving Primary Care*, Briefing Paper 7, King's Fund Institute.

Marmot, K.G. and McDowall, M.E. (1986) 'Mortality decline and widening social inequalities', *Lancet*, 2 August, p. 274.

Marmot, M.G., Syme, S.L., Kagan, A., Kato, H., Cohen, J.B., Belsky, J. (1975) 'Epidemiologic studies of coronary heart disease and stroke in Japanese men living in Japan, Hawaii and California: prevalence of coronary and hypertensive heart disease and associated risk factors', *American Journal of Epidemiology*, 102: 514–25.

Marsh, A. and McKay, S. (1994) *Poor Smokers*, London, Policy Studies Institute.

Martin, C.J., Platt, S.D. and Hunt, S.M. (1987) 'Housing conditions and ill health', *British Medical Journal*, 294: 1125–27.

Matthews, J.J. (1983) 'The communication process in clinical settings', *Social Science and Medicine*, 17, 18: 1371–8.

Maxwell, R.J. (1984) 'Quality assessment in health care', *British Medical Journal*, 288: 166–203.

Mayall, B. (1996) *Children, Health and the Social Order*, Open University Press.

McBride, H.M. (1983) *Tracing the Origins of Health Education*, South Bank Polytechnic.

McCarthy, M. (1982) *Epidemiology and Policies for Health Planning*, King Edwards Hospital Fund for London.

McCron, R. and Budd, J. (1981) 'The role of mass media in health education: an analysis', in Meyer, M. (ed.), *Health Education by Television and Radio*, Saur, Munich.

McKeown, T. (1976) *The Role of Medicine: Dream, Mirage or Nemesis*, Nuffield Provincial Hospitals Trust.

McKie, L. (1995) 'The art of surveillance or reasonable prevention: the case of cervical screening', *Sociology of Health and Illness*, 17, 4: 441–57.

McKinlay, J.B. (1979) 'A case for refocusing upstream: the political economy of illness', in Jaco, E.G. (ed.) *Patients, Physicians and Illness*, Free Press.

McKinlay, J.B. (1984) *Issues in the Political Economy of Health Care*, Tavistock.

McLeod, J. (1993) *An Introduction to Counselling*, Open University Press.

McLeod, J. (1994) *Doing Counselling Research*, Sage.

Medawar, P. (1984) *The Limits of Science*, Oxford University Press.

Medical Officer of Health (1896) *Annual Report for the City of Birminham*.

Mendelsohn, H. (1968) 'Which shall it be: mass education or mass persausion for health?', *American Journal of Public Health*, 58: 131–7.

Milburn, K. (1995) 'Critical review of peer education with young people with special reference to sexual health', *Health Education Research*, 10, 4: 407–20.

Mills, C.W. (1992) 'Language, logic and culture' in *Language in Education: A Source Book*, Routledge and Kegan Paul/Open University Press.

Milz, H. (1992) 'Healthy ill people: social cynicism or new perspectives?' in Kaplan, A. (ed.) *Health Promotion and Chronic Illness*, WHO.

Moore, J. (1989) 'The end of the line for poverty', speech delivered by the Secretary of State for Social Security, 11 May, DHSS.

Morgan, M., Calnan, M. and Manning, N. (1985) *Sociological Approaches to Health and Medicine*, Routledge.

MORI (1995) *Men's Health*, 95 Southwark Street, London SE1 OHX.

Murray, R.B. and Zentner, J.P. (1985) *Nursing Concepts for Health Promotion*, Prentice Hall, New York.

Naidoo, J. (1986) 'Limits to individualism' in Rodmell, S. and Watt, A. (eds) *The Politics of Health Education*, Routledge and Kegan Paul.

Naidoo, J. and Wills, J. (1994) *Health Promotion: Foundations for Practice*, Bailliere Tindall.

Naidoo, J. and Wills, J. (2000) *Health Promotion: Foundations for Practice*, (2nd edn), Balliere Tindall.

National Advisory Committee on Nutritional Education (NACNE) (1983) *Nutritional Guidelines for Health Education in Britain*, Health Education Council.

Nazroo, J.Y. (1997) *The Health of Britain's Ethnic Minorities: Findings from a national survey*, Policy Studies Institute.

Neaton, J.D., Broste, S., Cohen, L., Fishman, E.L., Kjelsberg, M., Schoenberger, J., (1981) 'The Multiple Risk Factor Intervention Trial (MRFIT). A comparison of risk factor changes between two study groups', *Preventative Medicine,*10: 519–43.

Nettleton, S. and Bunton, R. (1995) 'Sociological critiques of health promotion' in Bunton, R., Nettleton, S. and Burrows, R. (eds) *The Sociology of Health Promotion*, pp. 78–90, Routledge.

Nettleton, S. and Burrows, R. (1997) 'If health promotion is everybody's business what is the role of the Health Promotion Specialist within the NHS?' in *The Sociology of Health and Illness*, in press.

Nutbeam, D. (1992) 'The health promoting school: closing the gap between theory and practice', *Health Promotion International*, 7, 3.

Nutbeam, D. and Harris, E. (1995) 'Creating supportive environments for health', *Health Promotion International*, 10, 1: 51–9.

Nutbeam, D. and Harris, E. (1998) *Theory in a Nutshell: A Practitioner's Guide to Commonly Used Theories and Models in Health Promotion*, Sydney, National Centre for Health Promotion.

Nutbeam, D., Clarkson, J., Philips, K., *et al.* (1987) 'The health promoting school: organisation and policy development in Welsh secondary schools' *Health Education Journal* 46: 109–15.

Nutbeam, D., Smith, C. and Catford, J. (1990) 'Evaluation in health education: a review of progress, possibilities and problems' *Journal of Epidemiology and Community Health*, 44: 83–9.

O'Brien, M. (1995) 'Health and lifestyles: a critical mess? Notes on the dedifferentiation of health' in Bunton, R., Nettleton, S. and Burrows, R. (eds) *The Sociology of Health Promotion*, pp.78–90, Routledge.

Oakley, A.G., Bendelow, J., Barnes, M., Buchanan, O., Hussain, A.N. (1995) 'Health and cancer prevention: knowledge and beliefs of children and young people' *British Medical Journal*, 310: 1029-33.

Office for Public Management (1992) Health For All Evaluation Conference, Office for Public Management, London.

Office of Health Economics (1994) 'Health information and the consumer', No. 30, May 1994.

Oliver, M. (1993) 'Redefining disabiity', in Swain, J., Finkelstein, V., French, S. and Oliver, M. (eds) *Disability Barriers – enabling environments*, Sage/Open University.

Ong, B.N. and Humphris, G. (1994) in Popay, J. and Williams, G. (eds) *Researching the People's Health*, Routledge.

Open University (1992) *K258 Health and Wellbeing*, The Open University.

Open University (1998) D820 *The Challenge of the Social Sciences*, 'Issues in social research' Part 2, The Open University.

Parish, R. (1995) 'Health promotion: rhetoric and reality' in Bunton, R., Nettleton, S. and Burrows, R. (eds) *The Sociology of Health Promotion*, Routledge: 13–23.

Parlett, M. (1982) 'The new evaluation', in McCormick, R. (ed.) *Calling Education to Account*, Heinemann.

Parton, N. (1994) 'The nature of social work under conditions of (post) modernity', *Social Work and Social Sciences Review* 5 (2) 93–112.

Pattison, S. and Player, D. (1991) 'Health education: the political tensions' in Doxiadis, S. (ed.) *Ethical Issues in Health Education*, John Wiley.

Patton, M.Q. (1981) *Creative Evaluation*, Sage.

Pearson, M. (1986) 'Racist notions of ethnicity and culture in health education' in Rodmell, S. and Watt, A. (eds) *The Politics of Health Education: Raising the Issues*, Routledge and Kegan Paul.

Peberdy, A. (1993) 'Observing', in Shakespeare, P., Atkinson, D. and French, S. (eds) *Reflecting on Research Practice*, Open University Press.

Percy-Smith, J. and Sanderson, I. (1992) *Understanding Local Needs*, Policy Studies Institute.

Perkins, E.R., Simnett, I. and Wright, L. (1999) 'Creative tensions in Evidence-based Practice' in Perkins, E.R., Simnett, I. and Wright, L. *Evidence-Based Health Promotion*, Chichester: John Wiley & Sons.

Peto, R. (1994) 'Smoking and death: the past 40 years and the next 40' *British Medical Journal*, 309: 937–9.

PHA (Public Health Alliance and Radical Statistics of Health Group) (1992) *The Health of the Nation: are we on target?* PHA, Birmingham.

Pharoah, C. and Redmond, E. (1991) 'Care for ethnic elders', *Health Service Journal*, 16 May: 20–22.

Philips, C., Palfrey, C. and Thomas, P. (1994) *Evaluating Health and Social Care*, Macmillan.

Phillips, A. and Rakusen, J. (1978) *Our Bodies Ourselves*, Penguin.

Pill, R. (1990) 'Change and stability in health behaviour: a five year follow up study of working-class mothers' in The Health Promotion Trust *Lifestyle, Health and Health Promotion*, Proceedings of a Symposium, Chapter 5: 63–79, Health Promotion Research Trust, Cambridge.

Pill, R. and Parry (1989) 'Making changes - women, food and families', *Health Education Journal* 48: 51–4.

Pill, R. and Stott, N.C.H. (1982) 'Concepts of illness causation and responisbility: some preliminary data from a sample of working-class mothers' *Social Science and Medicine*, 16, 1: 43–52.

Pill, R. and Stott, N.C.H. (1985) 'Choice or chance: further evidence on ideas of illness causation and responsibility for health', *Social Science and Medicine*, 20, 10: 981–91.

Pill, R. and Stott, N.C.H. (1986) 'Looking after themselves: health protective behaviour among British working-class women', *Health Education Research*, 1: 111–19.

Popay J. and Williams, G. (eds) (1994) *Researching the People's Health;* Routledge.

Price, H. and Pry, J. (1995) *Helping People Change: Evaluating the Training Cascade*, Health Education Authority.

Prochaska, J. and DiClemente, C. (1984) *The Transtheoretical Approach: Crossing Traditional Boundaries of Therapy*, Daw-Jones Irwin.

Puska, P., Tuomilehto, J., Nissinen, A. *et al.* (1989) 'The North Karelia Project: 15 years of community-based prevention of coronary heart disease', *Annals of Medicine*, 21: 169–73.

Putnam, R.D. (1995) 'Bowling alone: America's declining social capital', *Journal of Democracy*, 6: 65–78.

Radley, A. and Billing, M. (1996) 'Accounts of health and illness: dilemmas and representations', *Sociology of Health and Illness*, 18, 2: 220–40.

Raleigh, V.S. and Balarajan, R. (1994) 'Public health and the 1991 census' *British Medical Journal*, 309: 287–8.

Rampling, A. (1996) 'Raw milk cheeses and salmonella' *British Medical Journal*, 312, 1: 67–8.

Rawson, D. (1992) 'The growth of health promotion theory and its rational reconstruction: lessons from the philosophy of science' in Bunton, R. and Macdonald, G. (eds) *Health Promotion: Disciples and Diversity*, Routledge.

Rawson, D. and Grigg, S. (1988) 'Health Education models and practice', *Health Education Journal* 47: 1.

Redelmeier, D.A., Molin, J.P., Tibshirani, R.J. (1995) 'A randomised trial of compassional care for the homeless in an emergency department', *Lancet* 345: 1131–4.

Redman, S., Spencer, E.A. and Sanson-Fisher, R.W. (1990) 'The role of the mass media in changing health-related behaviour: a critical appraisal of two models', *Health Promotion International*, 5, 1: 85–101.

Rennie, D. and Toukmanian, S. (1992) 'Explanation in psychotherapy process research' in Toukmanian, S. and Rennie, D. (eds) *Psychotherapy Process Research*, pp. 234–51, Sage.

Ribeaux, S. and Poppleton, S.E. (1978) *Psychology and Work: An Introduction*, Macmillan.

Roberts, H., Smith, S.J. and Bryce, C. (1995) *Children at Risk? Safety as a Social Value*, Open University Press.

Robertson, L., Kelley, A., O'Neill, H., Wixom, C., Eiswerth, R., Haddon, W. (1974) 'Controlled study of the use of television messages on safety belt use', *American Journal of Public Health* 64: 1071–80.

Rodmell, S. and Watt, A. (eds) (1986) *The Politics of Health Education*, Routledge and Kegan Paul.

Rogers, A., Pilgrim, D. and Lacey, R. (1993) *Experiencing Psychiatry*, Macmillan/MIND.

Rose, G. (1981) 'Strategy of prevention: lessons from cardiovascular disease', *British Medical Journal*, 6: 1847.

Rose, G. and Marmot, M.G. (1981) 'Social class and coronary heart disease', *British Heart Journal*, 45: 13–19.

Rotter, J.B. (1966) 'Generalised expectancies for internal versus external control reinforcement' *Psychological Monographs*, 80, 1.

Rovira, J. (1990) 'Economic aspects of AIDS' in Schwefel, D., Lendl, R., Rovira, J. and Drummond, M.F. (eds) *Economic Aspects of AIDS and HIV Infection*, Springer-Verlag.

Rowe, K. and Macleod Clark, J. (1993) 'Evaluating the effectiveness of coronary care nurses' role in smoking cessation' in Wilson-Barnett, J. and Macleod Clark, J. (eds) *Research in Health Promotion and Nursing*, pp. 197–203, Macmillan.

Sackett, D.L., Rosenberg, W.M., Muir, J.A., Gray, R.B., Haynes, W., Scott Richardson (1996) 'Evidence-based medicine: what it is and what it isn't', *British Medical Journal*, 312: 71–2.

Saltonstall, R. (1993) 'Healthy bodies, social bodies', in *Social Science and Medicine*, 36 (1): 7–14.

Sanders, D. *et al.* (1989) 'Randomised control trial of anti-smoking advice by nurses in general practice' *Journal Royal College of General Practitioners* 39: 273–6.

Schon, D. (1983) *The Reflective Practitioner* Jossey Bass, New Jersey.

Scott, D. and Weston, R. (1998) *Evaluating Health Promotion*, Stanley Thorne

Scott-Samuel (1992) 'Still got a long way to go: An international perspective' in PHA, *The Health of the Nation: Are We On Target?* PHA, pp. 7–18.

Scottish Office (1992) *Scotland's Health: A Challenge to Us All*, HMSO.

Scottish Office (1999) *Towards a Healthier Scotland: a White Paper on Health*, Edinburgh, HMSO.

Scriven, A. and Orme, J. (eds) (1996) *Health Promotion: Professional Perspectives*, Macmillan.

Secker, J., Wimbush, E., Watson, J. and Milburn, K. (1995) 'Qualitative methods in health promotion research: some criteria for quality' *Health Education Journal* 54: 78–87.

Seedhouse D. (1986) *Health: The Foundations for Achievement*, Wiley.

Seedhouse, D. (1988) *Ethics: The Heart of Health Care*, Wiley.

Seedhouse, D. (1996) *Health Promotion: Theory and Practice*, Wiley.

Seedhouse, D. (1997) *Health Promotion: Philosophy, Prejudice and Practice*, John Wiley and Sons.

Segal, J. (1991) 'Counselling people with multiple sclerosis and their families', in Davis, H. and Fallowfield, L. (eds) *Counselling and Communication in Health Care*, Wiley.

Shaper A.G., Pocock, S. J. *et al.* (1985) 'Risk factors for ischaemic heart disease: the prospective phase of the British regional heart study', *Journal of Epidemiology and Community Health*, 39: 197–209.

Shaw, M., Dorling, D., Gordon, D. and Davey Smith, G. (1999) *The Widening Gap: Health Inequalities and Policy in Britain*, The Policy Press.

Shiroyama, C., McKee, L. and McKie, L. (1995) 'Evaluating health promotion projects in primary care: recent experiences in Scotland' in *Health Education Journal* 34: 220–40.

Shrinkfield, A. (1983) 'Designing evaluations of educational and social progress by Lee. J. Cronbach: A Synopsis' in Madaus, G. *et al.* (op cit.) pp. 357–79.

Sichel, J. (1982) *Program Evaluation Guidelines*, Human Sciences Press, New York.

Sidell, M. (1985) 'A survey of Norwich well woman clinic', unpublished research report.

Sidell, M. (1995) *Health in Old Age: Myth, Mystery and Management*, Open University Press.

Silverman, D. (1987) *Communication and Medical Practice: Social Relations in the Clinic*, Sage.

Smaje, C, (1995) *Health, 'Race' and Ethnicity: Making sense of the evidence*, Kings Fund.

Smaje, C. (1996) 'The ethnic patterning of health: new directions for theory and research', *Sociology of Health and Illness*, 18, 2: 139–71.

Smith, G. and Cantley, C. (1984) 'Pluralistic evaluation' in Lishman, J. (ed) *Evaluation*, Aberdeen University Research Highlights No. 8.

Smith, J.K. and Heshusius, L. (1986) 'Closing down the conversation: the end of the qualitative-quantitative debate among educational researchers' *Educational Researcher*, 15: 4–12.

Smithies, J. and Adams, L. (1990) *Community Participation in Health Promotion*, HEA.

Smithies, J. and Webster, G. (1998) *Community Involvement in Health: from Passive Recipients to Active Participants*, Ashgate.

Society of Health Education and Promotion Specialists (SHEPS) (1993a) *Health Promotion at the Crossroads: a study of health promotion departments in the reorganized NHS*, SHEPS, London.

Society of Health Education and Promotion Specialists (SHEPS) (1993b) *Code of Practice*, SHEPS, London.

Speller, V., Learmonth, A. and Harrison, D. (1997) 'The search for evidence of effective health promotion', *British Medical Journal*, 315: 361–3.

Speller, V., Rogers, L. and Rushmore, A. (1998) 'Quality assessment in health promotion settings' in Davies, J.K. and MacDonald, G. *Quality Evidence and Effectiveness in Health Promotion*, Routledge.

Spratley, J. (1982) *Corby Healthy Choices Programme: A Report of an Evaluation*, CEREG paper 8, Centre for Continuing Education, The Open University.

Spratley, J. (1989) *Disease Prevention and Health Promotion in Primary Health Care, Team Workshops: an evaluation report*, HEA.

Springett, J. and Dugdill, L. (1995) 'Workplace health promotion programmes: towards a framework for evaluation', *Health Education Journal* 54: 88–98.

Stacey, M. (1994) 'The power of lay knowledge: a personal view' in Popay, J. and Williams, G. (eds) *Researching the People's Health*, Routledge.

Stainton Rogers, W. (1991) *Explaining Health and Illness: An Exploration of Diversity*, Harvester Wheatsheaf.

Stainton Rogers, W. (1993) 'From psychometric scales to cultural perspectives', in Beattie, A. *et al.* (eds) *Health and Wellbeing: A Reader*, Macmillan.

Stimson, G. and Webb, B. (1975) *Going to See the Doctor*, Routledge and Kegan Paul.

Sutherland, I. (1987) *Health Education: Half a Policy*, Allen and Unwin.

Sutton, S., Hallett, R. (1988) 'Smoking intervention in the workplace using videotapes and nicotine chewing gum' *Preventative Medicine*, 17: 48–59.

Sykes, W., Collins, M., Hunter, D., Popay, J and Williams, G. (1992) *Listening to Local Voices*, Nuffield Institute for Health, Salford Public Health Research and Resource Centre.

Tannahill, A. (1985) 'What is Health Promotion?' *Health Education Journal*, 44: 167–8.

Tannahill, A. (1990) 'Health education and health promotion: planning for the 1990s', *Health Education Journal* 49, 4: 194–8.

Tannahill, A. (1994) *Health Education and Health Promotion: From Priorities to Programmes*, Health Education Board for Scotland.

Tesh, S.N. (1988) *Hidden Arguments: Political Ideology and Disease Prevention Policy*, Rutgers University Press.

Thompson, J. (1992) 'Program evaluation within a health promotion frame-work', *Canadian Journal of Public Health* Supp.1.

Thorogood, M. and Coombes, Y. (2000) *Evaluating Health Promotion: Practice and Methods*, Oxford University Press.

Thorpe, M. (1988) *Evaluating Open and Distance Learning*, Longman.

Thunhurst, C. (1985) 'The analysis of small areas samples and planning for health', *Statistician*, 34: 93–106.

Tones, B.K. (1981) 'Health education: prevention or subversion', *Royal Society of Health Journal*, 101: 114–7.

Tones, B.K. (1983) 'Education and health promotion: new directions', *Journal of the Institute of Health Education*, 21: 121–3.

Tones, B.K. (1985) 'Health promotion - a new panacea?', *Journal of the Institute of Health Education*, 23, 1:. 16–21.

Tones, B.K. (1988) 'Devising strategies for preventing drug misuse: the role of the health action model' *Health Education Research*, 2, 4: 305–17.

Tones, B.K. (1995a) 'Making a change for the better', *Healthlines* November, 27: 17–19.

Tones, B.K. (1995b) 'Health education as empowerment', *Health Promotion Today*, HEA: 38–69.

Tones, B.K. (1996) 'The anatomy and ideology of health promotion: empowerment in context' in Scriven, A. and Orme, J. (eds) *Health Promotion: Professional Perspectives*, pp. 9–21, Macmillan.

Tones, B.K. and Tilford, S. (1994) *Health Education: Effectiveness, Efficiency and Equity*, Chapman Hall.

Towner, E., Dowsell, T. and Jarvis, S. (1993) *Reducing Childhood Accidents. The Effectiveness of Health Promotion Interventions: A Literature Review*, HEA.

Townsend, J., Roderick, P. and Cooper, J. (1994) 'Cigarette smoking by socio-economic group, sex and age: effects of price, income and health publicity', *British Medical Journal*, 309: 923–7.

Townsend, P. (1979) *Poverty in the United Kingdom*, Penguin.

Townsend, P., and Davidson, N. (1982) *Inequalities in Health: The Black Report*, Penguin.

Townsend, P., Davidson, N. and Whitehead, M. (1988) *Inequalities in Health: The Black Report and The Health Divide*, Penguin.

Townsend, P., Phillimore, P. and Beattie, A. (1987) *Health and Deprivation: Inequality and the North*, Croom Helm.

Tsouros, A., Dowding, G., Thompson, J. and Dooris, M. (1998) *Health Promoting Universities: Concept, Experience and Framework for Action*, Copenhagen, WHO.

Tuckett, D. (1979) 'Choices for health education: a framework for decision-making' in Sutherland, I. (ed.) *Health Education Perspectives and Choices*, Allen and Unwin.

Van Ryn, M. and Heany, C.A. (1992) 'What's the use of theory?', *Health Education Quarterly*, 19, 3: 315–30.

Van Teijlingen, Friend, J. Twine, F. (1995) 'Problems of evaluation: lessons from a Smokebusters campaign', *Health Education Journal*, 54: 357–66.

Vuori, H. (1982) *Quality Assurance in Health Services: Concepts and Methodology*, Copenhagen Regional Office for Europe, WHO.

Waitzkin, H. and Stoeckle, J.D. (1972) 'The communication of information about illness: clinical, sociological, and methodological considerations', *Adv. Psychom. Med.* 8, 180–215.

Wallace, S. (1993) 'Evaluation of the BBC/HEA Health Show', *Health Education Journal,* 52, 4.

Walters, R. (1995) *Primary Care Health Services in Health Education Authority: A survey of the UK Population Part 1,* HEA.

Watt, A. and Rodmell, S. (1993) 'Community involvement in health promotion: progess or panacea?' in Beattie, A. *et al.* (eds) *Health and Wellbeing: A Reader,* Macmillan.

Weale, A. (1988) *The Search for Efficiency. Cost and Choice in Health Care: the Ethical Dimension,* King's Fund.

Weare, K. (1992) 'The contribution of education to health promotion' in Bunton, R. and Macdonald, G. (eds) *Health Promotion: Disciplines and Diversity,* Routledge.

Weibe, G.D. (1951–52) 'Merchandising commodities and citizenship on television', *Public Opinion Quarterly,* 15: 679–91.

Weiss, R. and Rein, M. (1983) 'The evaluation of broad aim programs: experimental design, its difficulties, and an alternative' in Madaus, G. *et al.* (op cit).

Wellness Forum (1995) Press release and briefing notes, Wellness Forum (Great Peter Street, London).

Welshman, J. (1997) 'Bringing beauty and brightness to the back streets: health education and public health in England and Wales 1890–1940'. *Health Education Journal,* 56 (2): 199–209.

Welsh Office NHS Directorate: Welsh Health Planning Forum (1993) *Protocol for Investment in Health Gain: Healthy Living,* HMSO.

Which? (1996) May 1996: 58.

White, S.K. (1991) *Political Theory and Postmodernism,* Cambridge.

Whitehead, M. (1987) *The Health Divide,* Health Education Council.

Whittington, D. (1987) *Using Groups to Help People,* Tavistock/Routledge; cited in Burnard, P. (1992) *Effective Communication Skills for Health Professionals,* Chapman and Hall.

Wildavsky, A. (1995) *But is it true? A citizen's guide to Environmental Health and Safety Issues,* Harvard University Press, Cambridge Mass.

Williams, S.J., Calnan, M., Cant, S.L. and Coyle, J. (1993) 'All change in the NHS? Implications of the NHS reforms for primary care prevention' in *Sociology of Health and Illness,* 15, 1: 43–67.

Williams, G. and Popay, J. (1994) 'Researching the people's health: Dilemmas and opportunities for social scientists', in Popay, J. and Williams, G. (eds) *Researching the People's Health;* Routledge.

Williams, R.B., Boles, M. and Johnson, R.E. (1995) 'Patient use of a computer for prevention in primary care practice', *Patient Education and Counseling,* 25: 283–92.

Williams, R.G.A. (1983) 'Concepts of health; an analysis of lay logic', *Sociology,* 17, 2: 185–204.

Wohl, A. (1983) *Endangered Lives,* Croom Helm.

Woods, R. and Woodward, J. (1984) *Urban Diseases and Mortality in Nineteenth Century England,* Croom Helm.

Woolfe, R. (1996) 'Becoming a counsellor' in Hales, G., *Beyond Disability,* Sage.

World Health Organisation (WHO) (1948) Preamble of the Constitution of the World Health Organization, WHO.

World Health Organisation (WHO) (1977) *Health For All by the Year 2000*, WHO.

World Health Organisation (WHO) (1978) *Alma Ata Declaration*, WHO.

World Health Organisation (WHO) (1984) *Report of the Working Group on Concepts and Principles of Health Promotion*, Copenhagen, WHO.

World Health Organisation (WHO) (1985) *Health For All in Europe by the Year 2000, Regional Targets*. Copenhagen, WHO.

World Health Organisation (WHO) (1986) *Ottawa Charter for Health Promotion*. Geneva, WHO.

World Health Organisation (WHO) (1988) *Adelaide Recommendations on Healthy Public Policy*. Adelaide, WHO.

World Health Organisation (WHO) (1989) *Ethics and Health Promotion*, Copenhagen: WHO.

World Health Organisation (WHO) (1991) *Revised Targets for Health For All in Europe*, Copenhagen, WHO.

World Health Organisation (WHO) (1992) *'We Can Do It' Sundsvall Handbook* from the 3rd International Conference on Health promotion, Sundsvall, Sweden June 9–15, 1991, Stockholm, Karolinska Institute/WHO.

World Health Organisation (WHO) (1997) *The Jakarta Declaration on Health Promotion into the 21st Century*, WHO.

World Health Organisation (WHO) (1997a) *New Players for a New Era: Leading Health Promotion into the 21st Century*, Fourth International Conference on Health Promotion, Jakarta, WHO.

World Health Organisation (WHO) (1998) *Health 21 Strategy: The Introduction to the Health for All Policy for the WHO European Region*, Copenhagen: WHO Regional Office for Europe.

World Health Organisation (WHO) (1999) *Health Promotion Evaluation: Recommendations to Policy-Makers*, Report of the WHO European Working Group on Health Promotion Evaluation, Copenhagen: WHO Regional Office for Europe.

Wright, B. (1992) *Skills for Caring, Communication Skills*, Churchill Livingstone.

Wyllie, A. and Casswell, S. (1992) 'Formative evaluation of a policy-orientated print media campaign' *Health Promotion International*, 7, 3: 155–61.

Yen, L. (1995) 'From Alma Ata to Asda - and beyond: a commentary on the transition in health promotion services in primary care from commodity to control' in Bunton, R., Nettleton, S. and Burrows, R. (eds) *The Sociology of Health Promotion*, pp.24–40, Routledge.

Yin, R. (1989) *Case Study Research: Design and Methods*, Sage.

Young, I. and Williams, T. (1989) *The Healthy School*, Scottish Health Education Group, Edinburgh.

Zola, I. (1972) 'Medicine as an institution of social control', *The Sociological Review*, 20, 4: 487–504.

Zweig, F. and Mann, K. (eds) (1981) *Educating Policymakers for Evaluation*, Sage Research Progress Series, Vol. 9, Sage, Beverley Hills.

Index

PROMOTING HEALTH: KNOWLEDGE AND PRACTICE

PROMOTING HEALTH: KNOWLEDGE AND PRACTICE